THE BLACK DEATH
1346–1353
The Complete History

THE BLACK DEATH
1346–1353

The Complete History

Ole J. Benedictow

THE BOYDELL PRESS

First published 2004
The Boydell Press, Woodbridge
Reprinted 2004

ISBN 0 85115 943 5

The Boydell Press is an imprint of Boydell & Brewer Ltd
PO Box 9, Woodbridge, Suffolk IP12 3DF, UK
and of Boydell & Brewer Inc.
668 Mt Hope Avenue, Rochester, NY 14620, USA
website: www.boydellandbrewer.com

A CIP catalogue record for this book is available
from the British Library

Library of Congress Cataloging-in-Publication Data
Benedictow, Ole Jørgen.
  The Black Death, 1346–1353 : the complete history / Ole J. Benedictow.
    p. cm.
Includes bibliographical references and index.
  ISBN 0–85115–943–5 (Hardback : alk. paper)
  1. Black Death – History. 2. Plague – History.   3. Diseases and history.
4. Medicine, Medieval.   I. Title.
RC172.B46 2004
614.5'732 – dc22   2003024313

This publication is printed on acid-free paper

Printed in Great Britain by
Cromwell Press, Trowbridge, Wiltshire

Contents

Part Three
Patterns and Dynamics of the Black Death

Part Four
Mortality in the Black Death

Part Five
The Black Death: Its Impact on History

List of Maps, Figures and Tables

Maps

Figures

Tables

For my sons
ANDREAS and TANCRED

and for
MADAM GURÍ

and in memory of
PROFESSOR SIGVALD HASUND
who discovered the late-medieval crisis
and laid the foundations of the Norwegian
school of agricultural history

Preface

In this book, the term the Black Death is used to signify the huge plague epidemic that ravaged Europe, Asia Minor, the Middle East and North Africa in the years 1346–1353. Previous studies have mostly concentrated on the cultural, psychological and religious effects of the Black Death. The central reason for this imbalance is that little was known on the spread of the Black Death, and almost no demographic studies on mortality were available before 1960. In the last four decades of the twentieth century, many new studies on the local spread and mortality of the Black Death were published, which, taken together, provide a completely new opportunity to identify the territorial movement of the Black Death in Asia Minor, the Arab world and Europe, clarify its epidemiological characteristics, and even more importantly, to assess the great mortality caused by this huge plague epidemic, which is highly relevant to questions of its historical impact. The main objectives of this book are to study the epidemiology, the territorial spread and the mortality of the Black Death and to lay the foundation for more useful discussions of its historical impact. It is in these respects that this book's ambitious goal is to be a complete history of that epic epidemic (which should not be misunderstood to imply its final history).

Surprisingly, these many fine studies have not been collected, discussed and synthesized before, not even at the national level of analysis and synthesis. Ziegler's 1969 book on the Black Death in the British Isles is, in my opinion, still the best general study of the Black Death. Biraben gives a valuable brief overview of the Black Death's spread across Europe in his 1975 study, which, however, leaves much still to be said on the subject, while his discussion of mortality is really confined to some aspects of its French history. In the early 1970s, two Spanish scholars, Sobrequés Callicó and Ubieto Arteta, published valuable overviews of the spread of the Black Death across the Iberian Peninsula; at the end of the 1980s, Dubois presented a brief, but valuable summary of the Black Death's spread in France, but passes quite lightly over the question of mortality. I would also like to mention my own discussion of the Black Death in the Nordic countries in my doctoral thesis of 1992, which was published in a revised version in 1993, and reprinted in 1996. However, a serious attempt at producing a general synthetic study of the Black Death's epidemiology, territorial spread and mortality has not been attempted before. My book on the late-medieval plague epidemics in the Nordic countries is the only comprehensive and in-depth study of the Black Death covering national territories to have been published since Ziegler's study. The quite numerous new local studies and the opportunities they offer of expanded knowledge and insights have largely been neglected.

In the present book, no effort has been spared to collect, examine and synthesize the available studies on the Black Death's epidemiology, spread and demographic impact, from its origin in the lands of the Golden Horde in south-eastern Russia in 1346 until it petered out in central Russia seven years later, after having engulfed the Caucasus, Asia Minor, the Middle East, North Africa, and the whole of Europe excepting Finland and Iceland and, perhaps, a few small areas in addition. Why some areas or regions should have been spared is also an interesting question and has been allotted corresponding attention.

Most of the new studies have been undertaken by economic historians or historians of local history who have come across interesting source material that was also usable for analysis of the mortality suffered by the local population or some section of it in the Black Death. By implication, these studies quite often (but far from always) also contain information on the whereabouts of the Black Death in time and space.

The new data that have been forthcoming are usually only basic data. To develop them fully into epidemiological and demographic data requires a heavy input not only of the highly specialized knowledge of medievalists in relation to the understanding and treatment of the great diversity and intricacies of medieval source materials, but also of the insights of epidemiologists of plague, and of historical demographers. There is, of course, also a very demanding requirement with respect to access to the great diversity of European tongues in which the studies containing information on the Black Death have been written. This challenging set of scholarly requirements must be the reason that so far no real attempt has been made at collecting, examining and synthesizing the available data. Many of these studies have been published in local journals of history or in books on local history that can be quite difficult to identify and get hold of, especially in great numbers.

Uncertainty is inevitable in all attempts to produce demographic estimates on the basis of sources from 'pre-statistical' times – documents that never were intended to be used for this purpose. Margins of uncertainty and level of tenability are key terms. In the first half of the fourteenth century, some Italian city states developed registrations of their populations for various purposes that take on the character of censuses. However, generally the most important category of source used in these mortality studies is tax registers of various types that involve an array of source-critical issues relating to the proportion and social composition of untaxed population segments, care in registration, tax evasion, and so on. Only in England is the main type of source manorial records, which, of course, involve an array of source-critical issues of their own.

Endeavours to uncover the Black Death's pattern and pace of spread are too often dependent on notices in chronicles that are jotted down carelessly. Even worse, chroniclers quite often ignore the Black Death because epidemics were a peripheral subject to persons with classical education and classical models. It is often only possible to piece together a coherent basic outline of the Black Death's spread with great effort, too frequently involving substantial uncertainty in the concluding remarks.

Acknowledgements

I would like to use this opportunity to thank the Department of History, University of Oslo, the Faculty of Humanities at the University of Oslo, the Norwegian Research Council, and the Nansen Fund for grants to work at the National Library of Florence, the branch of the Library of the University of Marseilles in Aix-en-Provence, the University Library of Basle, the Library of the University of Barcelona and Biblioteca Cataluña in Barcelona in 1984 and 1987. These grants enabled me to collect and copy the studies of plague produced in these countries. My stay at Clare College, University of Cambridge, and at the Cambridge Group for the History of Population and Social Structure in the Lent term of 1993 gave me the opportunity to use both the Cambridge University Library and the library at the Cambridge Group. I would also like to express my gratitude to the librarians at Oslo University Library who made such splendid efforts to provide me with copies of papers and books from libraries in the Soviet Union/Russia in the east of Europe to the university libraries in Pamplona and in Madrid in the south-west. In 1997, the Association of Norwegian Non-fiction Writers and Translators gave me a grant for a three-month project-scholarship that enabled me to concentrate on planning and starting the writing of the present book. In April 2003 the Norwegian Research Council gave a grant to cover some of the costs of publication.

Maps 1 and 2 are reproduced by kind permission of Unipub AS, Problemveien 9, Postboks 84 Blindern, 0314 Oslo. All other cartography is by Joe Little, 12 Letcombe Walk, Grove, Wantage, Oxfordshire OX12 0BY.

Figures 1 and 2 are reproduced by kind permission of Unipub AS, Problemveien 9, Postboks 84 Blindern, 0314 Oslo; permission to reproduce figure 1 was also granted by Elsevier Science.

Glossary

Abscess Local inflammation of body tissue with deep suppuration (secretion of pus) caused by bacteria that destroy the cells in the centre of the area and leave a cavity filled with pus

Bacteraemia *See* primary and secondary bacteraemic plague

Boil Hard inflamed lymph node that may suppurate; often used in the past to indicate plague bubo

Bubo An inflamed, extremely tender swelling of a lymph node, especially in the area of the armpit or groin, that is characteristic of bubonic plague

Carbuncle Localized dead body tissue (gangrene) caused by plague bacteria (or staphylococci), usually by bacteria left in the site of a flea's bite

Case mortality rate *See* lethality rate

Case fatality rate *See* lethality rate

Endemic Sporadic cases of a disease in a human population, too few to be considered usefully designated as an epidemic, but which indicate that a particular type of contagion occurs in a population, are known as an endemic phase or situation

Entomology The discipline of natural science that studies insects.

Enzootic Sporadic incidence of contagious disease among animals (cf. endemic)

Epidemic Disease that spreads rapidly through a population or community for a period

Epidemiology Science of epidemics, especially how epidemics are spread and transmitted

Epizootic Disease spreading rapidly among animals, i.e., the term corresponding to the term epidemic among human beings

Expectoration Eject from lung airways by coughing

Fatality rate *See* lethality rate

Incubation period The period from infection to the outbreak of disease

Lethality rate The proportion of those who contract a disease who die from it. Also known as case fatality rate and case mortality rate

Lethal dose A measure of virulence. It is usually expressed as LD_{50}, i.e., the number of micro-organisms or micrograms of its toxin (*see* this term) with which human beings (or animals) must be infected in order to kill 50 per cent of them

Life table Life tables are based on series of age-specific death rates for each gender and show the probabilities of dying within particular age intervals according to various life expectancies at birth. Or, if focusing on the probabilities of surviving, life tables show life expectancies at each age level in societies with various life expectancies at birth

Morbidity Prevalence of disease (in an area)

Morbidity rate Proportion of a population that contracts a specific disease

Mortality The number of people who die within a particular period of time or on a particular occasion

Mortality rate The proportion of a population that dies, no matter what the causal factors. Plague mortality is the proportion of a population that dies from this disease in an epidemic

Pandemic Series of waves of epidemics. In European history, plague has ravaged populations and affected historical developments in two protracted series of waves of epidemics. The first (known) plague pandemic began in A.D. 541 and ended in 767, the other started in 1346 and lasted to c. 1650–1722 in most of Europe, longer in the Turkish Balkans and Russia. The Black Death is the first gigantic, particularly disastrous and notorious wave of plague epidemics of the second plague pandemic. A third plague pandemic was under way in the nineteenth and early twentieth centuries, but was stopped by countermeasures based on modern medicine and epidemiology

Pathogen Micro-organism than can cause disease

Pathogenicity The ability of micro-organisms to cause disease. *See also* virulence

Plague focus In many areas of the world where wild rodents live in great density, in colonies or otherwise, plague circulates continuously in the rodent population. Such a rodent population is called a plague focus

Primary bacteraemic plague When the infective material is passed directly on into the bloodstream without stoppage in a lymph node (and development of a bubo)

Primary pneumonic plague Patients with primary lung infections have been infected via the respiratory system. Droplets containing plague bacteria coughed up by persons that have plague infection in the lungs (pulmonary plague) are the source of infection (rarely also animals). (*See also* secondary pneumonic plague, and expectoration)

Secondary bacteraemic plague In about half of all cases of bubonic plague, bacteria at some point manage to overwhelm the lymphatic system and pass on into the blood stream, causing a bacteraemia that is secondary to the primary bubonic condition, cf. primary bacteraemic plague. These cases are almost invariably mortal

Secondary pneumonic plague In cases of bubonic plague in which plague bacteria pass on into the bloodstream (secondary bacteraemic plague) plague bacteria are transported to the lungs where they quite often consolidate and develop ulcers. These cause a frequent cough with bloody expectoration, a condition that is called secondary pneumonic plague, i.e., a pneumonic condition that is secondary to the primary infection of buboes. These cases are almost invariably mortal. Such cases are the origin of primary pneumonic plague

Sepsis, septicaemic In this book, the terms bacteraemia and bacteraemic are used with the same meaning. *See* primary and secondary bacteraemic plague

Toxin A poison produced by micro-organisms. Each specific type of pathogenic micro-organism produces its own toxin, which causes a particular disease when present in the system of a human or animal body.

Vector Carrier of disease, especially an insect that conveys pathogenic organisms from one person (or animal) to another

Virulence This term is closely related to the term pathogenicity, i.e., the ability of micro-organisms to cause disease, but introduces in addition the concept of degree. This makes it possible to differentiate between the disparate abilities of various pathogenic micro-organisms to produce disease and cause death in infected persons. Virulence is measured in terms of the number of micro-organisms or the micrograms of toxin needed to kill a given host when administered by a certain route. This is called the lethal dose. (*See* this term.)

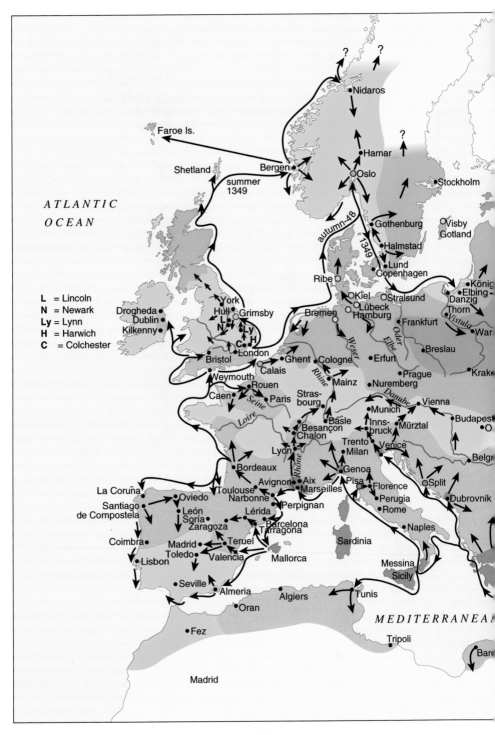

Map 1. Spread of the Black Death in the Old World, 1346–1353

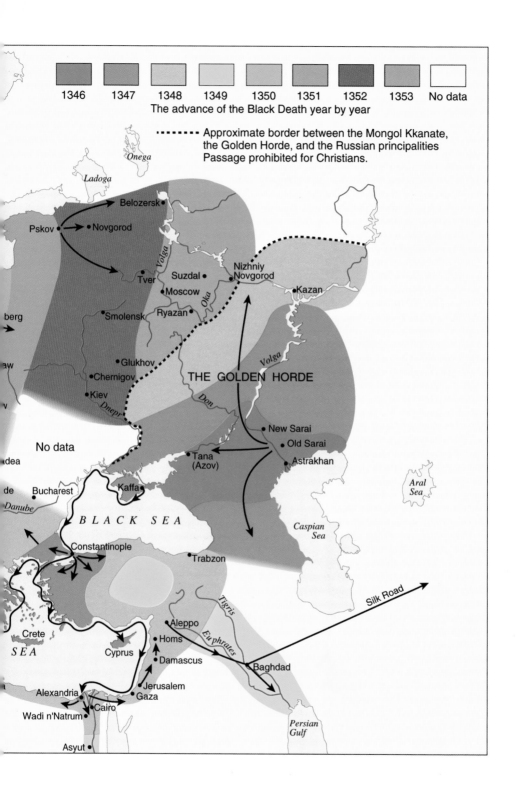

The advance of the Black Death year by year

| 1346 | 1347 | 1348 | 1349 | 1350 | 1351 | 1352 | 1353 | No data |

· · · · · · · Approximate border between the Mongol Kkanate, the Golden Horde, and the Russian principalities Passage prohibited for Christians.

Onega

Ladoga

Belozersk

Pskov → Novgorod

Volga

Nizhniy Novgorod

Suzdal

Tver

Moscow

Kazan

berg

Smolensk

Ryazan

Oka

Glukhov

Volga

Chernigov

THE GOLDEN HORDE

Kiev

Dnepr

Don

No data

New Sarai

Old Sarai

dea

Tana (Azov)

Astrakhan

Aral Sea

de

Bucharest

Kaffa

Danube

BLACK SEA

Caspian Sea

Constantinople

Trabzon

Silk Road

Crete

Tigris

SEA

Cyprus

Aleppo

Homs

Euphrates

Damascus

Baghdad

Alexandria

Jerusalem

Gaza

Wadi n'Natrum

Cairo

Persian Gulf

Asyut

Part One
What was the Black Death?

1

Why the History of the Black Death
is Important

The Black Death

Between the years 1346 and 1353, a terrible disease swept over Western Asia, the Middle East, North Africa and Europe, causing catastrophic losses of population everywhere, both in the countryside and in the towns and cities. In Florence, the great Renaissance author Francesco Petrarch wrote, dumbfounded, to a friend: 'O happy posterity, who will not experience such abysmal woe and will look upon our testimony as a fable.' It wrought such havoc among the populations that it earned, it seems, eternal notoriety as the greatest-ever demographic disaster. Because it was far more mortal and terrible than anything people had heard or read about, the memory of this disaster entered folklore and the writings of the learned alike. Thus, Petrarch erred in his belief that posterity would shrug off the accounts of the havoc it wrought as merely tall stories.

Many centuries later, Europeans began to call it the Black Death, a name that since has become the usual frightening name of this epic epidemic. The reason for this is probably a misunderstanding, a mistranslation of the Latin expression *atra mors*, in which *atra* may mean both terrible and black.[1] It has nothing to do with diagnostic symptoms, as persons seeking a rational explanation for this graphic name often believe.

People at the time knew nothing about bacteria, viruses and other microbiological agents of disease. The great majority believed that disease was God's punishment for their sins. The few physicians and other learned men who knew classical Greek medicine attributed epidemic disease to *miasma*. Miasma was corruption or pollution of the air by noxious vapours containing poisonous elements that were caused by rotting, putrid matter, and which were spread by wind. Miasma could enter persons by inhalation or through the skin. This miasmatic theory of infectious disease can be illustrated by writs from the king of England, who was deeply concerned about the dangers inherent in the unsavoury conditions in London. In 1349, Edward III wrote to the mayor of London and complained about all the filth that was being thrown from the houses so that

---

[1] D'Irsay 1926: 328–32.

the streets and lanes through which people had to pass were foul with human faeces and the air of the city was poisoned to the great danger of men passing, especially in this time of infectious disease.[2]

Edward also sent a writ on the same matter to the mayor and sheriffs of London in 1361. This was in the face of the second wave of plague, and, the writ contained, therefore, an analysis of the cause of plague and royal injunctions as to what should be done:

> Because by the killing of great beasts, from whose putrid blood running down the streets and the bowels cast in the Thames, the air in the city is very much corrupted and infected, hence abominable and most filthy stench proceeds, sickness and many other evils have happened to such as have abode in the said city, or have resorted to it; and great dangers are feared to fall out for the time to come, unless remedy be presently made against it. We, willing to prevent such dangers, ordain, by consent of the present Parliament, that all bulls, oxen, hogs, and other gross creatures be killed at either Stratford or Knightsbridge.[3]

In the Middle Ages, this miasmatic theory of epidemic disease was supplemented by an astrological dimension. In 1348, King Philip VI of France ordered the Medical Faculty of the University of Paris to produce a report on the causes of the Black Death and to what remedies one could possibly resort. The Faculty reported that at 1 p.m. on 20 March 1345 there was a conjunction of Saturn, Jupiter and Mars in the House of Aquarius. This was extremely potent with regard to the rise of epidemic disease because the conjunction of Saturn and Jupiter gave rise to death and disaster, while the conjunction of Jupiter and Mars disseminated pestilence in the air.[4] In this astrological theory of epidemiology, Jupiter was assumed to be warm and humid and to draw malignant vapours both from the ground and from water, while Mars was assumed to be hot and dry, and, therefore, had the capacity to kindle such malignant vapours into infective fire. Consequently, the rare conjunction of Jupiter, Saturn and Mars together presaged the most terrible epidemic disaster. In Shakespeare's words:

> a planetary plague, when Jove [= Jupiter]
> Will o'er som high-vic'd city, hang his poison
> In the sick air.

> when the planets
> In evil mixture to disorder wander,
> What plagues, and what portents, what mutiny[5]

In addition, miasmatic theory also assumed that volcanic outbreaks and earthquakes freed noxious vapours out of the ground.

Neither was there, according to this theory, much that man could do to prevent or cure epidemic disease, although it contained an encouragement to improve hygienic

---

2 Cited after Ziegler 1970: 161.
3 Cited after Gasquet 1908: 110.
4 Sticker 1908: 60–1.
5 Cited after Wilson 1963: 5–6.

conditions and to get rid of filth and dirt in the environment in order to prevent matter from rotting and producing miasmatic vapours in the vicinity of human settlement and habitation.

Actually, the Black Death was the first and particularly violent outbreak of this epidemic disease, and the following centuries witnessed frequent, often dramatic and disastrous outbreaks. But these pestilences never brought about the same dramatic level of demographic catastrophe. The capacity of plague to spread had been reduced, but its capacity to kill its victims wherever it arrived in local societies or towns, its *virulence*, was unabated. Contemporaries lived in constant fear of the next outbreak when their lives once more would be very much at risk.

They recognized that it was the same terrible disease that recurred. But because they had no theory of epidemic disease that could explain how many different epidemic diseases were caused by specific agents, they had no specific word for it. Physicians would use the classical Latin words *pestis* or *pestilentia*, with the general meaning of epidemic. It is an indication of the immense impact of the Black Death and ensuing epidemics of plague on the minds of the contemporaries that in many European languages these words eventually, in the form of *pest*, became a specific term for this disease.[6] However, in Northern Europe another word was immediately put into use, namely *plaga*, a name derived from the Latin word *plaga*, which means 'stroke'. King Magnus Eriksson of Norway and Sweden used this word about the Black Death in a royal letter as early as September 1349.[7] The Icelanders used it from the early fifteenth century at the latest, and in England this word came into use in the fifteenth century in the form of *plague*. The Black Death, then, is a particularly notorious epidemic of plague.

This book will concentrate on the Black Death itself. However, the historical significance of the plague epidemics will also be put in a long-term perspective. The magnitude of the demographic decline and the economic, social and cultural effects that can be ascribed to the total or cumulative impact of the late-medieval plague epidemics will also be discussed.

How the Black Death became important

The scholarly study of the Black Death began in Europe in the nineteenth century with the development of modern historiography, but most of the research has, as mentioned, been performed in the last four decades of the twentieth century. Much new knowledge is therefore now available, and it is possible to present a far broader and more profound and detailed picture than before of this greatest of all epidemic disasters and its demographic, economic, social and cultural effects.

At first, most scholars rejected the notion that any epidemic disease could have caused an enormous and lasting reduction of European populations. However, in the first half of the twentieth century, historians discovered that the Late Middle Ages was actually a period of large-scale and lasting decline in European populations both in the countryside and in towns and cities. This was first postulated by Sigvald Hasund,

---

[6] See, e.g., Herrlinger 1955.
[7] *Diplomatarium Suecanum (Svenskt Diplomatarium)*, Vol. 6, No. 4515, p. 156. This document is discussed in relation to the history of the Black Death both in Norway and Sweden.

the Norwegian agrarian historian, who, in 1920, published a small book, which he, using a term found in his sources, called *On the Great Mortality*. He showed that, in Norway, settlement contracted sharply, land rents plummeted, land prices were halved, and so on, and that this produced a new social scene that lasted throughout the Late Middle Ages. Summarizing his findings, he pointed out that all these developments would have to reflect a dramatic and lasting diminution of the population, and that only the Black Death and ensuing epidemics of plague could be the cause of a contraction of the population of this order of magnitude and duration.

Later, in 1935, the German scholar Wilhelm Abel published a more wide-ranging study comprising a much broader geographical perspective and more economic indicators, in which he succeeded in showing the same developments both in Germany and in several other European countries. In 1950, Michael Postan, the English economic historian, published a paper in which he managed to demonstrate definitively that this also was the case in England. Abel's and Postan's works (which were easily accessible in international languages) produced a breakthrough in the study of the Late Middle Ages. In the following decades, a great number of studies from almost all countries outside Eastern Europe disclosed the same pattern of developments. (For ideological reasons, the Communist regimes prevented the study of lasting demographic and economic decline and social transformation caused by disease.)

In addition, a large number of scholarly works have been published that show that the plague epidemics also had a profound impact on religious and cultural attitudes and their artistic expressions. There was a new obsession with death and the art of dying, a clear shift in the popularity of saints, (anti-)plague saints like St Rochus and St Sebastian becoming extremely popular. A vow to build a new and fine church was considered a powerful way of alleviating the wrath of the Lord and of preventing the threat of an approaching plague epidemic or reducing its ferocity. Church-building increased strongly and the building industry enjoyed a continuous boom in the Late Middle Ages.

It has also been shown that the Black Death and later plague epidemics affected political developments profoundly, primarily because it reduced sharply the incomes that kings and noblemen received from their manors and estates. The Hundred Years War, for instance, started in 1337 because of rivalries between the French and English kings, but lasted for more than a hundred years for other reasons: the Black Death and following epidemics caused a dramatic reduction in aristocratic and royal incomes. War gave rich opportunities for substituting lost agrarian incomes through the wages of war. The knights and squires of the shires enlisted for military service and were awarded with wages, spoils, ransoms for prisoners (especially for aristocratic élite warriors), with manors and fiefs in conquered areas, and so on. The kings used the opportunity to levy new war taxes, which to a large extent ended in the pockets of the warrior class as remuneration for their services or as profits for the merchants who happily sold provisions to armies that were more or less on a constant war footing. Thus, the social élites, the political classes, so to speak, had a strong interest in keeping the war going.

In Spain, the gentry, the 'hidalgos', had lost much of their income for the same reason, and had enjoyed the alternative opportunity for earning supplementary income by waging more or less continuous warfare against the Muslim Moors on behalf of the Spanish Crown. After the final victory in 1492, Columbus sailed off westwards and discovered Meso-America and South America on behalf of the Spanish Crown. Now it was the turn of the American Indians to face the greed, weaponry and martial art of the 'hidalgos', who earned fame or notoriety under the name of 'conquistadors', i.e., conquerors.

Thus, the arrival of the Black Death heralded a new historical period in which epidemic disease affected profoundly the structure and course of European society, from Norway to Spain, from England to Russia. Later research has shown that developments were quite similar in Arab countries in North Africa and the Middle East, and this appears also to be the case in Asia Minor and the Trans-Caucasian countries. This, then, is the reason the history of the Black Death is important: it made history.

2

Anatomy of a Killer Disease

What happened in India?

In 1993, the news that the Black Death had reared its grisly head in India hit head-lines of newspapers and the news programmes of TV channels all over the world. The centre of the epidemic was the city of Surat, about 200 km (125 miles) north of Bombay. Panic broke out, and reportedly one million inhabitants out of a total population of 2.5 million fled. The acute misery and the blind fear of the population despite the availability of modern curative as well as preventive technologies and the collapse of the local health administration made a lasting impression around the world. This panic struck an evocative chord in the minds of historians who had studied this type of reaction to plague in the past. Frightening reports about plague in Delhi, Bombay and other cities soon came pouring in.

However, in a few months it became clear that the health authorities in reality had managed to re-establish their functions quite rapidly and had succeeded in containing and combating the epidemic efficiently. In fact, the numbers of cases and fatalities proved to be quite small. Armed with a vast amount of modern knowledge about epidemic diseases in general and about the epidemiology of plague in particular, and equipped with efficient medication and useful hospital facilities, even the woefully inadequate health organization of a poor developing country had no real difficulty in preventing the incipient plague epidemic from exploding into a full-scale disaster and to force it into a hasty retreat.[1]

What journalists did not know and what people therefore were not told was that the anti-epidemic organization employed in 1994 by Indian health authorities had first been developed in Europe in the sixteenth and seventeenth centuries specifically to combat plague. In India, this type of anti-epidemic organization had first been established by the British colonial authorities in order to combat the great plague epidemics that broke out in 1896 and lasted for several decades. Nor was the public informed that much of the present knowledge about how plague is disseminated and transmitted had been discovered by British scholars in the decade 1905–14 in connection with these Indian epidemics. However, the first breakthrough in the study of plague had been achieved elsewhere a few years earlier.

---

[1] Quadeer, Nayar and Baru 1994: 2981–4.

The Discovery of the Enemy: *Yersinia pestis*

Shortly after the middle of the nineteenth century, missionaries and explorers reported from the Yunnan province in China, a remote western province on the borders of Burma and Vietnam, that true plague was rampant there.[2] To the consternation of the Chinese authorities it slowly but inexorably spread towards the coast. However, it was not before it reached Canton in 1894 that it attracted wider notice. The first plague case in Canton was reported in January. For special reasons, the endemic phase of a plague epidemic has an insidious character. For a time its presence is disclosed only by a few sporadic cases that ostensibly give no reason for grave concern. It was not until March 1894 that the epidemic flared up abruptly, the number of plague cases rose precipitously and the public and the authorities alike were shocked to acknowledge that they faced a powerful and dangerous epidemic of plague. In the course of the epidemic the plague killed between 40,000 and 100,000 persons in Canton: the collapse of the frail Chinese municipal organization in the face of epidemic disaster made more accurate figures impossible. Studies of samples of plague patients revealed that the plague had retained its lethal powers: the *lethality rate*, the proportion of those who died after having contracted plague, was 80 per cent, just as in old-time plague epidemics.[3] This means that of between 50,000 and 125,000 persons who had contracted the disease only between 10,000 and 25,000 survived. The Black Death was back in full strength.

Now the Europeans in China began to take the spread of plague seriously, because it threatened their commercial interests, and because they realized that, in the era of steamships and efficient international transport, the plague could be easily and unwitttingly spread with cargoes and passengers to Europe and the colonies. When plague broke out in Hong Kong in May, the Europeans were jolted into effective action to counter the threat. Shock waves spread through Europe, and the defence of Europe against the plague became a top priority for the great colonial powers that felt most threatened. Japanese authorities also feared that plague could be introduced into Japan and were on the alert. They sent their best medical scholars to Hong Kong to uncover the secrets of this disease and how it could be combated more efficiently and prevented from spreading further.

In addition to the acute epidemic situation that triggered the intense wish to acquire increased knowledge that could serve as a base for combating plague more effectively, there were two decisive factors that paved the way for rapid and real progress in the study of plague. First there was a breakthrough in modern, scientific medicine, especially bacteriology. Around 1870 it was discovered that contagious diseases were caused by specific types of micro-organisms. Many such categories of organisms could be discerned under the microscope. Others were too small, but additional techniques were developed to indicate their presence and their causal role in provoking disease. Most of them are viruses that cause such well-known diseases as smallpox, chicken pox, measles, mumps, influenza, the common cold, and so on. The pioneers of modern bacteriology gave the name *pathogens* to the micro-organisms that caused disease. Inspired by their new capacity to identify these enemies of human-

---

[2] See, e.g., Simpson 1905: 48–54.
[3] Benedictow 1993/1996a: 146–9.

kind that killed many millions of people every year, scientists went to their work with enormous energy and dedication; they became, as it were, St Georges determined to kill dragons.

The discovery of pathogenic micro-organisms also meant that it had become possible to study how the pathogenic agents of diseases were actually disseminated and transmitted, and, thus, to design specific, rational strategies to combat them. Bacteriological knowledge could serve as a basis for three main strategies of action: (1) development of vaccines, (2) development of medication and (3) development of anti-epidemic organizations and countermeasures.

The work to disclose the true nature of the Black Death began in earnest in Hong Kong in 1894 against the backcloth of an early medical revolution in the understanding of the nature of epidemic disease. Both the Japanese and the French governments dispatched leading bacteriologists to Hong Kong, S. Kitasato and A. Yersin, respectively. They arrived in the middle of June, and set to work in plague hospitals. They were rewarded with almost instant success. In a few weeks, they identified the same new type of bacterium in the blood and tissues of plague patients, and they also succeeded in isolating and cultivating it in culture. They also found the same bacterium in dead rats, a fact that confirmed suspicions raised by observations of dead rats both in Yunnan and in Canton and Hong Kong. These two men, then, produced the first important breakthrough in the modern efforts to combat plague: on the basis of modern medical knowledge and technology they succeeded in identifying the causal agent of the Black Death and its close association with rats and other rodents.

This achievement greatly facilitated further research and accumulation of knowledge on the mechanisms of dissemination and transmission of plague, which would make it possible to design more effective and accurate anti-epidemical measures, and to launch projects to develop a vaccine and medication.

The plague bacterium was named after Yersin, and is called *Yersinia pestis*; it could also have been named after Kitasato, who observed it some days earlier than Yersin, but Yersin gave it the more accurate description. Yersin drew also a very important conclusion from his findings concerning the role of rats in epidemic plague: 'It is probable that the rats constitute the principal vehicle.'

3

Bubonic Plague and the Role of Rats and Fleas

The Indian Plague Research Commission

The first breakthrough in the bacteriological study of plague did not have much immediate significance for the understanding of how plague was spread and transmitted, nor for the practical combating of plague. The distinguishing feature of the 1894 plague epidemic, like plague epidemics in the past, was that the great majority of the diseased developed one or sometimes two buboes, most often in the groin or on the thigh, but also quite often in the armpits, and occasionally also in other places. This ordinary form of plague was therefore called *bubonic plague*. It was understood that the buboes developed in places with a concentration of lymph nodes, which are a first-line defence of the body against invasion of micro-organisms, and that infection with plague bacteria was the reason that lymph nodes swelled into buboes. However, the identification of the plague bacterium did not explain how or why this characteristic diagnostic feature came about.

Neither did the discovery of the plague bacterium make a contribution to the concomitant efforts to contain the epidemic in Hong Kong. From this bustling Chinese port, plague travelled with steamships to India, Australia, the Americas, Indonesia, Madagascar, and even to England. As should be expected, it was in poor, underdeveloped India that plague fanned out in enormous epidemics, killing millions of people. The British colonial administration was unprepared for the task of combating large-scale plague epidemics, but employed at first, as best it could, traditional European countermeasures. However, these anti-epidemic countermeasures had only limited initial success in this vast and ethnically very complex and divided population containing a wide array of beliefs, cultures, systems of education, traditions of organization, and attitudes to local authorities and central governments that were very different from those found among populations in pre-industrial Europe.[1]

In 1905, the Indian Plague Research Commission was established to carry out a comprehensive research programme, and some of Britain's best medical scholars joined it. Significantly, the Commission recruited also a leading *entomologist*, i.e., a scholar who studies insects. This reflected the suspicion that there was a connection between plague among human beings and the repeated observation of dead rats in or

---

[1] Simpson 1905.

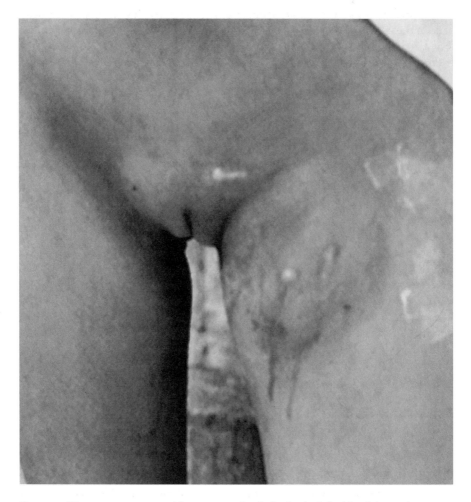

Figure 1. Vietnamese woman with a suppurating bubo in the left side of the groin

around human habitation, and that the agent of transmission, *the vector*, was the rat flea. In 1903, W. Glen Liston, the English entomologist, received a batch of fleas that had been caught on persons in a plague-infected block of overcrowded tenements in Bombay, and concluded that one half of them actually were rat fleas of the type having the black rat as its normal host animal. On the basis of descriptions of numerous rat deaths in the preceding period Liston concluded that great mortality among the rats had made it increasingly difficult for their fleas to find new rat hosts, and that starvation had made them turn on man instead. Actually, the inhabitants in the block complained that they had suddenly been so aggressively attacked by fleas that many had left their rooms to sleep in the veranda.[2] Two years later, Liston joined the Indian Plague Research Commission.

---

[2] Hirst 1953: 171–2.

The Indian Plague Research Commission produced a series of important discoveries and confirmations of earlier, more casual observations.[3] They proved definitely that plague was basically a rodent disease, and that infected populations of wild rodents functioned as reservoirs of plague contagion. Actually, in many areas of the world where wild rodents live in great density, in colonies or otherwise, plague circulates continuously in the rodent population. Such a rodent population is called a *plague focus*. Epidemics may break out when the plague bacterium is spread from a natural plague focus to populations of rats living in close contact with human beings.

In relation to human populations, the black rat plays a pivotal part because it likes to live in the immediate proximity of people, and this introduces rodent populations susceptible to plague into human environments, in houses, in granaries, mills, barns, and so on. The black rat has a great predilection for grain as a foodstuff, often living in the same rooms as its human hosts, earning its other name of the house rat. It is also the classic ship rat.

The presence of black rats constitutes an essential condition for the development of large-scale epidemics of bubonic plague. The Commission carried out a number of comprehensive experiments that proved that bubonic plague was transmitted only when the ordinary fleas of the rat were present, the *Xenopsylla cheopis*. This meant that human fleas, the *Pulex irritans*, which were swarming in the homes of ordinary Indians, did not play any role, or at least not a significant role. This finding, which implied that bubonic plague was not spread between human beings by cross-infection but was passed on from rats to people, presented itself to the Indian Plague Research Commission as the paramount problem to be resolved.

Plague bacteria in the blood

Fleas are bloodsucking insects, so the reason that rat fleas transmit plague while human fleas did not would most likely be associated with different properties of rat blood and human blood. Obviously, fleas would have to be infected with plague bacteria in order to become carriers of the disease and to be able to transmit plague bacteria, and, obviously, the infection would have to come from the blood of rats or human beings. Consequently, it was important to acquire knowledge about *bacteraemia*, i.e., the *incidence* with which blood from diseased rats and human beings contained plague bacteria, and the *level* of such infection.[4]

Even before the Commission set out to work, the blood of over one thousand plague patients had been examined at the time of admission to the Maratha Hospital in Bombay in 1902. It was shown that 43 per cent of patients had plague bacteria in the blood, and none of them recovered. Because admission to hospital tended to come late in the course of illness, it could be reasonably concluded that about half of all plague patients died without having bacteria in their bloodstream. Human plague cases without bacteria in their bloodstream could not be sources of infection for fleas. However, the level of bacteraemia was not studied.

---

[3]   The Indian Plague Research Commission's numerous pioneering studies are published in *The Journal of Hygiene* in the years 1906–14 (comprising also two Plague Supplements in 1912).
[4]   Known also by the more general term *septicaemia*, but in this book we are concretely dealing with bacteria, so the self-explanatory term bacteraemia/bacteraemic is used consistently.

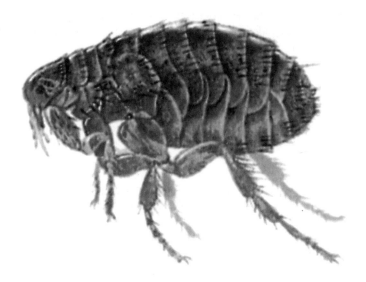

Figure 2. A female plague flea, *Xenopsylla cheopis*, about 2 mm in length

The Indian Plague Research Commission took up this line of research. They measured the feeding capacity of fleas, and concluded that fleas could, on average, accommodate in their stomach, when it was fully distended, about 0.5 c.mm (cubic millimetre). This meant that, in order to be infected with one plague bacterium, fleas would have to suck blood containing, on average, 2,000 plague bacteria per c.c. (cubic centimetre).

Next, the Commission carried out a systematic study of a sample of plague patients, regularly drawing samples of their blood during the course of illness, and testing the samples from each patient not only to see whether or not they contained bacteria and, thus, were *bacteraemic*, but also for the *level of bacteraemia*, i.e., the number of bacteria per c.c. of blood. Because there was no medication or other type of treatment available that could affect the disease, the researchers of the Commission could in all decency calmly study the course of developments in their patients until they died or, as happened in 18 per cent of the cases, until they recovered. The case *fatality rate*, i.e., the proportion of plague patients who died, was, thus, a shade above the average. In their study, the Commission found that 57 per cent of the patients developed bacteraemia at some point of the disease, a somewhat higher incidence of bacteraemia than in the study of patients at the Maratha Hospital. However, and most importantly, they also found that the levels of bacteraemia were very low. In fact, bacteraemia proved to be so low that it immediately became clear that human beings were very poor sources for infection of fleas. Only 14 per cent of the patients developed a degree of bacteraemia exceeding 10,000 plague bacteria per c.c. of blood, which would make the slightest possible infection probable at all. The Commission's similar study of bacteraemia in rats produced a radically different outcome: bacteraemia in rats was much more usual, and of crucial importance was the finding that, on average, bacteraemia in rats is roughly 500–1,000 times higher than in humans. The Commission's findings concerning bacteraemia in human plague cases have consistently been confirmed by later research, most recently in connection with the quite large plague epidemics in Vietnam during the 1960s (almost 6,000 registered plague cases in 1967), and in connection with studies of plague patients admitted to hospitals in the USA in recent decades.[5]

What happened in the gut of fleas?

There was, however, another conundrum to be resolved. What almost mystified the scholars was how plague bacteria in the fleas entered or were injected into the bite wound, or whether there were other possible routes to infection of human beings. They therefore developed a technique to find out how often there were plague bacteria in remnants of blood on the proboscis after fleas had sucked the blood of plague patients or diseased rats with bacteraemia, and, if so, how many. The findings were clear. Bacteria are so large that normally there were no plague bacteria left on the proboscis, and only rarely more than three bacteria when fleas had fed on highly bacteraemic rats. In addition, and what definitely excluded this possible route of infection, was that fleas that had had a meal normally did not feed again for at least a day or two, and plague bacteria on proboscises disappeared in a few hours.[6] The solution had to be something very different.

The Commission's scholars first thought of the possibility that plague was transmitted in the same way as another feared, insect-transmitted epidemic disease, *exanthematic typhus*. Lice play a crucial role in the transmission of the disease, but it had been discovered that transmission of the contagion did not take place by way of the bite itself. Instead, it was shown that the pathogen, which has many properties in common with virus, e.g., it is much smaller than bacteria, survived the passage through the alimentary canal of lice without loss of virulence. Consequently, the faeces of lice were highly contagious, and, importantly, lice like fleas very often defecate when they take in fresh blood. Exanthematic typhus is transmitted when persons, reacting to the bite, scratch themselves, because, at the same time, they scratch contaminated faecal material from the louse into the bite wound. Even dried faeces from lice contained virulent contagion, and could, in the form of dust, infect human beings by way of the mucous membranes.

However, again the Commission's researchers were disappointed. Plague bacteria could survive the passage through the alimentary canal of fleas, but they lost so much of their virulence that their potential for causing disease was greatly diminished. And plague bacteria were so much larger that they did not enter cuts in rat skin made to simulate bite wounds, at least not in sufficient numbers to cause disease even if the researchers did their best to scratch bacteria into the wound. They let guinea pigs crawl in heaps of unwashed bed linen from a plague hospital in order to find out if dust from dried infected material could cause disease. Although guinea pigs are extremely susceptible to plague disease, and 50 per cent will die if infected by 1–2

---

[5] All studies on bacteraemia in human plague cases and in rats are presented and discussed in Benedictow 1993/1996a: 242–64.

[6] These findings have later been confirmed both by American and Soviet research. See a presentation of this research in Benedictow 1993/1996a: 238–42. Bibikova 1977: 27; Bibikova and Klassovskiy 1974: 88–91.

plague bacteria, none of them contracted plague. The conundrum remained triumphant, the researchers became even more frustrated and puzzled.

Addressing these questions assiduously and systematically, exploring all known
patterns of pathogenic transmission, the Commission eventually, in 1914, was
rewarded with a breakthrough. The solution was closely connected to special features
of the flea's alimentary system. Fleas do not only have a stomach, a *ventriculus*, they
also have a *proventriculus*. The role of the proventriculus is to function as a valve,
permitting fleas to take in relatively large amounts of blood, because it prevents the
ingested blood from being driven out again by the high pressure in the distended
stomach. It was discovered that when fleas imbibe blood containing very high densities of plague bacteria, the bacteria proliferate faster in the stomach system than they
are passed on through the alimentary canal by the normal functions and movements
of the digestive organs. Gradually, an obstruction, called a block, is formed, consisting
of a mass of blood substance and bacteria. When a 'blocked' flea tries to feed, it is
forced to regurgitate the fresh blood back into the bite wound. In this process, bits of
the block containing thousands of bacteria tend to be injected into the host. Later
research has shown that partial blockage will also have much the same effect, the
point being that the stomach system must be sufficiently blocked to prevent the flea
from accommodating the feed and forcing it to regurgitate blood back into the bite
wound. It has also been shown that the number of plague bacteria present in the
regurgitant of a blocked flea tend to be of the order of magnitude of 25,000.[7] Thus, in
the case of plague, infection doses tend to be very high. Because a blocked flea is a
desperately hungry flea, it bites voraciously and repeatedly, and so tends to transmit
high infection doses repeatedly in quite a short time. This is an important explanation for the extreme mortality of plague disease.

The discovery that blockage in the stomach system of fleas was a necessary condition to make them able to transmit plague, meant that a sharp line had to be drawn
between *infected* and *infective* fleas: infected fleas do not become infective, function as
vectors and transmit plague unless and until their stomach system becomes blocked,
at least sufficiently blocked to cause blood to return into the bite wound when they
attempt to feed.

The Commission's findings also explained why human fleas did not, or at least
only rarely, transmit plague infection. Human beings do not develop a degree of
bacteraemia that can infect fleas with a sufficient number of bacteria to trigger the
growth of a blockage of the stomach system. Around 1970, Soviet researchers carried
out a study specifically designed to provide a more accurate notion of the level of
bacteraemia and the number of plague bacteria rat fleas would have to ingest in order
to develop blockage. It turned out that the required minimum dose was
50,000–500,000 bacteria (5.0×10^4–10^5), and such massive infective doses would only
produce blockage in about 20 per cent of rat fleas. In order to ensure development of
blockage, the researchers had to increase the infective doses considerably above this
level.[8] Within very wide margins of uncertainty, this outcome implies that only a very
few cases of bacteraemia so far observed in humans would provide blood with suffi-

---

[7]   Burroughs 1947: 382.
[8]   Benedictow 1993/1996a: 257–8; Bibikova and Alekseyev 1969; Bibikova and Klassovskiy 1974: 112.

ciently intense bacteraemia to cause even the occasional development of blockage in fleas.[9] This finding should be seen in the light of the fact that the rat flea has been shown to develop blockage more easily than other types of fleas.[10] Such levels of bacteraemia are, however, usual in rats, and these facts together produce a satisfactory explanation for why bubonic plague is conveyed by rat fleas, and why the outbreak of epidemics is dependent on the presence of the black rat.[11]

How was plague spread?

Plague could only be effectively combated following a thorough knowledge of how it was spread, i.e., the epidemiology of plague. In order to be able to stamp out plague the mechanisms and vehicles of dissemination would have to be identified so that effective countermeasures could be designed. The Commission launched a series of comprehensive research programmes to study how plague was introduced into communities, and how plague spread within and between communities and at various distances:

(1) the household level
(2) the neighbourhood level
(3) the local level
(4) the inter-local level

[9] These studies of plague bacteraemia in human beings are presented and discussed in Benedictow 1993/1996a: 242–64. It is clear that the level of bacteraemia in human beings is too low to infect fleas to a degree that may cause the development of blocks in the ventricular system of fleas that will make them infective – at least such developments will be very rare indeed. This is the reason the so-called human flea, *Pulex irritans*, does not play any (significant) role in the dissemination of plague contagion.

Alternative assertions to the effect that human fleas played a central role in plague epidemics and that inter-human spread was important have been put forward by some scholars, notably by Blanc and Baltazard who performed a study of a small plague epidemic (90 fatalities) in Morocco in 1940 (Blanc and Baltazard 1945). In my book *Plague in the Late Medieval Nordic Countries*, I have presented and discussed central aspects of this study and subsequent presentations of it quite thoroughly and explained why I consider it unsatisfactory and even fallacious. Furthermore, Blanc and Baltazard did not perform any studies of human bacteraemia and of blockage in fleas. See especially 1993/1996a: 247–50. See also Girard 1943: 4–43; Hirst 1953: 256–63.

There is also an independent line of argument: Blanc and Baltazard assert that plague spreads only endemically and episodically in the countryside, and that it was in the large cities of medieval Europe that the human flea took on an important and even dominating role by spreading plague directly between people, triggering off great epidemics driven by inter-human spread. Obviously, Blanc and Balthazard did not know that only a couple of per cent of Europe's population by any stretch of sociological imagination can be said to have lived in large cities, that no more than 10–12 per cent resided in urban environments at all, the great majority of them in quite small towns. It is clear, therefore, that Blanc's and Balthazard's theory of plague epidemiology, whatever its merits or demerits, cannot explain the Black Death's demographic effects, which, on the contrary, require exceptional powers of spread in the countryside. Actually, as shown below, this is the very special property of plague. See Benedictow 1987; Benedictow 1993/1996a: 234–6.

It is hard to understand why French plague research in Madagascar, which related to more than 40,000 plague cases and which was performed on a much larger scale and with a scholarly quality comparable to the achievements of the Indian Plague Research Commission has been so thoroughly neglected. In all important respects, the Madagascan plague studies confirm the Indian plague studies. Although the hovels and huts of the Madagascan natives swarmed with fleas, and lice, the French researchers never succeeded in confirming a single certain case of inter-human transmission caused by human ectoparasites. (More about this below.)

[10] Eskey and Haas 1940: 29–82.

[11] The grey or brown rat that is usual today in large parts of the world is also susceptible to plague and can theoretically constitute the rodent basis of plague epidemics or contribute to the dynamics of plague epidemics. However, it is important to note that this type of rat is not recorded in Europe before c. 1650, and in many countries not before c. 1800. In contrast to the black rat, the grey rat is shy and likes to live at a

(5) metastatic spread, i.e., spread by a leap at a considerable distance that causes the establishment of a new epicentre[12] of epidemic spread.

Liston had discerned some of the central elements of the first two types, the household and neighbourhood levels, in the block of tenements in Bombay. The Commission wished to broaden its understanding of this primary epidemic process: it launched a research programme designed to monitor the depletion of rat colonies when plague was introduced into a house in a village and triggered off contagious disease among the rats (i.e., a rat *epizootic*). As rats began to die, their consorts of fleas rapidly left their dead hosts as soon as their bodies began to cool off. Although rat fleas do not have such strong bonding to a specific animal host as many other types of fleas, they have a pronounced predilection for their ordinary hosts. They began, therefore, immediately searching for a new rat host, when people were also present. When the pool of rats had become strongly depleted, more and more fleas began to assemble on the remaining rats, which contracted plague and soon became too weakened by disease to make efforts to reduce the number of bloodsucking insects by scratching them off. Normally, black rats carry, on average, seven rat fleas, but the Commission noted with great interest that sick rats towards the end of an epizootic in a rat colony often carried 100–150 fleas. When these rats began to die, hundreds of dangerous rat fleas swarmed into the immediate environment of human beings, and because they now often did not succeed in finding a new rat host they would, desperately hungry, turn on them after about three days. How early in this phase rat fleas would, on average, find the opportunity to bite a human being is not really known, but presumably this would tend to happen fairly soon, after about half to one day.

The depletion of a rat colony in this way takes about 10–14 days. In addition, when people become infected about 3–4 days later it takes, on average, about 3–5 days before the infection develops into disease. This is the so-called incubation period, and in mortal cases the normal duration of illness is also about 3–5 days. The first human cases of plague illness will usually occur after 16–23 days, the first plague deaths after about 20–28 days, and within this range most often after about 24 days. These developments herald the endemic phase, characterized by a sprinkling of human cases that constitutes the transitional phase between the rat epizootic and the plague epidemic proper, typified by a rapidly increasing number of human cases. It was the very beginning of this transitional phase that the inhabitants of the plague-stricken block of tenements in Bombay had experienced, when they suddenly were so aggressively attacked by swarms of voracious rat fleas that many of them felt obliged to sleep in the veranda at night.

The characteristic features of this transitional phase explain the sudden and dramatic onset of plague epidemics with abruptly skyrocketing *morbidity rates*[13] and *mortality rates*.[14] This dramatic and explosive type of epidemic development is in itself a clear indication of plague. Epidemic diseases that spread directly between human

---

distance from human beings. Grey rats prefer to live in sewers and cellars or even as field rats and wood rats. The distance from human beings means that plague disease among grey rats will cause few direct casualties among human beings.

[12] The term epicentre normally signifies the centre of an earthquake.

[13] Proportion of a population that contracts a specific disease.

[14] Proportion of a population that dies in a specified unit of time no matter what the causal factors. The plague mortality rate is the proportion of a population that dies from this disease in an epidemic.

beings produce bell-shaped development curves that reflect the pace of a disseminative process based on human contact and the slow depletion of the pool of susceptible persons.

Very clearly, neighbours, relatives (inheritors), and other persons like physicians or priests who visited houses where people were sick from plague or people had died from plague, exposed themselves to grave danger. They would quite likely either be bitten by infective rat fleas that swarmed in the houses, or pick up such fleas in their clothing and bring them to their own home, where the fleas would seek out the rats and trigger a new plague epizootic. The connection would, however, be concealed because of the delay of approximately three weeks before the rat epizootic had run its deadly course and the incubation period of the first cases was ended.

In addition, the Commission launched a comprehensive project to study how plague was introduced from Bombay into surrounding villages, and also examined the process of spread within the villages. It was shown that plague normally arrived with persons unwittingly carrying infective rat fleas in their clothing or luggage, often natives of the village who had found work at the cotton mills in the big city, and now fled from the plague there. It was this pattern of panic and flight that to some extent repeated itself in India in the early 1990s, and caused grave concern that plague would slip out of control and explode into a disastrous full-blown epidemic.

In this mode of spread at a distance, rat fleas could play an important part for a special reason. There are two main types of fleas, *fur fleas*, which ride with their hosts, and *nest fleas*, which live in the nests of their hosts. The normal flea parasite of the black rat (*Xenopsylla cheopis*) is a typical fur flea. This means that these rat fleas are used to and adapted to riding with hosts, and therefore also ride easily in the clothing of human beings. For the same reason, they also tolerate light well. The human flea, on the other hand, is a typical nest flea that lives in the immediate surroundings of human beings, preferably in or around beds and other sleeping arrangements. They come out at night, feed on their hosts and seek out a usable place to digest the meal and lay eggs. The human flea is therefore not adapted to riding with its human hosts, and are very averse to light, so human fleas avoid riding with their human hosts. Examination of actively worn clothing did not, therefore, yield many human fleas even if human housing was greatly infested, as in India or North Africa. Human fleas typically move with furniture and bed linen and suchlike, i.e., they move with the 'nest'. For these reasons, human fleas will not under any circumstances be effective disseminators of plague infection, i.e., independent of the decisive point relating to the level of bacteraemia (septicaemia) in human beings and the level needed to produce blockage.

This finding has later been confirmed by another large-scale research project on plague performed by French scholars in Madagascar. Epidemics comprising more than 40,000 cases took place in the island in the 1920s and 1930s. Although the hovels and huts of the native population swarmed with human fleas, the researchers never registered a single case of bubonic plague spread from one person to another through the agency of the human flea.[15]

---

[15] Girard 1943: 4–43; Brygoo 1966: 42–4. Cf. Coulanges 1989: 10–11, 24, and n. 4 above.

Long-distance spread and grain-eating fleas

However, another crucial epidemiological question remained unanswered, namely the mechanisms of metastatic spread: how did plague leap abruptly for considerable distances, even hundreds of miles, to another region or country? Rats could of course travel in cargoes over long distances, but rats that were infected with plague would normally die in a few days, a fact that would finish any possible role they had as agents of spread. Again the solution was to be found with the rat fleas. The explanation proved to be another triumph for that amazingly creative process known as *evolution*, and the pivotal instrument of evolution called *survival of the fittest*.

Because the rat fleas were fur fleas adapted to riding with their hosts, they have for thousands of years fallen off, been scratched off or have left their dead hosts in the favourite environments of black rats. Because grain is the favourite food of black rats, their fleas have tended to be on their own in environments with grain or at least grain debris, in private grain stores, in the vicinity of querns (hand mills) where there is often grain debris on the ground, in the stores of local salesmen, in mills, bakeries, shipments of grain, and so on. It turned out that the fleas of the black rat had actually developed the ability to live off grain and grain debris, being dependent on blood only for laying eggs. The rapid turnover of generations and the great fertility that characterize fleas continuously produce a correspondingly huge number of mutant specimens, and therefore also at some point specimens that had this special property. The specimens that had acquired this property and their offspring would survive more often than rat fleas that did not possess this property, and in time this species of flea would be genetically adapted to this situation and have developed the ability to live off grain. This meant that infected fleas could travel over long distances, especially in climates that were not hot and dry so that they would not die quickly from desiccation. The humidity associated with voyages allows fleas to survive for many weeks, explaining why plague could be spread so easily by ship.[16]

In 1910, a plague epidemic broke out in England, in Latimer Cottages, a row of houses in the parish of Freston, five miles south of Ipswich, on the Shotley peninsula. Suddenly, people began to fall seriously ill and die, and it was thanks to an alert local family doctor that the epidemic was confined to a few cases.

Medical personnel also took a keen interest in two other outbreaks of dramatic illness in the area that they now suspected could have been plague cases. Again, long-distance transport of grain came to attention as the vehicle of spread of plague. Oceangoing ships on their way up the estuary leading to Ipswich would pause at anchor at Butterman's Bay to lighten their loads by transferring some of their cargo onto barges before proceeding upstream to Ipswich docks. Many of these ships were grain ships coming from foreign ports. This provided work for local labour and, thus, infected rat fleas could be brought ashore and trigger an epizootic in the rat populations.[17]

---

[16] Estrade 1935: 293–8; C.Y. Wu 1936: 260–1, 287.

[17] Zwanenberg 1970: 62–74; Howell and Ford 1986: 191–209. Because the house rat, i.e., the black rat, had disappeared and the grey rat, which lived at some distance from people, in sewers, cellars and as wood rats had supplanted it, contact between people and rat fleas was much reduced since medieval times, and plague took on an episodic and highly localized character.

However, the epidemiological point had been underscored, plague travelled easily with shipments of grain at a distance. The importance of grain transport was also noted by American epidemiologists in connection with the large plague epidemics in Vietnam during the war there, when plague arrived with shipments of rice.[18]

The Black Death and modern plague: Same or different?

This explanation of how plague spread at considerable distances based on notions of evolutionary change and adaptation through selection of mutant strains posed a new question: could one be certain that the plague studied in India actually had the same properties and spread in the same way as the Black Death? Was it really the Black Death that was the adversary, or had plague changed in substantial ways in the centuries that had passed since that medieval epidemic catastrophe?

It was well known that epidemic diseases change over time through evolutionary adaptation, usually becoming 'milder', tending to lose some of their pathogenic and lethal powers (*virulence*). The reason for this is clear: bacteria multiply by division, they divide often and their numbers are truly staggering. This means that there will be frequent mutations possessing a great variation of new properties. Some of these mutants will have acquired a property that is valuable for their survival and the survival of their descendants. Thus, new strains come into being that are better adapted for survival. In this evolutionary process, very dangerous strains will tend to kill off their hosts before they succeed in passing on their specific properties and, thus, will tend to become extinguished. Milder strains will tend to succeed in passing on their specific properties more often because their hosts survive or at least live longer, giving them more time to succeed in being passed on to a new host. In short, it is advantageous for parasites not to be too dangerous for their hosts.

The type of plague that challenged humankind and the resourcefulness of scholars around the turn of the twentieth century certainly appeared to possess full pathogenic and lethal powers. It also exhibited the typical clinical and diagnostic features of the Black Death and later plague epidemics as described by physicians and chroniclers in the past. That, then, represented in itself a problem, but it did not necessarily mean that plague had not changed in some important aspect(s) and was different from that old-time plague and the Black Death itself. In their laboratories, bacteriologists repeatedly discovered strains of plague with reduced virulence, i.e., weaker or milder strains. What happened to these strains?

The resolution of this problem was not found in India but in the former Soviet Union several decades later. It was discovered that there was a strong correlation between the virulence of the strains of plague and their ability to cause the growth of blockage in the ventricular system of fleas. This meant that, in contrast to other diseases, it was the virulent strains that would most often succeed in passing on their genetic material and special properties, while the milder strains would be at a disadvantage and would be mercilessly deselected by the evolutionary process.[19] This finding explained the apparent great stability in the clinical and diagnostic manifesta-

---

[18] Marshall, Joy, Ai et al. 1967: 604–5, 610.
[19] See my presentation of this research in Benedictow 1993/1996a: 241–2.

tions of plague and in its virulence and lethality. This made it clear that it was, indeed, for all practical purposes that old grisly disease, the Black Death, that had returned. This finding was of great significance for historians of medicine and demography because it meant that they could freely use the results of modern medical research in India, China, Madagascar, USA, Vietnam and Russia (the Soviet Union) in their studies of the Black Death and later epidemics of plague.

Rat history

Some scholars maintain that the Black Death could not have spread effectively and murderously in Northern Europe, because the black rat cannot live in cold climates. Without rats and rat fleas widely distributed in people's houses there could not be large-scale epidemics of bubonic plague.[20]

It appears, therefore, useful to present a short outline of the history of the black rat in the northern half of Europe, starting in the middle of Europe and moving northwards. Skeletal remains of the black rat dating back to Roman times have been found in Italy, in Roman Austria and all over Roman Germany to about the city of Cologne in the north-west (a Roman military camp called *Colonia* = settlement).[21] Two skeletal remains of the black rat have been found in excavations of a Roman villa near the city of Berne in Switzerland.[22] Finds of skeletal remains of the black rat dating back to the time of the Roman occupation have also been made in England, namely in York, London and Wroxeter in the north-east, south-east and west of England, respectively. In addition, up to 1984 there had been made six finds of skeletal remains of the black rat dating back to the Early Middle Ages, and 27 finds dating back to the 11th–15th centuries.[23] Subsequently, many new finds of remains of rats have been made in England.[24]

Thus, despite the fact that animal remains have only recently attracted the interest of archaeologists and osteologists (researchers on skeletal remains) it has been shown that the black rat was widely dispersed in England from Roman times and was distributed all over the country in the Middle Ages. The difference in established distribution between these two historical periods is probably due to the fact that there are fewer physical remains from Roman England than from medieval England that can be examined. Earlier archaeological excavations have inevitably destroyed relevant skeletal material. It could be suggested that the black rat was spread over the Roman Europe by the legions and through the market-oriented network that was established by the Roman Empire.

From the Roman border provinces the black rat could easily have been spread further into Germanic and Slavic territories by trade. Actually, remains of black rats dating back to late Roman centuries have been found in the excavation of a Germanic settlement at Waltersdorf in eastern Germany near present-day Berlin, and in Slavic settlements in present-day north-western Poland (Smuszewo) and on the eastern side

---

[20] See, e.g., Davis 1986.
[21] Armitage, West and Steedman 1984: 379.
[22] Stampfli 1965–6: 454–5.
[23] Armitage, West and Steedman 1984: 381.
[24] James 1999: 20–1; James 2001: 8–13.

of the Gulf of Gdansk (Tolkmicko). Thus, it is not surprising that quite numerous finds of skeletal remains of the black rat dating back to the early medieval period have been made in northern and north-eastern Germany, and in Poland, including sites on the Baltic Sea.[25] In the most important commercial centre in Northern Europe in the Early Middle Ages, namely the town of Haithabu situated north of present-day Hamburg, several finds of the skeletal remains of the black rat have been made.[26] From this important commercial centre, the black rat must have been distributed into the Nordic countries by ship transport, for the black rat is not only the house rat but also the classic ship rat.

However, the lines of trade and communication extended much farther in Northern Europe. Franks and Frieslanders traded with the Nordic countries in the Early Middle Ages and the Vikings sailed all around Western Europe, trading and plundering as they saw fit. In the 880s, the Norwegian merchant Ottar, who lived far north in northern Norway, visited King Alfred the Great of Wessex in England. He told the king about Norway and the other Nordic countries, an account that was included in the geographical section of the translation of the Roman author Orosius' *History of the World*, a project in which the king participated eagerly. Ottar's account produces a vivid picture of a network of trade by ship that interconnected the whole of Northern and north-western Europe in the ninth century.

Of course, if the black rat's physical constitution made it more or less impossible for it to live in regions with a cold winter climate and only moderately warm summers, no type of trade connection would make it possible for this type of rat to become so widely distributed in the Nordic countries that it could constitute the basis for large-scale plague epidemics. However, there is much evidence confirming the rural presence of rats in the Nordic countries in the medieval and modern period. The presence of the brown or grey rat was not commented on in Scandinavia before the 1750s, first in Norway. Until the 1790s, the black rat was the only rat in Sweden and Finland, the Nordic countries with the coldest winters. At the beginning of this century, the black rat was still found in a number of urban and *rural* areas in these countries,[27] and in Norway, it may still live in a few *rural* localities.[28] This fact undermines the climatological argument. It is usual to assume that the black rat was put on the defensive because, in the Early Modern period, new house-building techniques and materials and a new situation drove it out of people's houses, and it could not defend its territories against the larger and stronger grey or brown rat.

In Scandinavia, several finds of the skeletal remains of the black rat go back to the Late Viking Age and the early High Middle Ages that comprise both urban and rural ecological environments. Finds have been made in the cathedral city of Lund and a nunnery in Ny Varberg, both situated on the Sound, the sites of a monastery in Gudhem in western Sweden (south-western region of Västergötland), and Öland I. on Sweden's southern Baltic coast.[29] Large numbers of skeletal remains of the black

---

[25] Teichert 1985.
[26] Reichstein 1974 and 1987.
[27] Nybelin 1928: 850–7; Bernström 1969: 578–9, 584; Vilkuna 1969: 583–4.
[28] Personal communication from Rolf Lie, Zoological Museum, University of Bergen.
[29] See Bergquist 1957: 98–103; Lepiksaar 1965: 96–7, 1969: 38, 1975: 230–9; Boessneck and Von den Driesch 1979: 214–15. Lund and Varberg are today Swedish, but in the Middle Ages belonged to Denmark.

rat dating back to the thirteenth century and the late medieval period have recently been found during excavations in Stockholm.[30] The wide geographical spread and the substantial number of finds of medieval rat bones are quite remarkable not least because serious archaeo-zoological research is a relatively recent discipline.

There is also linguistic and literary evidence. In languages of Indo-European origin, e.g., Germanic languages, Latin and Romance languages, and Slavonic languages, the basic word in this connection is 'mus', in English mouse. In the past, people were not zoologists and had no scholarly or scientific training, and used this word to designate a number of animals that looked quite alike to them – mice, rats, stoats and polecats, for instance. For this reason, when this word mus or mouse was used, further information was needed to identify the specific sort of animal referred to. In the Norse language of the Vikings and the high medieval Nordic populations, a specific term came into use when people wished to identify the animal in question as a rat, namely völsk mus, which means Frankish mouse.[31] In view of what we know of the history of the brown/grey rat, there can be no doubt that this term refers to the black rat. The term Frankish mouse may contain some indication of the geographical origin of the black rats that spread in the Nordic countries, and that the time of introduction was the Viking Age, quite likely the ninth century when Viking fleets frequently sailed up the large French rivers, landing hosts of armed men that ravished the countryside and formed armies that besieged Paris.

There are references to rats in sagas and other literary works. A leading scholar in this field of study concludes: 'During the late medieval period, rats and mice are mentioned as generally known vermin in and around human buildings' in the Nordic countries.[32] There can be no doubt that there was a broad diffusion of the black rat in the Nordic countries in the Middle Ages, and that this constituted a sufficient biological base for large-scale plague epidemics.

It will also be clear from the presentation below of the spread of the Black Death in such Northern European countries as Norway and Sweden that the epidemics raged from spring to late autumn and were suppressed by cold weather. Actually, this seasonal feature can already be seen emerging in the case of its spread in Austria and Germany. The explanation for this seasonal pattern can only be that the Black Death was dependent on rat fleas for transmission and, therefore, required a murine basis in the form of the widespread presence of rats. This is in accordance with all the central modern monographs on plague based on the experience of medical researchers in India, China, Madagascar and elsewhere.

---

[30] Vretemark 1983: 294, 467.
[31] An Icelandic–English Dictionary 1975: 440; mýss valkar; Fritzner 1954: 755.
[32] Bernström 1969: 577–83, my translation from Swedish. Törnblom 1993: 367.

4

Plague: The Hydra-headed Monster

Bubonic plague

Plague made such an overwhelming impression on the researchers who studied it that they quite often resorted to classical Greek mythology in their descriptions. One leading researcher called plague the Hydra-headed monster, referring to the grisly monster-snake Hydra with nine heads, which eventually was killed by that great hero Hercules, who later used its blood as a lethal poison for his arrows. Like the Hydra, plague could appear in so many different forms and disguises.

The normal and basic process of transmission and infection of plague disease had been uncovered by the Indian Plague Research Commission:

(1) An infective, i.e., blocked, rat flea regurgitates ingested blood and fragments of the blockage containing thousands of plague bacteria into the bite wound.

(2) The inoculated plague bacteria are drained along a lymphatic tract to a lymph node, which swells into a bubo that may be of the size of a pea or, perhaps, an egg, and which is exquisitely tender. The site of the bite wound will decide where the bubo will develop: if the flea bite is on a leg, the infective material will normally be drained to the lymphatic nodes in the groin or on the thigh, and the bubo will develop there; because the legs constitute such a large part of the body surface and can be attacked by fleas also when people are sitting or walking, buboes develop most often in these areas of the body. However, buboes develop often also in the upper part of the body, especially in the armpits, and quite often in the neck, in the submaxillary area and behind the ears. Occasionally, buboes may also develop in many other parts of the body. This type of plague is called *primary bubonic plague*, because it starts with a primary infection of the lymphatic system. *Bubonic plague* is not only the basic form of plague, but also comprises the great majority of cases.

Occasionally, a blocked flea will insert its proboscis directly into a vein and regurgitate the ingested blood with bits of the blockage directly into the bloodstream; occasionally too, the infection dose will be so enormous that the lymphatic system is overwhelmed and a large number of plague bacteria will pass quite unimpeded on into the bloodstream. In the bloodstream, the bacteria will immediately start to multiply rapidly. This type of plague is called *primary* bacteraemic plague, because the infection of the blood stream is primary to all subsequent developments in the course of the disease. It is the most lethal of all types of plague; there are no survivors. In a study of more than 200 cases of primary bacteraemic plague in a plague epidemic in Colombo in 1914–15, it was shown that, on average, only 14.5 hours lapsed from the onset of illness to the death of the patient, some patients dying in a few hours. In the local population, the course of illness was described as fever in the morning, death in the evening.[1] This is the type of plague behind the terror-stricken accounts by medieval chroniclers of sudden death in the Black Death. In the past, physicians observed that plague without external signs was the most dangerous form. As one of them put it: 'that plague is the most dangerous/ which leaves no external signs/ attacking directly the spirits of life in the heart itself'.[2] In reality, primary bacteraemic plague is a fulminant type of bubonic plague where death occurs before a bubo has had time to develop.

In 50–60 per cent of plague cases, plague bacteria eventually succeed in over-whelming the lymphatic system and slip out of the bubo and into the bloodstream. This is called *secondary* bacteraemic plague in order to underscore that this type is developed from, and therefore secondary to, the primary infection of the lymphatic system, and, thus, is a form of bubonic plague. In the bloodstream, the plague bacteria multiply rapidly, and the patient's condition deteriorates rapidly. The Indian Plague Research Commission noted that all patients who developed bacteraemia, whatever the level, died. Later, a few survivors have been registered, but for all practical purposes bacteraemia in patients heralds imminent death.

In some of the bacteraemic cases, bacteria reach the peripheral blood circulation and capillary vessels where their tendency to clot and the weakening of the walls of the vessels caused by bacterial toxins can cause small haemorrhages under the skin.[3] These haemorrhages are the *petechiae*, the dark or purple spots or blotches, often described with terror in historical sources. In the case of the Black Death, these spots are described by the contemporary Florentine author Giovanni Boccaccio in the Introduction to his (in)famous book *Decameron*:

> [. . .] in men and women alike it [the Black Death] first betrayed itself by the emergence of certain tumours in the groin or the armpits, some of which grew as large as a common apple, others as an egg, some more, some less, which the common folk called *gavocciolo*. From the two said parts of the body this deadly *gavocciolo* soon began to propagate and spread itself in all directions indifferently; after which the form of the malady began to change, black spots or livid making their appearance in many cases on the arm or the thigh or elsewhere, now few and large, now minute and numerous. And as the *gavocciolo* had been and still was an infallible token of approaching death, such also were these spots on whomsoever they showed themselves [. . .]

This account of the clinical manifestations of the Black Death contains a characteristic part of humanist rhetorical exaggeration. It is not true that patients with bubonic plague invariably die, on average 20 per cent survive. It is not true, as Boccaccio appears to assert, that all cases of bubonic plague develop these dark spots, but it is for all practical purposes true that those who did invariably died. They were therefore called 'God's

---

1 Philip and Hirst 1917: 529–30, 534–5.
2 Block 1711: 21, 24–5. My translation from Swedish.
3 Chun 1936: 311–13, 316.

tokens' or, as a sign of familiarity, just 'tokens'. In the words of Shakespeare: 'the tokened pestilence where death is sure'.[4]

Could the Black Death have been an epidemic of primary pneumonic plague?

In cases of secondary bacteraemic plague, bacteria are also transported with the bloodstream to the lungs, where they may consolidate, multiply and cause pneumonia. In order to emphasize that the pneumonic inflammation is developed from, and therefore secondary to, a primary bubonic infection, this condition is called *secondary pneumonic plague*. This development occurs in about 10–25 per cent of bubonic cases.[5] Such patients often develop a cough and bloody expectoration (ejecting from the lung airways) containing plague bacteria, and these patients may occasionally infect others by droplet infection. Cases of pneumonic plague conveyed by cross-infection are called *primary pneumonic plague* in order to underscore that the patients have contracted this form of plague directly from another person by inhaling plagued-infected droplets, and not from a primary bubonic infection. Plague, then, is almost always transmitted in two different ways: by rat fleas that convey infection from rats to human beings, and by cross-infection between human beings through the inhaling of infected droplets.

Secondary pneumonic plague is often confused with primary pneumonic plague. Many historians appear to be poorly acquainted with secondary pneumonic plague and tend to assume automatically that the mentioning of bloody sputum (spittle and expectoration) in the historical sources refers to primary pneumonic plague. The clinical description of cases of the Black Death given by the Irish friar John Clyn of Kilkenny, for instance, has been misunderstood in this way:

> [. . .] many died of boils and abscesses, and pustules on their shins [= legs] and under their armpits; others frantic with pain in their head, and others spitting blood [. . .][6]

As can be seen, the references to buboes (boils) and to abscesses, pustules and carbuncles, which are local infections caused by remaining plague bacteria in infective fleas' bite sites, dominate the clinical description. John Clyn's observation that some died spitting blood cannot be taken as evidence to the effect that the Black Death was mainly an epidemic of primary pneumonic plague. On the contrary, the strongly restricted reference to the occurrence of cases with bloody expectoration indicates clearly the normal proportion of cases that develop secondary pneumonic plague in epidemics of bubonic plague. This statement, then, contains a good description (for the time) of an epidemic of bubonic plague, and, thus, is a good source to the medical and epidemiological character of the Black Death in England.

All standard works on primary pneumonic plague emphasize that primary pneumonic plague does not cross-infect easily, and, thus, does not spread according to the pattern of highly contagious viral droplet-conveyed diseases such as influenza or

---

4   MacArthur 1925–6: 358; Wilson 1963: 102.
5   Hirst 1953: 22. See also below p. 236, n. 6.
6   Hirst 1953: 13.

smallpox. There are several reasons for this important feature. The course of primary pneumonic plague is extremely fulminant. The patients live, on average, 1.8 days from the onset of the disease, the infective cough emerging, on average, after 24 hours. Cases of primary pneumonic plague that develop the contagious cough will, on average, be infective for only 19 hours. Actually, this type of plague is so fulminant and mortal that many patients die in the course of the first 24 hours, before developing any infective cough at all.

It is a general epidemiological tenet that diseases that kill off their victims quickly will have weak diffusive powers because they will have little time to achieve transmission. Such ferocity may even put their survival as a species, and the types of diseases they convey, in danger of extinction. In the case of primary pneumonic plague, this problem is very much exacerbated by two other important factors:

(1) The plague pathogen is a bacterium, and as such it is very much larger than viruses. For this reason, plague bacteria will need to be spread by much larger droplets than viruses, which, nonetheless, can only contain a few bacteria at the most, and do not go far.

(2) The large or largish size of droplets containing plague bacteria has also another important consequence: often, the droplets will not get into the lungs even when they are inhaled. Larger droplets tend to impinge on the upper respiratory tract, particularly in the tonsillar region. Here the infected droplets occasion infection of the pharynx and, next, when plague bacteria move on into the bloodstream, they cause primary bacteraemic plague.

Thus, in a strange way, primary droplet infection actually quite often gives rise to bubonic plague, albeit in such a fulminant form that the patients die before a bubo has had time to develop. Also these patients die without developing an infective cough, and, thus, do not contribute to the continued spread of primary pneumonic infection. Because these cases constitute a sizeable proportion of all cases of primary pneumonic plague, leading authorities underline that they have a marked deleterious effect on the diffusive powers of primary pneumonic plague.[7]

In this way several important medical and bacteriological factors interact to produce the characteristically weak powers of spread of pneumonic plague, and ensure that outbreaks usually die out fast. This disease can exist on its own for only a short time, and it is dependent on bubonic plague to emerge again. Typically, primary pneumonic plague occurs in small, episodic outbreaks, usually at the family or neighbourhood levels, and outbreaks comprise rarely more than a few tens of victims.[8] In the words of an American scholar in a modern textbook of bacteriology:

> Primary plague pneumonia occurs primarily in persons in close and prolonged contact with another person with pneumonic plague. Hence, respiratory transmission occurs most frequently to medical personnel or household contacts who are directly involved with the care of the patient.[9]

---

[7]   L.-T. Wu 1926: 189–90; Chun 1936: 318–19; Pollitzer and Li 1943: 212–16.
[8]   L.-T. Wu 1913: 243–7; L.-T. Wu 1926: 9–97, 187–95; L.-T. Wu 1927–8: 55–70; Klimenko 1910: 659–61; Chun 1936: 317–20; Pollitzer and Li 1943: 212–16; Pollitzer 1960: 347; Meyer 1957: 712–14; Meyer 1961: 249–61; Poland 1983: 1230.
[9]   Poland 1983: 1230.

Because women all over the world carry the main responsibility for the nursing of the sick in the household, they are at particular risk of contracting epidemic diseases by cross-infection, and this is also the case with primary pneumonic plague. In 60 primary pneumonic outbreaks in Upper Egypt from 1904 to 1924, 'women constituted 71 per cent of those who contracted the disease, a fact well in accord with the familial character of lung plague in Upper Egypt'.[10]

In 1910–11, the greatest known epidemic of primary pneumonic plague spread in Manchuria with offshoots into northern China and the adjacent Vladivostok area in Russia's Pacific region. Because there was no anti-epidemic organization in this distant province, the epidemic ran its course without being significantly affected by anti-epidemic countermeasures.[11] In the end, it killed about 60,000 persons. As the population of Manchuria at the time is estimated to have been about twelve million persons, the 50,000 fatalities there constituted a population mortality of 0.4 per cent, illustrating the poor diffusive powers of this particular disease.

In 1912, Chinese authorities established the North Manchurian Plague Prevention Service (NMPPS) to acquire more knowledge about the epidemiology of primary pneumonic plague and to have a permanent organization prepared to combat the disease on the basis of modern western medicine. Most of our knowledge on primary pneumonic plague is based on the results of the comprehensive research that NMPPS performed on the past epidemic, and in connection with a pneumonic epidemic that broke out in 1920, but which the new sanitary organization contained quite successfully (9,000 cases).

One should, however, note that the ability to spread in the Manchurian epidemic was, in fact, greatly strengthened by extremely favourable circumstances for the dissemination of this particular disease compared with any medieval or early modern scenario in North Africa, the Middle East or Europe. In the first place, the railway played an important role, transporting infected and infective persons rapidly over long distances. This repeatedly gave rise to new effective epicentres of spread. However, it was also observed that gravely sick persons had travelled over long distances coughing and sneezing in overcrowded compartments, evidently without occasioning a single case of transmission.[12]

Secondly, the social circumstances were exceptionally favourable to such a spread. The demographic composition of the population at risk was extraordinary, consisting for a large part of seasonal and migrant workers. Chinese peasants working in the mines and along the Sungari and Amur rivers constituted at the time a large part of the Manchurian population. Some hunted tarabagans for their valuable fur. These were largish rodents living there in such great numbers that plague circulated continuously among them without eradicating the population, in what is called a plague focus (see above); some hunters became infected, and they were the source of the epidemic. These workers stayed mostly in highly overcrowded inns and lodging-houses: 'Two, and sometimes three, tiers of berths for the lodgers are present, there being just room enough between the tiers for a man to sit up.' An ordinary lodging-house of this type could be 15 ft square and 12 ft high, i.e., 20.9 sq.metre and 76.4 cu.metre. This

---

[10] L.-T. Wu 1926: 34.
[11] L.-T. Wu 1913–14: 237–90; L.-T. Wu 1926; L.-T. Wu 1934: 1–3.
[12] L.-T. Wu 1926: 71.

space would be packed with three tiers of berths, one above the other, accommodating more than 40 persons, each having at his disposal less than 1.9 cu.metre of
space. For protection against the severe winter cold when the temperature in
Manchuria 'as a rule reaches minus 30°C to minus 40°C', the lodging-houses were
constructed either entirely underground or at least partly underground. The windows
were closed during the winters, and 'even in May the rooms were ill-ventilated and
stuffy'.[13] These men were evidently breathing, sneezing and coughing in the immediate proximity of the next man. The population density structure was close to ideal for
the spread of diseases by droplet infection, far more favourable in fact than in any
normal medieval European or Arab population.

Summing up, it is clear that primary pneumonic plague cannot play a major independent epidemic role and that the Black Death cannot have been wholly or mainly
an epidemic of this kind, as assumed by some historians.

Prominent medical scholars in plague research underline that the dynamics of
primary pneumonic plague are not manifestly weaker in hot and dry areas than in
cold and wet areas. Upper Egypt, Madagascar and Java are areas where this disease
spreads more readily than in other places. The reason for this is prevalent social
customs and norms, which require that relatives and friends have comprehensive
close and physical contact with the diseased, hugging, comforting, massaging,
collecting in their hands bloody expectoration coughed up by the patients, and so
on.[14] This behaviour provides much close contact between uninfected persons and
patients, satisfying the basic requirement for cross-infection to occur with more than
episodic frequency. Behavioural factors are decisive, the role of climate being of
minor significance. In the words of the director of the NMPPS and its leading
researcher Wu Lien-Teh: 'in our opinion, an overwhelming majority of cases receive
infection through being in the direct range of a cough'.[15]

Recent American experience bears upon this point. In America, several veterinarians and their assistants have contracted primary pneumonic plague after contact
with pet cats that had killed plague-infected ground squirrels and had become
infected by droplet infection. Sixty-one persons who had had face-to-face contact with
one of the veterinarians after he began coughing, were considered to be at risk,
including family members, office associates, members of staff and fifty-five hospital
contacts. A middle-aged woman with primary pneumonic plague had contact with c.
180 persons before her three-day course of illness ended fatally. Plague was not diag-
nosed until four days after her death. Nonetheless, no case of infective transmission
had occurred in any of these two case histories,[16] attesting to the low communicability
of primary pneumonic plague.

Cases of primary pneumonic plague and of primary bacteraemic plague often
develop intense bacteraemia, and there has been some speculation that such human
cases could infect human fleas sufficiently to cause development of blockage and
therefore the rise of a concurrent epidemic of bubonic plague disseminated and
transmitted between humans. This is not supported by evidence. Such evidence was

[13] L.-T. Wu 1913: 248–9.
[14] L.-T. Wu 1926: 33, 62, 165; L.-T. Wu 1936c: 413, 416; Wakil 1932: 98, 102; Brygoo 1966: 64–71.
[15] L.-T. Wu 1926: 165, 180–1, 301–2.
[16] Leads 1984: 1400; Poland 1983: 1231.

diligently sought by the NMPPS. Although the inns and lodging-houses where the Chinese workers lived swarmed with human fleas and other types of bloodsucking insects, no such case was recorded in connection with the pneumonic epidemic of 1910–11, which, as mentioned, comprised 60,000 cases.[17]

In Madagascar, plague was rampant after 1920; 40,000 cases of plague were registered in the following two decades, about 20 per cent of the cases were classified as primary bacteraemic plague and another 20 per cent as primary pneumonic plague. Although the huts and hovels of the natives swarmed with fleas, not a single certain case of inter-human transmission by the human flea was ever recorded, and the human flea could at most only have played an episodic role.[18]

However, these types of *mixed epidemics* of plague could be a fruitful model to have in mind in the study of the Black Death. In some areas the Black Death could have taken on this form.

Can it be true that plague spreads more effectively in the countryside than in urban areas?

The question of the relationship between the identity of the Black Death and modern plague was also highlighted by another fascinating observation by the Indian Plague Research Commission that constituted a seemingly impossible epidemiological conundrum. The central tenet of modern scientific epidemiology is that: 'no matter by what method a parasite passes from host to host, an increased density of the susceptible population will facilitate its spread from infected to uninfected individuals'.[19]

However, to their amazement plague in India seemed to defy this obvious epidemiological 'truth'. Actually, this strange phenomenon was discovered by another British medical scholar working in India, namely E.H. Hankin. In 1905, the same year as the Indian Plague Research Commission was formed, he published data on the correlations between plague mortality and population density in the Bombay area that were as clear as they were inexplicable (Table 1).

Table 1. Population density and plague mortality per thousand inhabitants in Bombay Presidency 1897–8

Locality	Population size	Death rate (per 1000)
Bombay	806,144	20.1
Poona	161,696	31.2
Karachi	97,009	24.1
Sholapur	61,564	35.0
Kale	4,431	104.9
Supne	2,068	102.5
Ibrampur	1,692	360.5

[17] L.-T. Wu 1926: 185–6.
[18] Brygoo 1966: 44, 47.
[19] Burnet and White 1972: 11.

Hankin was so intrigued by his finding that he wished to test it on historical plague data. He turned to the few data on the late-medieval plague epidemics in England that were available at the time, and, in fact, succeeded in producing interesting evidence to the same effect. This underpinned the validity of his enigmatic finding of inverse correlation between mortality rates in plague epidemics and population densities, but he was at a loss to explain it.[20]

Hankin's study intrigued also the Indian Plague Research Commission. A few years later its member Major Greenwood reached the same 'curious and interesting' conclusions in his statistical studies of plague in the Punjab: 'the rate of plague mortality tends to increase as the absolute population of the infected community diminishes'. Greenwood too gathered and analysed studies of plague in England in the Late Medieval and Early Modern periods. Again his conclusions confirmed Hankin's findings.[21] Almost thirty years later, Wu Lien-Teh reached the same conclusion for China: 'the smaller the community the greater the rate of mortality'.[22]

Although this finding appeared untenable and inexplicable, it was of the utmost importance. Only a disease with great powers of spread in the countryside and in thinly populated areas in general, could, in fact, have the demographic effects that the Black Death was supposed to have had. On the eve of the arrival of the Black Death in medieval Europe, about 90 per cent of the population lived in the countryside, with at most a couple of per cent in urban centres with more than 10,000 inhabitants. Their findings provided, therefore, an intriguing and important support for the view that it was actually the Black Death that had returned, and that, therefore, the results of modern research were applicable to the analysis of that notorious grisly wave of plague epidemics in the Near East, the Middle East, North Africa and Europe.

Recent research has produced strong confirmation of this view both in the form of data on morbidity and mortality rates caused by plague epidemics in human communities with different levels of settlement density, and in the form of an epidemiological explanation. These data reflect the patterns of spread of plague epidemics that raged in Italy in the years 1630-2 and in southern France in the years 1720-2, respectively. The information is summarized in Figure 3,[23] which shows very clearly indeed that these large plague epidemics actually caused much higher morbidity rates in small villages and in rural areas than in towns and cities. Not even the metropoles, the largest cities of the time, with well above 100,000 inhabitants, seem to have suffered comparable morbidity rates.[24]

The status of plague research would be weakened if these findings could not be well explained or rejected. Fortunately, it appears that this epidemiological conundrum has now been resolved satisfactorily. The basic epidemiological principle about the relationship between the powers of spread of epidemic diseases and population density is absolutely valid for diseases spreading directly between human beings. In

[20] Hankin 1905: 48-83.
[21] Greenwood 1911: 62-151.
[22] L.-T. Wu 1936c: 396-9.
[23] The specific French population data: small village = 74-109; village = 213-450; large village = 540-850; small town 1 = 1,000-1,750; small town 2 = 2,000-3,000; town 2 = 4,200-6,000; city = 22,500-24,000; metropolis = 100,000. The specific Italian population data: village = 190-640; town = 2,025-3,900; city = 12,000-76,000; metropolis = 130,000-140,000.
[24] Benedictow 1987: 403-21; 1993/1996a: 178-80.

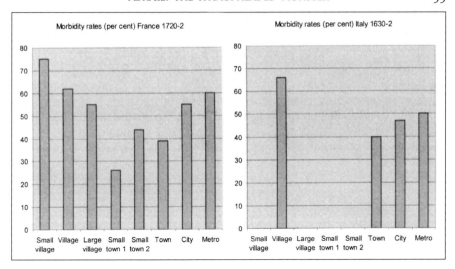

Figure 3. Population density and morbidity: France 1720–2 and Italy 1630–2

the case of diseases spread by cross-infection, the density pattern is, so to speak, one-dimensional, comprising only human beings; then, the density of susceptible human beings will at least for the most part determine the powers of spread. However, epidemics of plague among human beings are secondary to epizootics among commensal rodents, the contagion being transmitted by rat fleas to human beings. In the case of rat-based plague, the density pattern is three-dimensional, comprising the density not only of human beings, but also of rats and rat fleas. The latter two density factors will tend to co-vary strongly and to override the significance of the density of humans.

Rats are social animals that define and defend their territories. This means that in the countryside at least one rat colony will normally be co-resident with a household, whereas in urban areas several households will usually crowd together within the territory of a rat colony. The ratio of human beings to rats and their fleas will tend to be lower in urban environments than in rural, i.e., there will be more persons to share between them the dangerous rat fleas released from the dead rats of an afflicted rat colony.[25]

This epidemiological model provides a basic explanation for how plague may wreak havoc after having arrived at some small-scale residential unit, and why, in the case of plague, severity of impact on human population does not increase with mounting density of human settlement. This finding is of crucial importance: in the mid-fourteenth century, around 90 per cent of the population in Europe, the Middle East or North Africa lived in the countryside with but a small fraction of present-day density; and only an epidemic disease with these disseminative properties could have caused the dramatic population decline in the Late Middle Ages.

However, the identification of these epidemiological properties of plague does not explain *how* plague was spread between local societies, from settlement to settlement,

[25] Benedictow 1987: 423–9.

and from holding to holding in thinly populated areas, producing extreme local mortality rates.

It will, therefore, be an important task in this book to identify and analyse the pattern of mortality rates in relation to population densities caused by the Black Death in order to determine whether or not it conforms to these observations and the explanation given. It will also be an important task to examine patterns of local spread in order to explain the extraordinary capacity of the Black Death to blanket the countryside of medieval Europe.

5

The Territorial Origin of Plague and of the Black Death

A short history of plague before the Black Death

The origin of such an overwhelming epidemic disaster as the Black Death is a question that has fascinated scholars and amateur historians alike. This question of origin really comprises two questions, namely (1) where did plague originate as a disease, where was its ancestral homeland, so to speak; and (2) where was the area of departure of the Black Death?

Plague being a disease that does not leave any mark on the human skeleton, the study of the history of plague is entirely dependent on written information. It is not possible to penetrate deeper into the past than allowed by the history of writing and available documentation. And the deeper into the past we venture, the fewer records remain for our examination.

Historically, early records are necessarily associated with the early sites of civilization that covered only tiny parts of the Earth's surface. Plague is basically a disease circulating among wild rodents, and it will in all probability have originated elsewhere and have a long history before contact was made with some early civilization and written information came into being. Early written records containing references to epidemic disease were produced by people who had no, or only peripheral, genuine medical knowledge and real diagnostic interest. Epidemic disease would normally be viewed as an expression of God's or the gods' wrath and punishment or as unleashed by specific astrological constellations. Medicine would be based mostly on magic and religious rituals. Because of this non-rational causal understanding or interpretation of disease, the chroniclers of that distant past refer normally only vaguely to 'pestilences', without providing specific information that allows modern identification. And when descriptive words are used, their meanings are often difficult to grasp unless they occur many times in different connections.

Fortunately, in the case of plague, written information goes further back in time than could reasonably be expected. The exceptional ferocity of plague epidemics is, of course, one important reason; another is that it is the only epidemic disease that exhibits buboes as a standard diagnostic feature. Blood spitting is also a quite characteristic diagnostic feature of plague that catches people's imagination and will quite often be mentioned.

Quite likely, the earliest account of plague is given in the Bible. I Samuel 4–6 and the

Septuagint[1] contain dramatic accounts of war between the Philistines and the Israelites which took place in the twelfth century B.C., more than three thousand years ago. The Philistines won a great victory and captured the Ark of the Covenant from the Israelites. However, terrible epidemics ravaged the cities to which the Ark was taken: 'the head of the Lord was against the city [Gath] with a very great destruction; and He smote the men of the city, both small and great, and they had emerods in their secret parts [. . .] the hand of God was very heavy there'. In the *Septuagint*, I Kings 5, we read: 'And the hand of the Lord was heavy upon Azotus [Ashdod], and he brought evil upon them, and it burst upon them in the ships, and mice sprang up in the midst of their country, and there was great and indiscriminate mortality in the city.' We are also told that 'mice' 'marred the land'. In the end, the Philistines were so desperate that they handed the Ark back to the Israelites and, in addition, sent as propitiatory offerings five gold images of the buboes and five gold images of the 'mice which ravage the country', one for each of the five Philistine cities and chiefdoms.

There are several problems of translation that must be elucidated in order to reach a more convincing identification with plague. The word 'emerods' is closely related to 'haemorrhoids'. However, the Hebrew word that is translated with 'emerods' is *ofalim*, which means swelling or bubo, and the choice of word reflects a certain shyness in relation to the sexual connotations associated with the groin. Another expression of this shyness is the strange reference to ships in the *Septuagint*; the Hebrew word *ilfa* = ship has also the meaning 'the entire pelvic region',[2] and this word is probably also related to *ofalim*. This double meaning of the word 'ship' introduces at least an intriguing element of ambiguity, but, then, of course, the writer could have both possible meanings in mind.

Meanwhile it has been asserted by some scholars that the phrase 'emerods in their secret parts' refers to piles caused by bacillary dysentery. In his excellent standard work on plague, *The Conquest of Plague*, L.F. Hirst, who had served as an army physician during the First World War, dismisses this view out of hand:

> The present writer worked for two years on military epidemics of bacillary dysentery. He never heard of haemorrhoids as a complication of the acute phase of the disease, and they are very rarely, if ever, seen even as an accompaniment of chronic bacillary dysentery [. . .] Bacillary dysentery is not a very deadly disease among Oriental communities, except in infancy, whereas plague mortality usually exceeds 80 per cent. If dysentery broke out among Oriental armies, it was unlikely that that it seriously impeded their operations.

W.P. MacArthur, who likewise served as an army physician during the First World War, has independently made a statement to the same effect.

> I cannot follow the reasoning which has led to the identification of the Biblical epidemic as dysentery and piles [. . .] The disease does not cause

---

[1] The *Septuagint* or the Alexandrinian translation of the Old Testament was produced by Greek-speaking Jews in Alexandria around the middle of the third century B.C., and is the oldest extant translation of the Old Testament into Greek. It contains a number of parts (*apocrypha*) that were later excluded from the Old Testament by Palestinian Jews on the grounds that they had come about after the time the divine inspiration, which governed the making of the Old Testament, had ceased.

[2] In colloquial Norwegian called 'mid-ship'.

piles, people do not die of piles and an epidemic of piles in any circumstances is to my mind incredible; rectal prolapse is an occasional complication but it is not common enough to colour the general picture of the disease.

Both these physicians spent much of their lives studying and combating plague, and both think that the Biblical description fits well with their experience. Hirst calls it 'the first of all indubitable plague epidemics'.[3]

Next, one should note that people in the past were not zoologists; they tended to call animals that looked alike to them by the same name. Thus, the Hebrew word 'akbar' was used both about mice, voles and rats, in exactly the same way that, in Indo-European languages, the basic word mus, in English mouse, meant rat as well as mouse and is often used also about a number of other animals with some likeness to these two animals (see above). One should note that remains of black rats have been excavated at archaeological sites in Palestine that go back to Neolithic times some 2000–3000 years B.C., and there is therefore no doubt about the presence of the black rat.[4] Zoological studies of Palestine's animal life in the first decades of the twentieth century found that black rats were also usual in the countryside, and sometimes in amounts that made them 'a real pest', fitting nicely with the reference to 'mice which ravage the country'.[5] The propitiatory offering consisted of five gold buboes and five gold rats (probably). Taken together, this makes a quite good case for assuming that the epidemic that ravaged the Philistine cities was bubonic plague.[6] Votive offerings that represent rats and others that appear to represent buboes are also known from Roman Antiquity.[7]

Unquestionable references to plague are found in classical and Hellenistic Greek medicine.[8] Plague is mentioned in several places in the so-called Hippocratic corpus of medical books and writings.[9] The Greeks themselves ascribed these medical writings to a great physician called Hippocrates, allegedly born on Cos I. off the coast of Asia Minor in 460 B.C. Modern philological studies have shown that the various books and writings ascribed to Hippocrates must have been written over a period of several hundred years by a number of different physicians. In fact, it has not been possible to ascribe any of the books or writings to a specific person by name of Hippocrates who must, consequently, be considered a mythical person.

However, like the mythical Hippocrates, the leading Greek physicians of antiquity actually came from Greek colonies along the coasts of Asia Minor, or in the Middle East or North Africa. The greatest medical school of antiquity developed in Alexandria on Egypt's Mediterranean coast in the Hellenistic period (323–30 B.C.), where medicine was taught and practised on the basis of the Hippocratic corpus. The famous library of Alexandria was central in the flowering of medicine there. The references to clear cases of plague must be assumed to reflect actual observations in the areas where Greek physicians were

[3] Hirst 1953: 9; MacArthur 1952: 210.
[4] MacArthur 1952: 209–12, 464; Bodenheimer 1960: 20–1, 110, 128, 177, 179.
[5] Bodenheimer 1935: 96.
[6] MacArthur 1952: 210–11; Hirst 1953: 6–9; Blondheim 1955: 337–45.
[7] MacArthur 1952: 209.
[8] In Greek history of the antiquity, the Classical Period runs from 500 to 323 B.C., the Hellenistic Period from 323 to 30 B.C.
[9] Sticker 1908: 19–20.

active, and the collection and discussion of these observations in the learned medical circles associated with the medical school.

The presentations of plague in the *Hippocratic corpus* have a peculiar feature, in that they all refer to episodic occurrence, the odd case, and, thus, appear to reflect endemic plague, not epidemic plague.[10] This means that these Greek physicians were familiar with areas where wild rodents lived in such great density that plague could circulate continuously among them, at least for quite longish periods, without reducing their density below the level that could sustain the spread and, thus, become extinguished; as we have seen, such areas that function as reservoirs of plague in nature are called *plague foci*.[11] In such areas, herdsmen, hunters, children playing and others occasionally came across a rodent sick or dead from plague, were attacked by hungry fleas, and contracted the disease. Such areas are also today found in North Africa, and within the areas of modern Iran, Iraq and Syria where small epidemics and episodic human cases of plague are still reported.

However, it is unusual that such plague foci do not occasionally give rise to plague epidemics when plague contagion is passed on to domestic rats. This feature of the references to plague in the *Hippocratic corpus* remains, therefore, intriguing. This point is underscored by the fact that indisputable accounts of serious plague epidemics in the Hellenistic period are found in other medical writings. Rufus of Ephesus, who lived around A.D. 100, renders comments on serious, clearly identified, outbreaks of plague reported by the pupils of Dionysius (the Hunchback) in North Africa and the Middle East around 300 B.C. (in texts that are no longer extant):

> The buboes that are called pestilential, are very acute and very fatal, especially those which one may encounter unexpectedly in Libya, Egypt, and Syria, and which they say were accompanied by high fever, agonizing pain, severe constitutional disturbance, delirium, and the appearance of large, hard buboes that did not suppurate [secrete pus], not only in the usual regions of the body, but also at the back of the knee and in the bend of the elbow, where, as a rule, similar fevers do not cause their formation.

One should note that, in antiquity, the geographical term Libya meant North Africa and that the geographical term Syria comprised also most of present-day Israel, 'Palestine' and Jordan. Rufus mentions also subsequent epidemics reported by Posidonius and Dioscorides in Libya, i.e., North Africa, about 50 B.C.[12] Around year A.D. 100 Aretaeus of Cappadocia (a south-eastern region in Asia Minor), a Greek physician living in Alexandria, describes epidemic plague in no uncertain terms: 'the epidemic buboes in the groin are caused from the liver; they are very malign'.[13]

In view of the enormous amounts of grain that from the time of Caesar were shipped from Egypt to Rome[14] to cover the free distribution of grain and flour to the

---

[10] See Glossary or above, p. 18.

[11] See Glossary or above, pp. 13, 29.

[12] Dioscorides was a Greek army surgeon in the service of Emperor Nero (A.D. 54–68).

[13] Sticker 1908: 21–2. That the growth of malignant buboes in the groin originated in the liver is a recurrent medical opinion in Hippocratic medicine. It is inferred from its humoral theory of human physiology, which is based on a notion to the effect that the human body contained four chief fluids, the so-called *cardinal humours*, namely blood, phlegm, choler and, lastly melancholy or black choler.

[14] More accurately, the grain was shipped to Rome's seaport town Ostia whence it was transported into Rome.

Roman proletariat, it is almost inconceivable that plague should not have been shipped as well. As has been mentioned, grain is the favourite food of the black rat, which is an important reason that it is known not only as the house rat but also the classic ship rat. This is also the reason that its normal flea species has developed the capacity to live off grain (see above, p. 20). In a country like Egypt, where plague broke out at least episodically, plague-infected rats should be expected to enter ships headed for Rome at least occasionally,[15] and grain containing plague-infected fleas would be distributed among the Roman population. In fact, disastrous epidemics are reported in the second half of the second century and in the third century A.D., but the accounts contain no useful diagnostic information that can permit identification of the type of disease. It is clear that these epidemics caused considerable diminution of the Roman population, which undermined the tax basis and military manpower basis of the Western Roman Empire, and, consequently contributed to hastening its decline and fall.

The Black Death was not the first clearly identified great wave of plague epidemics to spread around the Mediterranean and over large parts of Europe, to be followed by a number of smaller waves of epidemics over a protracted period of time. As mentioned above, such series of waves of epidemics are called *pandemics*. The *first plague pandemic* swept into Europe and Asia Minor from Egypt in A.D. 541 and epidemics recurred in Europe until 767, comprising in all fifteen successive waves of epidemics.[16] This first plague pandemic is often called the *Justinian(ic) pandemic* after the Eastern Roman emperor at the time of the first ferocious outbreak in Constantinople in (541–)542. The Black Death that is the subject of this book was the first disastrous wave of epidemics of the next *plague pandemic*.

The chroniclers give some interesting information on the geographical origin of the first wave of plague epidemics of the first plague pandemic, the Black Death of the Justinian pandemic, so to speak: they either point to Egypt whence it was obviously shipped abroad, but it is also stated that it originated in Ethiopia. We should probably understand this as south of Ethiopia, because there is a plague focus of long standing in the southern parts of Africa, particularly in the areas of present-day Uganda, Kenya and Tanzania where plague cases still regularly occur. The reference to Ethiopia should probably be seen in the light of a lack of knowledge about African geography south of Ethiopia. However, it is also suggested that the pandemic started in south-western Arabia, and there is actually a small plague focus north of Yemen that is probably of a long standing. There is an account of a local plague epidemic in Yemen in 1157 that spread on all the way into Egypt.[17] Possibly, therefore, the Justianian plague pandemic could have originated there, have travelled with camel caravans northwards to Egypt or been transported over the Red Sea at its narrow southern end to present-day Djibouti or Eritrea and have travelled with camel caravans northwards through Ethiopia, Sudan and into Egypt, eventually reaching the great commercial seaport cities of Pelusium and Alexandria.[18] In a medical compendium produced by the Arab physician Ali ibn Rabban in A.D. 850, the origin of plagues is placed in Sudan. In the

---

[15] Or more accurately, for Rome's seaport Ostia.
[16] Biraben and Le Goff 1969: 1491–1508. Biraben and Le Goff overlooked that the Justinian pandemic reached as far north as England. MacArthur 1949: 169–88; MacArthur 1959: 423–39.
[17] Dols 1977: 33.
[18] See also Sticker 1908: 24–35.

thirteenth century, the distinguished Arab physician Ibn Nafis describes plague buboes and reports that plague often occurred in Ethiopia.[19]

This implies that the plague epidemics mentioned in classical antiquity could have been triggered by importation of plague contagion from the large plague focus in southern and south-eastern Africa or the small plague focus north of Yemen. On these occasions, plague contagion could have contaminated populations of wild rodents in North Africa and the Middle East and have given rise to the establishment of temporary local plague foci. These plague foci seem to be unstable because plague epidemics generated within these regions apparently disappeared completely for centuries from North Africa and the Middle East, for instance in the centuries before the Justinian pandemic began in 541, and between 1057 and 1348. In other words, the plague history of these regions appears to tend to exhibit a cyclical character. This suggests that the susceptible wild rodents in these regions did not live in sufficient density to constitute bases for permanent plague foci; their numbers and density tended to be depleted by plague disease to the point where they could not sustain the continuous circulation of plague infection. The disappearance of plague would allow the wild rodents to reconstitute their numbers and density, and, thus, their capacity for being re-established as plague foci on the next incursion of plague.

It is often wondered why, from the second half of the seventh century, the waves of epidemics in this first (known) plague pandemic rapidly lost much of their capacity to spread, because nothing of consequence was really done to stop their spread. The general reasons that this pandemic waned and petered out in Europe are, nonetheless, quite clear. The gradual breakdown of the Roman Empire in the west and the great unrest caused by the migrations of Germanic peoples undermined urban life and commerce. The economy retreated into an almost universal manorial system based on subsistence farming aimed at self-sufficiency in foodstuffs and other products of everyday consumption. These developments ended or greatly reduced travel and transport of goods, and, thus, the mechanisms by which plague contagion could be spread. Another decisive development was the triumph of Islam in North Africa and the Middle East in the seventh and eighth centuries, which broke off almost entirely the exchange of goods and persons over the Mediterranean, and, hence, transportation of plague contagion from these areas to Europe.

Summing up, there can be no doubt that plague had been established for substantial periods both in North Africa and in the Middle East at least 1,700 years before the outbreak of the Black Death, and probably for almost 2,500 years. It is also clear that there were plague foci of long standing in southern parts of Africa and north of present-day Yemen.

However, these findings in the western parts of the Old World do not prove that plague could not have a long history also in other parts of the Old World. In China, an Imperial encyclopaedia was produced and published under orders of Emperor Kang-Hsi in 1726 that also contains a complete list of epidemics registered in Chinese medical works, literature, historiography and documents. The list comprises a time span of 2,000 years, beginning in 221 B.C. and ending in A.D. 1718. In this list, outbreaks

---

[19] Dols 1977: 15.

of epidemic plague are mentioned only twice, in the seventh century and in the seventeenth century.

Although Chinese sources contain many accounts of severe or disastrous epidemics, chroniclers and other authors usually only mention them in an unspecific way as 'pestilence', without furnishing diagnostic information that allows modern identification. Even more significantly, also the old Chinese medical classics fail to describe plague, although they clearly describe, for instance, cholera. Wu Lien-Teh points out that he has

> failed to find any mention of the word plague, rendered in Chinese *Shu-yi* (rat pest), in any ancient Chinese medical publication [. . .] In spite of years of patient search among such books [. . .] no reference to plague, *shu-yi* or any malady showing any signs or symptoms similar to it could be obtained until we reached the year A.D. 610, when a certain book called *Ping-yuan* or 'Sources of Disease' by Ch'ao Yuan-fan appeared. Here we find mention of E-hê meaning 'malignant bubo' which disease is described as 'coming on abruptly with high fever together with the appearance of a bundle of nodes beneath the tissues. The size of the nodes ranges from a bean to a plum. The skin and muscles around are dry and painful. The nodes may be felt to move from side to side under the skin. If prompt treatment is not given, the poison will enter the system, cause severe chill and end in death.'

Significantly, this source does not refer to epidemic plague, and appears to reflect endemic plague, the sporadic incidence of plague cases contracted by casual contact with diseased wild rodents.

Sun Szu-mo, a noted physician who died in A.D. 652, mentions plague in his book *Valuable Prescriptions*. He uses the term 'malignant bubo' together with a description of the disease that is similar to that given by Ch'ao Yuan-fan. He provides the extra interesting piece of information that plague 'was common in Ling-nan (i.e., the modern province of Guangdon [the southern coastal province containing Canton and Hong Kong]), rarely in interior provinces'. Plague is then not mentioned again for almost a thousand years until, in 1642, when, in a *Treatise on Epidemics* by Wu Yu-k'e, it is called

> bubo epidemic, which was described as widespread, many persons being attacked at the same time and some dying within a few hours after the onset of symptoms. This disease was characterized by the appearance of 'tumours' in various parts of the body, such tumours being movable under the skin.[20]

What about the plague focus in the Yunnan province that was the area of origin of the *third plague pandemic* in the second half of the nineteenth century?[21] Conspicuously, it is not mentioned even in Chinese sources before 1792. One may, thus, cautiously take this as an indication that it was established in connection with the plague epidemics in the first half of the seventeenth century.[22] Also, conspicuously, plague was not mentioned again in the Guangdong province until 1894 when the pandemic that was on its way from Yunnan arrived. It appears that this area did not have sufficient

---

[20] L.-T. Wu 1936a: 10–13. Essential data from the list of epidemics compiled under orders of Emperor Kang-Hsi are given at the end of that chapter and at the end of McNeill 1979.
[21] See above, p. 9.
[22] L.-T. Wu 1936b: 12.

density of rodents to entertain plague continuously, and that, as in North Africa, the pool of rodents eventually became so depleted that diseased rodents would, on average, infect less than one healthy rodent each; plague among these rodents would, consequently, peter out and become extinguished. This is the reason that there has not been a permanent plague focus within China that would cause endemic cases and occasional outbreaks of epidemics, and hence would catch the attention of physicians and be included in medical works (until the focus in the Yunnan province was established much later).

There are, therefore, a number of indications to the effect that plague has not been an old epidemic disease in China, and that there have only been a few incursions of plague throughout this ancient civilization's impressive and relatively well-recorded history. First, it is certainly interesting to note that plague is not mentioned in the classic Chinese medical books. Secondly, it is noteworthy that the first mention of plague is as late as the seventh century, a thousand years later than the information on plague provided by Greek physicians in the classical medical literature of antiquity.[23] Thirdly, it is conspicuous that there actually are only two references to plague in the seventh century, and, then, there is no further mention for a thousand years. Is it really likely that this can be the case in this great Chinese civilization with its great literary tradition and enormous respect for knowledge and history if severe and disastrous waves of plague epidemics repeatedly had ravaged it? Although no final conclusions can be drawn on the basis of this material, it certainly indicates that plague has been a rare disease in Chinese history, and it appears not to have affected Chinese society in the seventh century or in the seventeenth century in the profound way that, for instance, European society was affected by the two first plague pandemics (and, perhaps, also the Western Roman Empire). Perhaps China has been shielded from importation of plague by the Great Wall and the Chinese mandarin leadership's very strong inclination to reject every kind of foreign influence, shut out foreign merchants and prohibit trade abroad by Chinese nationals? In short, intensive isolation could have protected China from plague except for rare and temporary incursions that did not lead to the establishment of a permanent plague focus until it was introduced into the remote province of Yunnan at some time, as it seems, in the seventeenth century.

The plague history of that other great Asian civilization, India, resembles the Chinese pattern. Plague is not identified in Indian sources before the eleventh century A.D. According to Arab chronicles, India was ravaged by plague in 1031. An old sacred Hindu book written in that century, the *Bhagavat Purana*, describes plague both in man and rats and gives instructions to Hindus on the precautions to be taken in the event of its appearance. One of these precautions is that people should abandon houses in which dead rats are found.

It is often said that plague epidemics were recorded in India from the eleventh to the end of the seventeenth century when the disease appears to have disappeared completely. However, a closer look at the sources reveals that they are unspecific and refer only to 'pestilences', i.e., epidemics that, in principle, could be any serious infectious disease.

---

23 The much older and probable account of plague in the Bible may be considered a special case, but not necessarily an irrelevant case in this context.

Although this does not preclude plague, no specific, substantiating evidence can be adduced. It is of special interest in our context that this also means that there is no significant evidence for the Black Death in India.[24]

This conclusion includes also a Russian source. Some scholars have used a brief notice in the *Chronicle of Pskov* to argue for an origin in India:

> This mortality lasted in Pskov all summer; it started in the spring and held on in the autumn, and did not cease until the winter [. . .] Some said that this epidemic came from India, from Sun City.

As can be clearly seen, even the chronicler indicates that this is only rumour and hearsay. The reference to an origin in Sun City in India is clearly pure myth, and even a confluence of myths: Sun City is a translation of a Greek name of an Egyptian city, namely Heliopolis, which lay in the north-eastern part of the present-day Egyptian capital of Cairo. The Greek name reflects that one of Alexander the Great's generals, Ptolemy, took over Egypt and founded his own dynasty. Actually, it is the same old Egyptian city that Egyptians many centuries earlier called On. The chronicler cannot provide any concrete testable piece of information, not even hearsay about any outbreak along the long route from India to the Crimea. Obviously, this source is unusable for the question of the territorial origin of the Black Death.[25] It could also be compared to the Arabic writer Ibn al-Wardi's assertion that the Black Death had originated in the 'Land of Darkness', where it had raged for fifteen years before it moved on (see below).

Specific evidence of plague in India is not provided again until 1615 when the disease broke out in the Punjab and spread to other parts of India in the following years. Recurrent plague epidemics occurred until the end of the seventeenth century, when plague appears to have disappeared completely. In 1812–21, there were local plague epidemics in a small area in the Gujarat province in north-western India, and also in the conterminous province Sindh in present-day Pakistan. Then, plague disappeared completely for some years until, in the years 1836–8, there was a small outbreak some 300 km (200 miles) north-east of the centre of the outbreak in Gujarat.[26] It should be noted that these outbreaks were believed by some to be due to importation of infection from Persia. This may have been the occasion when a plague focus was established on the southern slopes of the Himalayas.[27] However, this development could conceivably have taken place in the previous plague period, and the local outbreaks in the first half of the nineteenth century could therefore possibly have originated there. The quite strong objection is that a plague focus in this area ought to have manifested itself in episodic cases and outbreaks that should at least occasionally have been recorded in some way.

Then the plague disappeared from India again, or at least nothing is heard of it, and it did not reappear until it was introduced from abroad, specifically by ship from Hong Kong in 1896 as part of the third plague pandemic that originated in the Yunnan province in China (see above).

---

[24] Cf. Dols 1977: 44.
[25] *Pskovskaya Letopis'* 1837: 31. My translation from Russian. The same meaning is briefly mentioned in *The Chronicle of Nikon.*
[26] Simpson 1905: 41–7.
[27] L.-T. Wu 1936b: 5.

Summing up, we must emphasize the fact that the earliest references to plague in India are almost 1,500 years younger than in the West. This must primarily reflect that there was no plague focus within India that could sustain plague continuously, at least not until plague obtained a permanent foothold on the southern slopes of the Himalayas at the beginning of the nineteenth century, or just possibly some centuries earlier. There is no evidence for the Black Death.

Also in the case of India, therefore, it is possible to discern a pattern that indicates that the presence of plague is considerably later than in Africa and the Middle East. It also appears likely that there was no plague focus within the Indian territory until the first decades of the nineteenth century. Like China, India was invaded by plague in the seventeenth century. This may, then, refer to a common origin in a wave of plague spreading out of, perhaps, the Central Asian plague focus. Importantly, there is no evidence for plague epidemics in India during the first half of the fourteenth century, which, in our context, is the crucial period if the Black Death were to have originated in this part of Asia.

In the Middle East and North Africa, wild rodents appear not to have lived in sufficient density to constitute permanent plague foci: plague tends to reduce their numbers and their density below the necessary level to sustain the continuous circulation of plague infection, and, consequently, after some time these plague foci disappear. This allows the wild rodent populations to reconstitute their numbers, and the plague foci can be reactivated when the next incursion of plague into these areas occurs.

Quite likely, therefore, the early plague activity in the Middle East and in North Africa was linked to the ancient plague focus in south-eastern parts of Africa which, consequently, stands out as the likely candidate for the doubtful honour of being the ancestral homeland of plague. However, the small plague focus north of Yemen must also be considered in this context. It must be underscored that this conclusion with respect to the question of the ancestral homeland of plague does not exclude other possible areas of origin, only that it can be better substantiated by presently available evidence than any alternative.

Where did the Black Death come from?

In 1347, Italian merchant ships brought the Black Death from the Crimean seaport Kaffa (today called Feodosiya) on the Black Sea to Constantinople and to seaports along the coasts of the Mediterranean. This was the crucial event that unleashed the Black Death's disastrous spread throughout Asia Minor, the Middle East, North Africa and Europe. The Black Death could, of course, have originated far away, moving out of its plague focus many years earlier, and travelling thousands of kilometres before it reached Kaffa. Where was the Black Death's area of origin? When and why did the Black Death break out of its plague focus? Along which route and by what means of transport did it reach Kaffa?

The conclusion reached in the previous chapter on the probable ancestral homeland of plague has great significance for a discussion of the geographical origin of the Black Death. The history of plague in North Africa and the Middle East is much older than any other historical information on plague from any other region of the Old

World. It is at least 1,700 years older than the Black Death, and quite likely almost 2,500 years older. On the basis of contagion picked up in south-eastern parts of Africa or north of Yemen, plague was present in these regions both in the form of plague foci of considerable duration and more episodically as plague epidemics. This means that plague probably spread eastwards throughout the Old World from North Africa and the Middle East: modern research has discovered a string of plague foci stretching almost continuously from the Middle East and the Caucasus to Manchuria[28] in the east (see Map 2, p. 46).

Some of these plague foci can easily be ruled out as the Black Death's area of origin. There are small plague foci on the southern slopes of the Himalayas, and in the Chinese provinces Yunnan and Guangdon and in Vietnam that are probably of quite recent origin. Starting to the west of Baku, the capital of Azerbaijan, one plague focus runs south-westwards along the south-western shores of the Caspian Sea and further on through northern Iran all the way into southern Iraq, where it suddenly turns north-westwards and eventually ends up in Syria. It is known that the Black Death spread southwards into the Caucasus (see below), so the Caucasian–Middle East plague focus cannot, therefore, have been the area of departure of the Black Death.

However, three remaining plague foci must be taken into account as possible areas of origin of the Black Death: (1) a plague focus that runs from the north-western Kazakh and Russian shores of the Caspian Sea into southern Russia in the direction of the Crimea; (2) a huge plague focus that spreads out from the eastern shores of the Caspian Sea, covering much of the steppes of Central Asia (Kazakhstan, Uzbekistan, Turkmenistan), and sending a long tongue eastwards up to the eastern shores of L. Balkhash in eastern Kazakhstan; a probable extension of this focus is located along the conterminous border areas of China and the three Central Asian republics Kazakhstan, Kirgizstan and Tadzhikistan; (3) a vast plague focus that comprises parts of the Russian Siberian border areas on the Republic of Mongolia, most of Mongolia itself, and northern parts of the present-day Chinese provinces of Outer Mongolia and Manchuria.

However, were all three plague foci in operation in the fourteenth century, and, therefore, possible areas of origin of the Black Death? We know that plague was present in North Africa and the Middle East at least 1,700 years before the Black Death and probably 2,500 years earlier, and that plague probably spread eastwards from these areas throughout the Eurasian continent. Thus, in order to penetrate further into the problem of the geographical origin of the Black Death, it is necessary to acquire some concrete notion of the continental pace of spread of plague in wild rodent populations with more or less assistance from human activities. This will provide an indication as to which of the three plague foci can reasonably be assumed to have been in function at the time of the Black Death.

Let us take as the point of departure for discussion and clarification of this question a similar event, when plague entered a new continent, namely North America, in San Francisco in June 1899. What was plague's subsequent pace of spread eastwards over the North American continent among wild rodent populations consisting mainly of ground and rock squirrels, prairie dogs, chipmunks and deer mice?

[28] Manchuria is today the easternmost province of China, but used to be the land of the Manchurian Mongols.

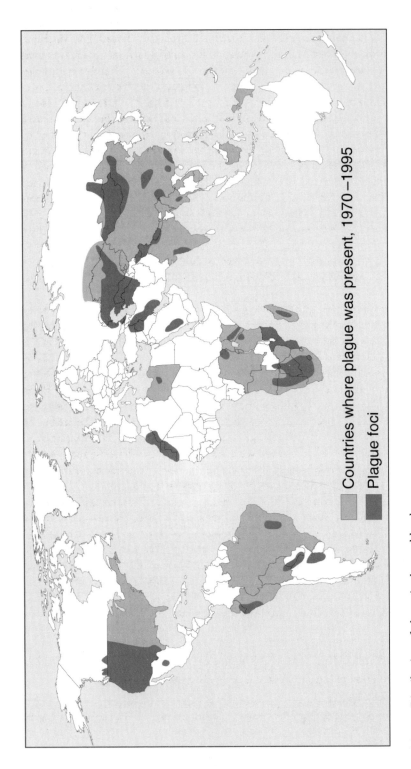

Map 2. Distribution of plague in the world today

Countries where plague was present, 1970–1995

Plague foci

Seventy-five years later, plague had penetrated into 12 states[29] and had crossed the middle of the USA at 100° longitude, a distance of more than 2,000 km (1,250 miles) from its point of departure, and had also invaded Canada in the north and Mexico in the south.[30] In the words of McNeill: 'Such a vast area of infection, in fact, is equivalent to any of the long-standing plague foci of the Old World.'[31] This also means that the average pace of spread eastwards over the continent had been of the order of magnitude of 25 km (16 miles) a year. This pace of spread was mainly owing to natural processes of spread caused by animal behaviour: contact between diseased and healthy rodents, sick rodents being caught by birds or beasts of prey and carried at a distance to nests or lairs, perhaps being lost on the way, bloody remnants infecting scavenging rodents by infective droplets, and so on.[32] Clearly, human beings also played a part, in that they transported plague-infected rodents or their infected fleas at a distance into new areas, causing metastatic spread and giving rise to new effective centres of spread. Nonetheless, McNeill who discusses this problem with great insight and precision concludes that 'the geographic spread of plague infection in North America occurred naturally' in the sense that it was basically passed on between colonies of ground-burrowing rodents, and that 'the spread of plague in North America, while affected by such [human] acts, did not depend on human intervention'.[33]

At a similar pace of spread, plague would have moved the roughly 7,000 km from the Middle East to Manchuria in about 300 years. The assumptions with respect to pace that underlie this estimate can be substantially inaccurate without affecting the validity of the point that is being made: that plague could easily, or rather would inevitably, have spread from an ancestral homeland in south-eastern Africa or the south-western Arabian Peninsula via the Middle East and Western Asia and all the way across Central Asia to Manchuria within the indicated time horizon. Because the basic dynamics of the process of spread are derived from the natural behaviour of rodents and fleas, it is not really important that huge areas of the Eurasian land masses that would need to be covered were very sparsely inhabited by men, mostly by nomadic groups travelling about with their herds of cattle and horses, or by simple peasants living intensely localized lives in widely dispersed villages.

Movement of goods and people across these enormous distances did take place from an early time. However, only luxury goods could repay the extreme costs of transportation over such distances on pack horses or camels. Such goods would tend to be poorly suited for transportation of rodents or their fleas, and the very long duration of transport would leave such sources of infection minimal chances of survival. An additional factor is that the caravan routes ran through large areas of desert or semi-desert with a climate that would rapidly kill fleas in goods or luggage by desiccation (sea transport of fleas is an entirely different matter). The most important vehi-

[29] Washington, Idaho, Montana, Oregon, Wyoming, California, Nevada, Utah, Colorado, Arizona, New Mexico, Texas.
[30] WHO Expert Committee on Plague 1970: 6; Barnes, Quan and Poland 1984: 9SS–14SS.
[31] McNeill 1979: 145.
[32] Pollitzer and Meyer 1961: 458; Poland 1983: 1230. Cf. McNeill 1979: 145, who states that the rodent system 'allows for the propagation of infection from one rodent community to another across as much as ten to twenty miles per annum'.
[33] McNeill 1979: 145–6.

cles of transportation of plague-infected fleas were undoubtedly camels, because camels are susceptible to plague infection. Camels can, therefore, function as vehicles of spread and represent some risk of infection both to man and other susceptible animals.[34]

Of course, the modern American data on the pace of territorial spread of plague in wild rodent populations cannot be used without necessary cautions and reservations for inference to similar events in the distant past. However, *wherever plague's ancestral homeland was*, 1,700–2,500 years should be ample time for plague to spread all the way over the Eurasian continent on the basis of natural processes of spread and the occasional contributions of human transportation, long before the time of the Black Death.

Did the Black Death start in the Far East or in a plague focus nearer Europe and the Middle East? This question has been discussed by several scholars. In the complete list of epidemics mentioned in Chinese historical and medical sources and registered in the great Chinese encyclopaedia of 1726, it is not possible to identify a plague epidemic before the 1640s. It is true that plague was first mentioned in the seventh century, but it was in terms of a diagnostic description without any reference to an epidemic of plague. Nonetheless, the theory of a Chinese origin of the Black Death has long fascinated scholars, and not only western scholars. Although Wu Lien-Teh underscored that plague was barely mentioned at all in Chinese sources, he was, nonetheless, fully convinced that the Black Death originated in China. In a translation of the complete list of historical epidemics published in the 1726 encyclopaedia, he actually interpolated, i.e., inserted, a note to the effect that the Black Death started in China in 1346.[35]

In this discussion, a report by Daniel Chwolsen, the Russian archaeologist, has served to play a confusing part. In 1885, he studied two large Nestorian cemeteries,[36] which had been discovered near Issyk-kul in present-day northern Kirghizstan (close to China's western border). Some 330 headstones contained the names of more than 650 persons who had been interred in the period 1186–1349; 106 of these persons are specifically said to have died in the years 1338–9, and it is stated that about ten of them, according to Chwolsen, had died of 'plague'. Several scholars have taken this piece of information as good evidence showing that a plague epidemic had occurred at Issyk-kul and have inferred quite reasonably that this epidemic must have been the Black Death on its westwards march from China.[37] This ruled out Wu Lien-Teh's interpolated statement to the effect that the Black Death started in China in 1346. Moreover, it has been shown that the word Chwolsen translated as 'plague' in reality only has the general meaning of 'pestilence', i.e., 'epidemic'.[38] This means that there is no specific historical information indicating in a specific way any outbreak of plague in the Far East for hundreds of years before and after the Black Death. Thus

---

[34] Fyodorov 1960a: 275–81; Christie, Chen and Elberg 1980: 724–6.

[35] L.-T. Wu 1936a: 47.

[36] The Nestorians were a Christian sect holding that Christ had both distinct human and distinct divine persons and hence that the Virgin Mary should not be called 'Mother of God'. This theological view was condemned by the Councils of Ephesus (431) and Chalcedon (451), and disappeared from the Greek Church, but lived on in Persia, Syria, Mesopotamia and some other areas.

[37] Pollitzer 1954: 14; McNeill 1979: 155.

[38] Norris 1977: 10.

the theory of a Chinese origin of the Black Death must (for the time being) be given up as unsubstantiated by historical data.

There is also a decisive independent line of argument that relates to the political situation along the caravan routes. The caravan routes from China to the Crimea had been established as important trade links in the aftermath of the Mongol conquests that took place in the first decades of the thirteenth century under the leadership of Jenghiz Khan, and, later, by his grandson who conquered southern Russia in 1236–40. The Mongol conquests united China, Central Asia, Persia and southern Russia (including the Crimea) into a giant empire, which allowed the establishment of overland caravan routes and the safe passage of goods and merchants all the way between China and towns on the Black Sea and Sea of Azov. This is the political background of the flourishing trade between China and Europe in the second half of the thirteenth century. In 1266, the Mongol leaders of the Golden Horde ceded land to the Genoese at Kaffa in the Crimea, and later to both the Genoese and the Venetians in Tana on the Sea of Azov, with permission to build a consulate and warehouses and, thus, to establish trading stations. The Italians soon fortified the towns to make goods and profits more secure.[39]

However, the political and religious developments in the Mongol Empire in the decades preceding the Black Death had very disruptive effects on trade and travel. There was a wide-scale conversion to Islam and the empire broke up into a number of warring Muslim states. This process involved increased religious fervour and fulminating anti-Christian attitudes, and the presence of Christian merchants was considered increasingly intolerable.

This was also the case with the Kipchak Khanate of the Golden Horde, the Mongols who ruled over the vast steppes of southern Russia, the land of ancient Scythia, and had reduced the Russian principalities to subjugated tribute-paying dependencies. In 1313, the Kipchak Khanate converted to Islam, which also triggered a process of conversion among the local Tartar populations that supported the Mongols. In the end, in 1343, Janibeg, the Kipchak Khan over the Golden Horde, took military action to throw the Italians out of their trading stations in Kaffa and Tana in order to put a definite end to trade with Christians in the lands of the Golden Horde, and, at the same time, he severed the trade link between China and Europe along the caravan routes.[40] The Italians were driven out of Tana in 1343, and were besieged in their fortified town of Kaffa in the same year, and again in the years 1345–6. It was, indeed, during the second siege of Kaffa, that plague broke out in the Mongol army and in some manner was passed on to the besieged Italians (see also below, Chapter 23).

Under these circumstances, it must be considered highly unlikely that plague could have been passed on by trade and travel from China to the Italians in the Crimea. No merchants in their senses would risk precious goods and expensive and dangerous transport over thousands of kilometres to the Christian Italian merchants through Muslim states that were intensely hostile to trade and contact with Christians. The rulers of the Muslim states along the caravan routes would eagerly seize the

[39] Dols 1977: 48–52.
[40] See, e.g., Norris 1977: 13.

goods, claiming them to be meant for illegal trade with Christians. At the end of the caravan route, the ruler had actually gone to war to drive away the Christian merchants, and the towns of destination were under siege.[41]

The Black Death has made a profound impression on the scholars who have studied it and discussion of the origin has, apparently, appealed to their sense of the extraordinary and exotic. Usually, scholars would approach the problem of origin on the basis of the principle of proximate origin, because the shorter the distance to be covered, the fewer obstacles to dissemination: accordingly, the proximate plague focus would be preferred for an initial working hypothesis on origin. According to the principle of proximate origin, then, the plague focus closest to the area from where the Black Death was shipped to Europe, i.e., Kaffa in the Crimea, should be considered the most likely area of origin.[42] It is therefore very significant that Russian chroniclers state in no uncertain terms that, in 1346, plague broke out in the areas containing the plague focus, which stretches from the north-western shores of the Caspian Sea into southern Russia in the direction of the Crimea. The most informative chronicle gives this account:

> In the same year [1346], God's punishment struck the people in the eastern lands, in the town Ornach [on the estuary of the R. Don], and in Khastorokan, and in Sarai, and in Bezdezh [at an arm of the R. Volga], and in other towns in those lands; the mortality was great among the Bessermens, and among the Tartars, and among the Armenians and the Abkhazians, and among the Jews, and among the European foreigners,[43] and among the Circassians, and among all who lived there, so that they could not bury them [sic].[44]

Significantly, the quite detailed information provided in this chronicle is credible and compatible with other information on the Black Death in this region, and it constitutes a meaningful history of origin in a known plague focus. It also provides a geographical outline that contains a logical progression of spread from this plague focus into the surrounding lands of the Golden Horde, then southwards into the Caucasus and westwards into the Crimea. Along the western route, the Black Death reached the Crimea and the Mongol-led Tartar army that beleaguered the Italians in Kaffa, and along the southern route it ravaged the lands of the Circassians, the Abkhazians and the Armenians on its march along the eastern shores of the Black Sea and through the Caucasian region, eventually gaining the ground that would allow it to spread further into Asia Minor, the Middle East and Persia [Iran]. Obviously, the author has had good informants. There is no satisfactory evidence to the effect that

---

[41] Norris 1977 and 1978.
[42] Fyodorov 1960b.
[43] The original meaning of the word 'fryazy' is 'the French', but it is used in the chronicle in the usual general meaning of European foreigners, in this case the Genoese and the Venetians.
[44] Vasil'yev and Segal 1960: 28. My translation from Russian. The Abkhazians and Circassians are peoples living along the eastern coasts of the Black Sea and adjacent areas. The Bessermens are a small population living in north-eastern Russia and do not fit into the pattern. However, there is great ethnic diversity in the Caucasian region, and the author may have had in mind some other people, or possibly the people of Bezdezh.

this terrible disease started far away and caused havoc anywhere along the thousands of kilometres of the caravan route.[45] The outbreak is narrowly and unambiguously associated with the area of the plague focus that stretches from the north-western shores of the Caspian Sea into southern Russia.

Several scholars have formerly suspected and suggested that the Black Death originated in this area, but did not know the Russian sources that provide important support for this view.[46]

Other contemporary sources also state that the Black Death originated in this area. Nicephoros Gregoras, the Greek historian who lived in Constantinople and witnessed the ravages of the Black Death there in 1347, wrote that in the spring of 1346 plague came from 'Scythia and Maeotis and the mouth of the Tanais [R. Don]'. Scythia is the ancient, classical name of the area that at the time was ruled by the Golden Horde. Spring is a very likely season for the start of a plague epizootic among rodents that will translate into an epidemic among human populations. Also the Byzantine Emperor John VI who abdicated in 1355 in order to write a history of the Byzantine Empire maintained that the Black Death started in Scythia (among the 'Hyperborean Scythians').[47]

Then there was the Arab writer Ibn al-Wardi, who collected information on the early phase of the Black Death from Muslim merchants returning to Syria from the Crimea. First, he makes the more or less mythical statement that the plague started in the 'Land of Darkness', and that it had been raging there for fifteen years before it moved on. No specific geographical indication of cities or areas ravaged by the disease in these years is provided, and nothing can therefore be learned from it. However, the merchants also told Ibn al-Wardi that the epidemic was rampant in the land of the Uzbeks, at the time a name for the territory of Golden Horde, in October–November 1346, that it emptied the villages and towns of their inhabitants, and that it next spread to the Crimea and to Byzantium.[48] Although Ibn al-Wardi's account is not unambiguous in regard to the question of the origin of the Black Death, the concrete information that he provides agrees completely with an origin in the land of the Golden Horde in present-day southern Russia. It agrees also with the Russian sources that the Black Death spread out of the central parts of the Golden Horde that contain the local plague focus westwards to the Crimea. The time perspective of the epidemic events in his account indicates that the outbreak around Kaffa occurred probably in early 1347. This rough outline of the movement of the Black Death in time and space accords well with the sparse information on what happened next.

The most detailed and dramatic account is related by Gabriele de Mussis of Piacenza (in northern Italy). Like Ibn al-Wardi, he did not witness these events himself, but gathered information from returning merchants. Because his account cannot be tested properly and contains doubtful, exaggerated and dramatizing elements, it should be taken with a pinch of salt.

Also according to de Mussis, the Black Death started in 1346 in the lands of the

---

[45] As for the mythical reference in *The Chronicle of Pskov*, see above under the discussion of plague in India.
[46] See, e.g., Burnet and White 1972: 226; Norris 1977 and 1978.
[47] Bartsocas 1966: 395–6.
[48] Dols 1977: 41, 51–2.

Golden Horde ('among the tribes of Tartars and Saracens'), and subsequently attacked the Mongol army that besieged Kaffa:

> [...] It seemed to the besieged Christians as if arrows were shot out of the sky to strike and humble the pride of the infidels who rapidly died with marks on their bodies and lumps in their joints and several parts, followed by putrid fever; all advice and help of the doctors being of no avail. Whereupon the Tartars, worn out by this pestilential disease, and falling on all sides as if thunderstruck, and seeing that they were perishing hopelessly, ordered the corpses to be placed upon their engines and thrown into the city of Kaffa. Accordingly were the bodies of the dead hurled over the walls, so that the Christians were not able to hide or protect themselves from this danger, although they carried away as many dead as possible and threw them into the sea. But soon the whole air became infected, and the water poisoned, and such a pestilence grew up that scarcely one out of a thousand was able to escape.[49]

De Mussis starts his account by giving a religious interpretation of the outbreak of plague in the Mongol army: arrows from the skies are a much-used symbol for epidemic manifestations of divine wrath, which in this case struck the 'infidel' who had dared to attack the Christians. Next, he provides an unmistakeable description of plague symptoms, buboes and the dark and purple spots or blotches that appear in the skin of a variable but often substantial proportion of plague cases (see above, p. 26). However, his assertion with respect to mortality, that hardly one in a thousand survived, is greatly exaggerated, since actually about 20 percent of plague patients survive the disease.

Because de Mussis gave in to the Christian temptation to explain the outbreak of the plague epidemic in the Mongol-led Tartar army as the Lord's punishment of the pagan Muslims for attacking the Christians, he finds himself in a very awkward position when he must explain to his Christian audience how it could be that also the Christians subsequently became victimized by the same disease. Now, of course, religious explanation is unusable. He turns, therefore, to the non-religious epidemiological theory of classical medicine, the miasmatic theory of epidemic disease (see above, pp. 3–5): plague was passed on to the townspeople because the Mongols and Tartars, in their pagan Muslim barbarism, catapulted the corpses of plague-stricken men over the walls of the town. This would certainly make any good Christian shudder: Christians believed according to the Catholic Church's teachings that salvation also depended on being interred in a consecrated cemetery. They would, therefore, never consider disposing of their dead in a way that would mean perdition and eternal punishment in Hell. In this manner, de Mussis succeeds in maximizing the contrast between the barbaric pagan Muslims and the Christians.

Many scholars have taken this story at face value and understood it as the first instance of bacteriological warfare. However, this is impossible, since neither the Mongols or Tartars nor the Arabs or the Christians knew anything of bacteria, but they did share the notion of miasma. In principle, we could be dealing with an

---

[49] Translation from Latin into English in Simpson 1905: 137–8. The Latin text is published in Haeser 1882: 157–61.

episode of miasmatic warfare to which the Mongols could resort because they did not have the religious restrictions that prohibited Christians from acting in such a manner. Although miasmatic warfare could conceivably be the motive, it is improbable that it actually worked out according to intentions. Miasma would only develop in rotting matter, and consequently, newly dead persons would not represent any appreciable danger, and the townspeople would have had time to dispose of the dead bodies before they developed dangerous miasmatic properties. For the Mongols to achieve their end according to miasmatic epidemiological notions, they would have had to postpone catapulting plague victims over the walls until they had 'matured' into at least an incipient miasmatic stage as revealed by a telling smell. This would not really represent a grave danger to the Mongols who were already stricken by plague, only for the townspeople. Tragically, the pagan Muslims succeeded in their evil intentions despite the townspeople's heroic efforts to get rid of the corpses: soon 'the whole air became infected, and the water poisoned' and a gruesome epidemic broke out among the townspeople.

According to our modern medical knowledge of plague epidemiology, de Mussis's explanation is untenable. Corpses of persons dead from plague are not contagious whatever the form of plague. According to de Mussis and other informants, the Black Death in Kaffa was an unambiguous epidemic of bubonic plague, which means that the patients were uninfective. Since bubonic plague is transmitted by rat fleas, effective transmission of plague into the town by the catapulting of corpses would be dependent on infected rat fleas being hidden in the clothing of the dead. However, fleas start leaving dead animals or persons as soon as they notice a diminution of temperature. For the Mongols and Tartars to have succeeded in passing on plague to the townspeople in this way, they would have to catapult plague victims over the wall as soon as they had expired and retained almost normal body temperature; and this they would not have done (if not for religious considerations) precisely because, in their miasmatic way of thinking, it would have been ineffectual. But, then, of course, the story may not be true at all, but could have been constructed in order to resolve the painful religious enigma inherent in the fact that the Black Death was passed on from the pagan beleaguering army to the Lord's own Christians in Kaffa, and next with their unwitting help was passed on to Christian Europe itself where it was causing unthinkable havoc at the time de Mussis wrote his account.

An epidemiological explanation of how plague entered Kaffa based on modern medical knowledge will have to focus on a process that was unobtrusive to beleaguerers and beleaguered alike. What the besieged would not notice and could not prevent was that plague-infected rodents found their way through crevices in the walls or between the gates and the gateways. This would trigger an epizootic among the town's house rats that after some weeks would translate into the beginning of a plague epidemic among the townspeople.

The outbreak of plague in the military camp surrounding Kaffa, and, next, in the town itself had both local and far-reaching historical consequences. The besieging army disintegrated under the impact of plague, and the Kipchak Khan had to lift the siege. According to de Mussis, the Genoese and Venetians fought on bravely for some time and managed to organize a blockade of the coasts of the Golden Horde with their warships, events that must have taken place in the first half of 1347. De Mussis also notes that some of the Genoese fled in their ships and on the voyage back to Italy unleashed the plague in the Byzantine capital Constantinople and, subsequently, in Italy. The flight of the Italians probably reflects the fact that the coming of warmer spring weather meant that the plague epizootic that had been developing slowly in Kaffa during the winter months rapidly took on the character of a fulminating disastrous epidemic that persuaded many Italians to flee in panic and head for their home cities in Italy. As we shall see, Constantinople was probably contaminated at the end of May, which fits very well into the general picture of the events.

One can hardly blame the merchants and their crews who under the impact of the plague epidemic desperately sought refuge in their ships and sailed away with enormous relief, counting themselves lucky to have escaped from imminent and gruesome death. Instead, they would soon discover that plague had entered their ships, and those who survived this desperate voyage would soon come to realize that their flight had triggered probably the greatest disaster in human history.

However, the population living in the lands of the Golden Horde where plague had been spreading since spring 1346 also had equally desperate reasons to flee from the terrible epidemic catastrophe that unfolded around them. Plague was the unobtrusive companion of people who fled to save their lives, often in vain, unwittingly bringing catastrophic death of epic proportions to their fellow men in other towns, areas and regions.

The official religious conversion to Islam of the khanate and the zealotry of new converts that led to the military campaign against the presence of Christian merchants and the prohibition of trade with Christians must to some extent have been directed also against Russian tradesmen and merchants. Only an intermission or temporary sharp reduction in the trade relations between the Russian principalities and the Golden Horde can explain that the Black Death did not invade Russia from the south-east. Instead, it launched its Russian campaign, after it had spread all the way across Europe from the Crimea to the Baltic countries, whence it moved into the Russian areas from the north-west in late 1351. For this reason, the history of the Black Death in Russia will form the end and not the beginning of the Black Death's European history, a solid proof of the crucial importance of contact, trade and travel for the dissemination of epidemic disease in general as well as in the specific case of the Black Death.

Part Two
Spread of the Black Death

6

The Caucasus, Asia Minor, the Middle East and North Africa

Introduction: Some central epidemiological and sociological concepts
We now come to the issue of the territorial spread of the Black Death. The understanding and analysis of a complex and huge epidemiological process that comprises such vast territories and enormous numbers of people is dependent on good analytical tools, and useful epidemiological and sociological concepts. Additional analytical concepts will be presented and discussed in the introduction to the chapter on the spread of plague in Europe.

In order to describe and discuss the pattern and pace of spread of the Black Death in ways that will produce valuable insights, clear concepts for various types of human settlements, adapted to medieval social realities, are needed. The concepts of city and town are not unambiguous in ordinary parlance. In the Middle Ages, urban populations were generally much smaller than we are used to today. In this book, the concept of town will be used to signify urban centres with 1,000–9,999 inhabitants, the concept of city will be used to signify urban centres with 10,000 and up to around 100,000 inhabitants. The very few cities with 100,000 inhabitants or more were the metropolises of the Middle Ages. The concept of city is also associated with any urban centre with a cathedral and resident bishop, whatever its size. In some cases, the use of this concept will be made clear by the term cathedral city.

Assertions with respect to the time of the outbreak of the Black Death in various communities are mostly found in chronicles (annals).[1] In this connection, an important general point must be made on the time horizon of the associated epidemiological and sociological processes from the introduction of contagion into a local community, town, city or metropolis until the presence of plague becomes obvious and recognized by the chronicle-producing social élites. These epidemiological and sociological processes comprise a number of phases: (1) plague among rats (the enzootic and epizootic phases); (2) the endemic phase: the first sprinkling of human cases, often concentrated in a few houses, and also including the incubation period,

---

[1]   In other languages than English, the word 'annal' is used in singular with the same meaning as chronicle, which means that both specific chronicles and scholarly journals employ 'annal' in this way.

n the infective bite to the time a person falls ill, and the average duration of e in mortal cases; (3) the development of the epidemic proper. The time izon of these epidemiological phases is well known: it takes (as mentioned) 10–14 days, on average 12 days, from the introduction of contagion into one or more colonies of house rats before the rat population is so decimated that their fleas have difficulties in finding new rat hosts and begin to turn on human beings in their immediate proximity. Rat fleas have a clear predilection for their natural hosts and will usually transfer to men only when they have not succeeded in finding another rat host to feed on after about three days, and are becoming increasingly desperate.[2] It is assumed that infective rat fleas would then find the opportunity to bite a human being quite soon, usually after about 0.5–1 day. When the rat fleas begin to turn on men, the epizootic translates into the endemic phase, which starts unobtrusively with the incubation period, which lasts, on average, 3–5 days before infected persons fall ill.[3] The course of illness in mortal cases usually also lasts 3–5 days;[4] taken together, the incubation period and the period of illness in mortal cases last, on average, eight days.[5] This means that the first human cases would occur after 16–23 days, the first plague deaths after about 20–28 days, and within this range most often after about 24 days, from the introduction of plague into a community until its presence is reflected in the form of the first endemic deaths.

The occurrence of a few deaths by disease would not cause much concern in a time when general mortality was many times higher than today; deaths were routine occurrences and mortality crises caused by epidemic disease were frequent events for which people were mentally and culturally prepared. In the endemic phase, the plague became observable, but remained usually unrecognized as the incipient phase of an epidemic disaster.

As an increasing number of rat colonies became infected and depleted, a growing number of people were exposed to hungry, aggressive rat fleas, an increasing number of persons would become infected, and after about a week, the mortality would reach a level that heralded the transition from the endemic to the epidemic phase. Thus, the epidemic phase started about four weeks after the first rat colony had been contaminated. The early epidemic process would normally have gained momentum for at least a week before it had developed into a clear epidemic form with numerous human cases, which with terrifying rapidity and incidence died, and the true grisly nature of the unfolding epidemic disaster began to impress itself on people.

The time horizon of these developments taken together is normally 12 days (epizootic) + 3 days (fasting rat fleas) + 0.5–1 (before first infective transmission), 7 days (endemic), + 8 days (incubation and illness for the last endemic cases) + 8 days (incubation and illness for the early epidemic cases infected during the endemic phase), in all 39 days, or 5.6 weeks. At this point of the developments, the presence of a serious epidemic disease would be recognized in small transparent communities, villages, townships, perhaps also in small towns.

This analysis is based on a vast amount of general epidemiological knowledge on

2   Pollitzer 1954: 485.
3   Pollitzer 1954: 409–11.
4   Chun 1936: 313.
5   Pollitzer 1954: 418; cf. also p. 485.

plague and suggests that the early process of contamination and spread follows a quite stable pattern of development. This pattern represents, therefore, general or standard empirical information on this type of epidemiological process. As such it can be used as a generalized analytical tool, a rule of thumb, or, as it will be called here, a standard assumption. Standard assumptions will not always conform completely or very closely to the actual shape of events in the individual cases of a capricious reality. However, plague develops according to a quite strict epidemiological pattern. For this reason standard assumptions will usually conform to or approach quite closely the factual structure of events and will serve to facilitate the disclosure and identification of the general character of epidemiological developments and the culturally conditioned human responses. As such they function as sociological concepts aimed at gaining generalized synthetical insights. In this book, a number of standard assumptions will be developed for similar analytical purposes.

The chronicle-producing social élites lived mainly in large towns and cities. Significantly, as members of the upper classes they did not live in the harbour areas, or in the quarters of the poor. Severe epidemics could have been spreading for some time among the poor before they came to the attention of the upper classes. City authorities would often shut their eyes to the awesome fact of a developing plague epidemic long after its presence had become quite obvious, perhaps fearing that official recognition of this fact would persuade their trade partners and customers in the countryside to break off trade and stay away, causing calamitous unemployment, drastic misery and combustible social situations. The great hesitation of city authorities in admitting the presence of plague even in the seventeenth century has been vividly demonstrated in a number of studies.[6] This attitude served the upper classes' economic interests, but was also in the general interest of the poor and would tend to delay recognition of presence of the Black Death.

The upper classes were quite used to epidemic outbreaks among the poor classes; it was a sad fact of life. The spread of a serious epidemic among the poor would not draw much attention before it began to threaten the residential areas of the upper classes, or it caused such havoc that it would attract notice. This point can be substantiated: in several instances later in this book when chroniclers give disparate assertions on the commencement of the Black Death in a specific town or city, and there is available independent material for testing them on the basis of modern knowledge of plague epidemiology, the earliest dating can without exception be shown to be correct or most likely to be closest to the factual developments. When there are no alternatives, the dating in a chronicle will quite likely be late. With this background, it appears that the presence of the Black Death will not be noted by chroniclers before the epidemic phase has lasted about a week and developed a more substantial epidemic form.

Summing up, the time lag between the time of contamination and the recognition of the presence of the Black Death as noted in chronicles will depend on the size of the community, about 5.5–6 weeks in villages and townships, 6–7 weeks in towns, seven weeks in cities, and quite likely a week longer in the few metropolises of the time with about or over 100,000 inhabitants.

---

[6] See, e.g., Cipolla 1973, 1976, 1979, 1981; Benedictow 1985b: 182–93.

In the case of plague winter weather will tend to slow down or stop the epidemiological processes, often meaning that epidemic activity disappears and the presence of
plague will revert to a mainly epizootic phase caused by a rapid depletion of the
number of fleas,[7] a strong diminution of bacteraemia in infected rats, a much slower
reproduction rate of bacteria in the fleas' stomach system and a correspondingly
much less frequent development of blockage in fleas. The slowdown in areas with
cool winter climate can readily be observed in France, for instance, while the temporary seasonal break with cold winter weather can be observed in the Tyrolese mountains, in northern Germany, and in the Nordic countries.

The conquest of Constantinople and Asia Minor

From its origin in the lands of the Golden Horde and, secondarily, in Kaffa, the Black
Death could mainly move on by two main routes: by land southwards and by ship
across the Black Sea into the Mediterranean Sea. It could not easily move to the west
or north out of the Golden Horde's area, because of the hostility to trade and contact
with the Christians among the Mongol leadership at the time. Obviously, that would
also have to include the Russians, although it did move some distance up the R. Volga
and also a short distance along the R. Don.

Nicephoros Gregoras states that the plague had broken out at the estuary of the R.
Don in spring 1346, while Ibn al-Wardi had gathered information to the effect that
the epidemic raged in the lands of the Golden Horde in October–November 1346.
These pieces of information give a rough, credible outline of the early epidemic
events: the first phase relates to the start of the epidemic, the second relates to a
highly developed phase after months of spread. No accurate information on the
progression of plague southwards across the Caucasian region is available, and this
makes it difficult to assess the pattern of spread in Western Asia and Asia Minor and
further into the Middle East. According to the Russian chronicler cited above, in
1346–7 the Black Death moved southwards and south-westwards through the lands of
the Golden Horde in southern Russia across the Caucasus, ravaging the Trans-
caucasian region. A Persian source mentions a serious plague epidemic in nearby
Azarbaijan in 1346–7.[8]

The epidemic forces that spread along the southern route across the Caucasus
formed one arm of a great pincer movement, to use a military concept, in which the
Black Death moved by land and along the riverine commercial routes. The other arm
of the pincer was constituted by epidemic forces that had been landed in urban
centres on the coasts of Asia Minor and the Middle East from which they advanced
into the surrounding regions. Spreading slowly but relentlessly, this pincer movement would in time surround and gradually engulf Asia Minor and the Middle East
in a staggering epidemic catastrophe.

The Mongol-led Tartar army that besieged Kaffa disintegrated under the impact of
plague, and the Kipchak Khan had to lift the siege. De Mussis relates that the Genoese

---

[7]   Benedictow 1993/1996a: 160–71.
[8]   Dols 1977: 45.

and Venetians fought on bravely for some time and managed to organize a blockade of the coasts of the lands of the Golden Horde with their large ships, events that must have taken place in the first half of 1347. He also notes that some of the Genoese fled in their ships and on the voyage back to Italy unleashed the plague in the Byzantine capital Constantinople, one of the few metropolises of the time. The plague in Constantinople began to unfold in early July in such a way that its presence was recognized,[9] which, according to the standard assumption on the time horizon of this process, indicates that Constantinople was probably contaminated seven or eight weeks earlier, i.e., in the first half of May. This supposition makes it clear that the contagion cannot have come from its movement through the Caucasian region. The timing of the outbreak reflects probably that the plague epizootic that was slowly developing in Kaffa in the early winter of 1347 exploded with the coming of warm weather in the spring, persuading many of the Italians to flee in panic and head for their home cities. The first stop on their return voyage would be Constantinople, where there was also an Italian trading station.

As the contagion continued to spread among the rat colonies in wider parts of Constantinople, the Black Death raged with increasing force. In September, it had acquired the character of a vast epidemic, raging simultaneously in large parts of the city, yet still gaining force. The full brunt of the epidemic occurred in the late autumn.[10] As the Black Death raged with increasing violence among the population, people with means or with relatives in other places who would receive them began to flee the city. This increasing movement out of the contaminated metropolis furnished the Black Death with enormous fresh power to spread. During the autumn, the Black Death succeeded in covering the whole western coast of Asia Minor and also gained a foothold on the European side of the straits. These invasions, which probably began in the late summer, were important for the spread of the Black Death, because the straits between the Black Sea and the Mediterranean Sea and the principal sea lanes leading further on along the western coast of Asia Minor were some of the busiest commercial routes in this part of the world.

The origin of the plague epidemic that broke out in Trebizond, an important commercial centre on Asia Minor's eastern Black Sea coast in September, is more uncertain.[11] It could, of course, have arrived with Italian ships coming from Kaffa. However, this would be quite a detour for homebound Italian ships, implying that the merchants and crews on board were not in much of a hurry to get home, which under the circumstances appears unlikely. It is therefore more likely that the Black Death's arrival in Trebizond was due to a metastatic leap brought about by contaminated refugees from the Black Death. These refugees could have come from two directions: as refugees from the plague front that moved through the Caucasus' Black Sea regions in the first half of 1347, and had engulfed most of the Transcaucasian region by the summer of 1347, or conceivably as refugees from Constantinople. Thus, having reached the border areas of Asia Minor, Mesopotamia [Iraq] and Persia [Iran] during the spring of 1347, the Black Death had apparently started to penetrate Asia Minor in

---

[9] Biraben 1979: 32.

[10] This information on the epidemic developments in Constantinople is based on the accounts of de Mussis and G. Villani, see Biraben 1975: 53.

[11] Biraben 1979: 32.

a typical way by late summer: riding in the gut of rat fleas hidden in the goods or clothing of merchants, tradesmen or refugees who acted as passive porters, it sent a metastatis to an important urban centre with a wide commercial network. In the autumn, plague had gained a bridgehead around Trebizond.

From the important points of introduction in Constantinople and Trebizond the Black Death continued its slow but relentless spread through Asia Minor. It covered a band of roughly 100 km inland on the western coast in the course of 1347; the following year it covered roughly the same distance, but now moving in from all sides; and, finally, in 1349, it conquered the upper mountain region, the Anatolian Plateau, where Turkish Muslim people now reigned.

From Constantinople to Alexandria[12]

Areas that at the time were dominated by Muslim religion and culture played an important part in the history of plague transmission. Muslim culture and historiography has its own historical chronology. Nonetheless, for several practical reasons it has been decided to use consistently European chronology, including the term medieval, throughout this book, including when referring to Muslim countries in the Middle East, North Africa and elsewhere: (1) because the great majority of the readers of this book will only be familiar with European chronology; (2) because the Black Death's history in Europe is far more comprehensively represented by sources and discussed in scholarly works; (3) because the study of this epidemic is far more developed in European historiography. The term medieval refers to the first phase of the new European civilization following the breakdown of the Western Roman Empire, the period from c. A.D. 500 to about 1520. This historical period is subdivided here into the Early Middle Ages spanning the years A.D. 500–1000, the High Middle Ages A.D. 1000–1350 and the Late Middle Ages A.D. 1350–1520. When the start of the Late Middle Ages is set at 1350, this is an expression of the notion that the Black Death and ensuing plague epidemics moulded the last phase of the Middle Ages in a decisive way, an indication of the importance of the subject of this book. An in-depth discussion of this perspective is undertaken in Part 5 below.

The study of the Black Death's transmission from its original homeland in the land of the Golden Horde produces strong evidence for the importance of ship transport in its dissemination. The commercial sea lanes that began in the Italian settlements in the Crimea also saw quite a comprehensive trade between the land of the Golden Horde and the Mamluk Empire in Egypt. This was a trade route spanning three continents: it started in the south-easternmost corner of Europe, led across the Black Sea to Constantinople in Asia Minor for rest and fresh supplies of food and drink, then followed sea lanes through the straits, along the western and southern coasts of Asia Minor and the Middle East, eventually to end in the great city of Alexandria in Africa. The establishment of such a demanding trade route testifies to the rapid progress in European shipbuilding and trade organizations that made such voyages possible on a regular basis and to the aggressive and adventurous entrepreneurial mentality of

---

[12] For the presentation of the spread of the Black Death in the Middle East and North Africa I am much indebted to Dols 1977: 45–67.

Italian medieval business culture. In particular Russian and Tartar slaves, horses, furs, hides and wax from the land of the Golden Horde were in much demand in the Mamluk Empire.[13]

The lively commerce between the Golden Horde and the Mamluk Empire in Egypt is the reason the Black Death reached Alexandria by a major metastatic leap as early as the early autumn of 1347, no more than two months after the outbreak in Constantinople. Alexandria was by far the largest commercial city in this part of the world, with widespread and far-reaching exchange of goods and merchants both by land and by ship. This was the decisive event in the spread of the Black Death in this region, shaping the pattern of its spread in time and space.

The Arab chronicler Al-Maqrzi describes the arrival of a slave ship that had put to sea from a Black Sea port with 32 merchants, and 300 men, slaves and crew on board. It had been boarded by the Black Death either in the port of departure or in the harbour of Constantinople, and when the ship put into port in Alexandria, only four merchants, one slave and about 40 sailors were still alive, and these survivors died in the port. The mortality is obviously considerably exaggerated: since lethality in plague is about 80 per cent of the diseased, among 332 men, 60–70 persons would be expected to survive even if they all contracted the disease. This is a 'tall story' feature, which is staple fare in medieval accounts of the Black Death both in the Muslim world and in Europe. The story is, nonetheless, important because it may serve to explain why contaminated ships managed to sail on despite great mortality on board: these large ships that engaged in long-distance transport of slaves and other valuable or precious goods had very large crews, both because rowing was still an important source of propulsion, and because they also comprised a military contingent with defensive functions against pirates. Thus, even in the case of plague, there would be enough survivors to carry on the voyage to the destination.

One should also note that high mortality and epidemic disease were facts of life in shipping not only in the Middle Ages but also in the Early Modern period. The crews on the sailing ships that transported slaves from West Africa to the New World suffered as high (or higher) mortality rates as the slaves, which meant that mortality rates were at least 20 per cent in the seventeenth and early eighteenth centuries, but abated somewhat to about 12 per cent in the following period. Merchants and crews were accustomed to look death in the eye and regarded the outbreak on board of severe epidemics and deaths with great fatalism.

The conquest of the Middle East

Precisely because Alexandria was a great and bustling commercial city, it also functioned as a mighty epicentre for the dissemination of epidemic disease. The urban layout of Alexandria was that of a great sprawling town dominated by small single-floored or two-storied buildings covering a vast area. It took quite some time before plague had spread widely among the innumerable rat colonies, and the epidemiological process had translated into a widely diffused and clear epidemic presence in this great city. This characteristic developmental pattern of plague in large cities is

[13] Dols 1979: 56–7.

the reason that the Black Death did not really begin to move forcefully out of Alexandria along the principal commercial routes before the late autumn. In April, it had covered much of the lower Nile Valley and had reached Gaza to the east. It is stated that, in Gaza, the Black Death raged in full force from 2 April to 4 May 1348, a suspiciously short period of time, which suggests that only partial information on the event has been passed on to posterity.

Gaza was the gateway to Palestine and Syria (which at the time also comprised present-day Lebanon). The renowned Muslim traveller Ibn Battutah relates that he stayed in Aleppo (north-western Syria) in June when he first heard about the plague in Gaza. Moving southwards, he met the Black Death first in Homs, a town situated about halfway to Damascus (which again was about halfway to Gaza). He continued his journey to Damascus, where he arrived in July. He must have been an extraordinarily courageous man even as a medieval traveller and adventurer: for Damascus was in the grips of the Black Death. We are told that people were fasting and arranging processions to persuade Allah to raise the plague epidemic. This conforms to the contemporaneous religious notion of the cause of epidemic disease both in the Muslim world and in Christendom, that it was unleashed by Allah or the Lord, respectively, to punish people for their sins. Logically, the only effective way to stop an epidemic was to please the Almighty by demonstrating profound remorse and contrition.[14] When Ibn Battutah somewhat later went on to Jerusalem, the Black Death appears to have subsided there. Because the Black Death moved northwards while Ibn Battutah moved southwards his account provides an inverse outline of the progression of the Black Death through Palestine and Syria.

About the same time as the Black Death arrived in Alexandria by ship, the Black Death sent another important metastatis from the Transcaucasian plague front into the Middle East by another usual method, the human folly of war. A Persian source relates that, in 1347, an army that besieged Tabriz in present-day northern Persia near the border of Azerbaijan moved on to besiege Baghdad in Mesopotamia, the capital of present-day Iraq. However, plague broke out in the army and soon penetrated into the city.[15] The great walls and valiant efforts that kept out brave and inventive beleaguerers did not prevent plague-infected rodents from entering the city. Large-scale transport of provisions to a beleaguering army exposed it greatly to plague contagion, especially because grain would have to be the most important source of food and calories for the men. As explained above, grain is the black rat's preferred type of food and is, at the same time, also most suitable for transport of infected rat fleas, which had developed the ability to live on grain and grain debris. This is, then, already the second case of a type of event described in connection with the siege of Kaffa: that armies attract plague contagion, and the onslaught of plague causes armies to disband in disarray, thus strengthening its powers of spread.

As the Black Death moved northwards along this route it becomes increasingly difficult to decide whether it was the original plague front that had moved through the Caucasus and been brought to Baghdad in late 1347 or the plague coming out of

---

[14] It was also argued in Islamic scholarly literature that plague was only a divine punishment for 'infidels' and impious gravely sinful Muslims, while for the pious Muslim, plague was a mercy and a martyrdom, so that they would be certain to go directly to Paradise. Dols 1982: 69.

[15] Dols 1979: 45.

Alexandria that made the new conquests. This question arises, for instance, in the case of Aleppo, an important commercial centre in north-western Syria, which was attacked in October 1348. It could also be the case with Antioch to the west of Aleppo, although this city might as well have been contaminated by ship transport. The final stage of the spread of Black Death in this part of the world was a process of engulf-ment, in which plague moved in on the remaining uncontaminated territories from different directions, ravaging the cities and towns mercilessly and blanketing the countryside.

The Black Death's transmission into Arabia is little known. It was brought by pilgrims to Mecca in 1348. Pointedly, a contemporary Arab chronicler comments that plague spread among the pilgrims that year, and another chronicler adds that many students and inhabitants of Mecca died. This outbreak caused a lively discussion between Muslim scholars, because Muhammad should have promised that the holy cities of Medina and Mecca would not be attacked by any serious epidemic disease. The fact that the Black Death did not spread to Medina was seen as a miracle, while the ravages of plague in Mecca were explained as Allah's wrath because the city authorities had permitted the presence of unbelievers, namely Jews.[16] This is an instance of the same sort of thinking that unleashed persecution of Jews in Europe.

In 1348–9 the Black Death gained a major bridgehead around Mecca and Jiddah on the Red Sea coast, but it is not known whether it penetrated further inland from this base.

The Black Death was brought from Egypt to Yemen in 1351 by the king of Yemen and his entourage when they returned from imprisonment in Cairo. And this appears to be the last hurrah of the Black Death in the Middle East.

The conquest of North Africa

The Black Death began its westwards march out of Alexandria into North Africa at about the same time as it began to advance eastwards, reaching the town Barqa (Barce), present-day Al Marj in present-day western Libya, about the same time as it reached Gaza to the east.

However, the Black Death also acquired an early foothold in the city of Tunis by ship transport from Sicily. This metastatic leap reflects that the town of Messina in Sicily had been contaminated with the Black Death already around 20 August 1347 (see below). It also reflects the short distance between Sicily and Tunis and the substantial commercial contacts between Sicily and this part of the African continent, grain being, notably, the main product exported from Sicily.[17] The Black Death appears to have broken out in Tunis at the latest in April 1348 and still raged violently in June. A local poet expressed his despair in this way:

> Constantly, I ask God for forgiveness.
> Gone is life and ease.
> In Tunis, both in the morning and in the evening –
> And the morning belongs to God as does the evening –

[16] Dols 1977: 63.
[17] Wolff 1959: 156. With respect to the role of grain in the dissemination of plague, see above, pp. 20–1.

> There is fear and hunger and death,
> Stirred up by tumult and pestilence . . .[18]

The poet holds the usual opinion of his time that epidemics are Allah's punishment for sins, and the only effective way to stop an epidemic is to earn forgiveness by adequate religious action.

The invasion of Tunis permitted the Black Death to attack present-day Libya both from the east and the west; Tripoli was in all likelihood invaded from the Tunisian offshoot.

From Tunis, the Black Death also moved further west and south-west into Algeria and Morocco. Military events also affected the pattern and pace of spread of the Black Death here in North Africa. The Marinid ruler of Fez in Morocco attempted to conquer Tunisia, but was decisively defeated in April 1348. The reason for this, according to the prominent contemporary Tunisian historian Ibn Khaldun, was the outbreak of the Black Death. The retreating army disseminated plague along its route. It has proved desperately difficult to trace the movement of the Black Death across this region. We are informed that one of the defeated Marinid ruler's councillors returned from the campaign to Tlemcen in present-day Algeria, close to the border of present-day Morocco, where he died of plague in 1348. Ibn al-Khatib relates that he learned in 1349 that his mother had died of plague in Taza, a town situated near Fez. An alternative source for importation of plague to Morocco in 1348 was Mallorca and southern Spain where the Black Death broke out in March and April, respectively, an area which conducted extensive trade with Morocco.[19]

The Black Death moved also southwards from Alexandria up the Nile Valley and into Upper Egypt. In 1348, it first entered Cairo at the end of the Nile Delta, about 125 km south-east of Alexandria, but it did not attain its maximum intensity in this great city until the last three months of the year.[20] Next, it spread almost to the town of Asyut on the R. Nile about 250 km further south, and it also hit the great complex of monasteries in Wadi n-Natrum in the desert south-west of Cairo, where pilgrims again obviously played a part in the dissemination of the Black Death. In 1349, the Black Death first invaded Asyut and then moved on to Luxor, almost 250 km to the south of Asyut as the crow flies, although the great bend of the Nile at Quena increases the distance to be covered on the ground significantly. In February 1349, the plague epidemic spread with devastating effects in Upper Egypt.[21] The Black Death seems to have needed about a year and a half to wreak 'havoc throughout Egypt from Alexandria in the north to the outskirts of Aswan in the south'.[22]

In North Africa, as elsewhere, the Black Death was disseminated at a distance by the same types of movement of goods and people, by merchants and tradesmen, refugees and pilgrims. Short-distance, inter-local and intra-local spread would here, as elsewhere, mostly be brought about by the peasant population's normal activities, bringing produce to and from local markets, taking care of their diseased family

[18] Cited after Dols 1977: 64–5.
[19] Dufourcq 1970–1: 52–4.
[20] Dols 1977: 182.
[21] Dols 1977: 161.
[22] Udovitch 1971: 124.

members and relatives, and inheriting dangerous things like clothing, bedding and mattresses from deceased relatives.

One would expect that the Black Death spread further into Africa, southwards along the Nile and the caravan routes into south-eastern Africa, and from North Africa via the caravan routes leading to West Africa, another important source of slaves for North Africa and the Middle East. However, there is no evidence to this effect that can transform this opinion from hypothesis to valid inference. It could be that camel caravans moving southwards with luxury goods to be exchanged for slaves were poor means for dissemination of plague contagion. This should not be taken to mean that plague could not be transported at a distance by caravans, only that it would tend to occur quite rarely.

Ibn al-Khatib noted to his amazement that nomadic Arabs in North Africa who lived in tents and moved from place to place were not hit by the plague. This sharp contrast between the fate of the agricultural and urban populations, which suffered immensely from the onslaught of the Black Death, and the nomads, which avoided the disease almost completely, reflects the fact that rural and urban populations were greatly exposed to rats and rat fleas, while the nomads were not. This, then, is important evidence to the effect that the Black Death in North Africa had the same dynamic basis in rats as elsewhere, in consonance with the findings in India, China, Madagascar and in other developing countries in the twentieth century.

7

Mediterranean Europe

Introduction

The armies of the Black Death spread simultaneously in many directions in many countries and regions, employing, as it were, various tactics and strategies relevant to specific environments, available means of transport and local cultures. The simultaneity and complexity of the movements of the Black Death's triumphant armies of bacteria, rats and fleas are difficult to grasp and present. The best approach, everything considered, is to give a fully integrated account of its history in individual large countries like France and Italy or within the framework of two or more countries that also form natural territorial entities in an epidemiological perspective, like the Iberian Peninsula (Spain, Portugal and the Muslim Kingdom of Granada), and the British Isles. This approach lends itself to systematic study of the patterns of spread in time and space in various areas and regions that in some important respects were bound together by political, economic and communication systems. Such systems always contain specific patterns of interaction within national territories and their regional and administrative subdivisions that affect the spread of epidemic diseases in crucial ways, in the Late Middle Ages, including the Black Death. Countries bound together by special ties such as, for instance, Spain and Portugal, England and Ireland, will also tend to develop economic and social relationships that will be suited to the exchange of contagion; they will, in other words, tend to function as epidemiologically integrated territories.

This Part 2 on the spread of the Black Death is followed in Part 4 by a section on mortality presented according to the same territorial principle. This should make it fairly easy to piece together the territorial pattern and pace of spread and the demographic impact of the Black Death for various national and territorial contexts. It is hoped that this approach will provide national readerships of today with a satisfactory overview of this most dramatic event in their country's history.

As the history of the Black Death moves northwards and eastwards in Europe, with the exception of England, the sources become progressively fewer and less informative and consist increasingly of notices in chronicles of generally deteriorating quality. It becomes increasingly difficult to outline its pattern of spread and its demographic, economic and social impact.

The arrival of the Black Death in important European seaports on the Mediterranean Sea was a momentous and sinister event in the history of Europe. This was the initial phase of the Black Death's conquest of Europe, when it secured bridgeheads of vital strategic importance. It prepared the ground for the Black Death's multi-pronged invasion of the European continent, causing the death of a much larger part of the population than any other murderous event in this part of the world, including the terrible tragedies of the twentieth century, the two world wars and Hitler's and Stalin's enormous totalitarian atrocities.

We will never know whether the Black Death was transported to Mediterranean seaports directly from Kaffa or whether it had also contaminated other Genoese and Venetian merchant ships in Constantinople. One may wonder how a ship with plague on board in those times could have completed such long voyages, from Kaffa or Constantinople to Genoa or Venice in northern Italy, before the crew and oarsmen had been depleted to a point that would prevent the ship from continuing. The reason was probably that the large commercial ships involved in long-distance trade contained not only large numbers of sailors and oarsmen, but also a substantial military contingent, which, supported by the crew, would defend the precious goods against pirates. This means that sufficient numbers would often survive or avoid the disease to keep the ship going to its destination, an achievement upon which the crew would be dependent for receiving their wages, and the merchants for avoiding great losses and earning great profits. A chronicler's description of the large number of persons on board such a ship at the time was rendered above in connection with the early arrival of the Black Death in Alexandria.

Giovanni Villani, the Florentine merchant and administrator, and one of the most reliable and informative medieval chroniclers, commented also on the coming of the Black Death:

> Having grown in vigour in Turkey and Greece and having spread thence over the whole Levant and Mesopotamia and Syria and Chaldea and Cyprus and Rhodes and all the islands of the Greek archipelago, the said pestilence leaped to Sicily, Sardinia and Corsica and Elba, and from there soon reached all the shores of the mainland [. . .] And many lands and cities were made desolate. And the plague lasted till –[1]

Giovanni Villani left some blank space at the end of this account that he intended to fill in when the Black Death eventually had gone away. However, he was to be one of the Black Death's myriad victims and never completed it.

The first part of Europe to be attacked by the Black Death after it left the Crimea with Italian galleys was the small European part of Constantinople. In the autumn, the Black Death spread south-westwards in quite a narrow strip from this point of intrusion into Europe all along the shores of the straits that lead to the Aegean Sea, the arm of the Mediterranean Sea between Greece and Asia Minor.

As indicated by Giovanni Villani, during the late summer and autumn of 1347 the Black Death managed to cover the whole or at least large parts of southern and central Greece, a fact that suggests that the Black Death was introduced both over land and by sea and expanded and gained territory via a number of separate routes. Greek nationals and Italian galleys fleeing from Constantinople would be a forceful

[1] Schevill 1961: 239–40.

combination that exposed Greece greatly to early attacks. The Italian galleys would normally follow the coasts of Greece, putting into selected harbours for rest and provisions of food and drink.

We will never know whether or not the invasion by the Black Death of the small European part of Constantinople and its spread along the shores of the straits and the incursion to Greece could have served as a territorial base for a further spreading into Europe, because other events overshadowed completely its disseminative potential. The crucial events were the introduction of the Black Death in important seaports and commercial centres further west. These urban centres functioned as the bridge-heads and areas of deployment for the armies of the Black Death. Within a few weeks, the awesome invisible armies of murderous epidemic death began to march out of these coastal cities and towns and conquered the whole of Europe within a few years.

The Italian galleys sailed on along Greece's western coasts, but while the Venetians continued northwards into the Adriatic Sea, the Genoese galleys would cross over to Italy in the narrow strait between present-day Albania and Italy's heel, and sail on along the shores of the sole of Italy's geographical boot, so to speak, until they came to Sicily. Here they would call at the harbour of the island's principal port Messina for rest and provisions before setting sail for the final stretch of the long voyage back to their beloved Genoa, their *patria* as they called it. However, this time the Black Death had put into the harbour of Messina with the Genoese:

> At the beginning of October, in the year of the incarnation of the Son of God 1347, twelve Genoese galleys were fleeing from the vengeance which our Lord was taking on account of their nefarious deeds and entered the harbour of Messina. In their bones they bore so virulent a disease that anyone who only spoke to them was seized by a mortal illness and in no manner could evade death [. . .]

Thus, the Franciscan friar Michael of Piazza describes the arrival and outbreak of the Black Death in Messina in an account that is often and widely cited without much hesitation or source criticism. He wrote his account a decade after the event, and one should note that a contemporary commentator dates the outbreak in Messina to the end of September, which is considered the correct date of this historical event, because it fits better with the subsequent events.[2] According to the standard assumption on the time lag between the time of contamination and the time of recognition by chroniclers, Messina was probably contaminated by the Black Death about six weeks earlier, in the second week of August.

One should also disregard the number of galleys that conform to the set of magical and mythological numbers of which medieval people were so fond and which they preferred over tedious and vulgar empirical observations. This mentality can also be seen in the fanciful descriptions of the extreme inter-personal contagiousness of the plague, which is without foundation in observable medical fact but not, of course, in the miasmatic epidemiological theory of classical Greek medicine. Educated medieval people preferred to hold the tenets of miasmatic theory above the principle of empir-ical observation; the accounts should conform to lofty classical theory, not to the

---

2   Del Panta 1980: 111–12.

vulgar factual observation that any ignorant person would be able to make. Their opinions and statements were more shaped to enhance their social standing by demonstrating education and learning than by establishing empirically tenable and testable knowledge. This mentality of the educated and learned classes permeates their accounts and make considerable demands on modern scholars who endeavour to glean facts from fiction, and is the reason these accounts so often contain little useful factual material.

In Messina, which was quite a large town, the Black Death soon revealed its true nature, subjecting the inhabitants to an incomprehensible epidemic catastrophe. The panic that unfolded is also vividly rendered by the friar:

> When the catastrophe had reached its climax the Messinians resolved to emigrate. One portion of them settled in the vineyards and fields, but a larger portion sought refuge in the town of Catania, trusting that the holy virgin Agatha of Catania would deliver them from their evil. But flight was no longer of avail. The disease clung to the fugitives and accompanied them everywhere they turned in search of help [. . .] The population of Catania was so godless and timid that no one among them would have intercourse or speak to the fugitives [. . .] Thus the people of Messina dispersed over the whole island of Sicily and with them the disease, so that innumerable people died.[3]

No wonder the Messinians took to their heels when the Black Death revealed its awesome powers of epidemic carnage and fled in panic from the catastrophe, unwittingly spreading the Black Death all over Sicily. Large parts of Sicily and all the major towns were embroiled with the armies of the Black Death in the course of October and November.

Soon people also fled in panic from Sicily, taking the Black Death with them. In December, plague raged in Sardinia, Corsica and nearby Elba I., close to the lush and beautiful coastline of Tuscany. The Black Death was poised to strike into the densely populated industrial heartland of Italy, only about 130 km from Florence itself as the crow flies.

Inevitably, at the end of the year, the Black Death crossed the narrow Strait of Messina and established its reign of death in the town of Reggio di Calabria. The Black Death had invaded the Italian mainland and had acquired, so to speak, a foothold on Italy's toe.

As should be expected, ships returning from the Crimea or Constantinople also unloaded the Black Death in Genoa itself. It arrived with three galleys loaded with spices, and we are told by a chronicler that these galleys had spread the plague in many places along the long voyage from the Crimea. The outbreak appears to have been recognized in the very last days of 1347, which, according to the standard assumption and in view of the cool weather, implies that the contamination was introduced into the city about seven weeks earlier, in the second week of November.[4]

At the middle of January it became evident that the Black Death had managed to cross from Sardinia or Elba over to Pisa, where it was making its murderous way

---

[3] Nohl 1961: 7–9, renders Michael of Pizza's account almost complete in English translation.
[4] Sticker 1908: 49; Del Panta 1980: 111–12.

through this small city on the coast of Tuscany, 60 km west of Florence.[5] In view of
the delaying effects of cool winter weather on the epidemic processes, the fact that the
outbreak had reached a stage that caught the attention of the chronicle-producing
Pisan upper classes at the middle of January implies that the contagion was probably
introduced about seven weeks earlier, at the end of November 1347. Pisa was Florence's port of export and import; from this bustling commercial hub the Black Death
could easily ride unnoticed with goods or people to Florence and other places in
Tuscany. The Black Death was thus linked to the main European communication
networks of trade and travel by land.[6]

The Venetian galleys that sailed impatiently homewards up the Adriatic Sea also
carried the Black Death on board and spread the contagion along the Dalmatian
eastern coasts of the Adriatic Sea where many of the islands off the coast and a few
bridgeheads in seaports belonged at the time to the city state of Venice (today they
belong to the Republic of Croatia). First, it went ashore in Spalato (present-day Split)
where the outbreak was noticed on Christmas Day 1347, and it broke out in Ragusa
(present-day Dubrovnik) before 13 January. This implies that Spalato was probably
contaminated around 10 November, Ragusa at the very end of that month.

On 25 January, the epidemic presence of the Black Death was noted in Venice
itself.[7] In this great metropolis, it would, under ordinary circumstances, take about
eight weeks from the time of the contamination until the outbreak was recognized.
However, at that time, the epidemiological processes would probably be slowed
down by cool winter weather. This means that Venice was probably contaminated
around 25 November, which fits well with the time of contamination of Spalato and
Ragusa. The invasion of this metropolis, the largest commercial centre in Italy, with
wide-flung commercial contacts,[8] was a momentous event in the early history of the
Black Death's conquest of Europe.

However, a chronicler asserts that the Black Death had already broken out in the
city of Marseilles in south-eastern France by 1 November 1347. Although later dates
of the recognized outbreak are given by other chroniclers, the earlier dating appears
trustworthy because the Black Death broke out in Aix-en-Provence, 25 km to the
north, around 1 December,[9] and in other towns and cities in the region within a time
pattern that accords with this dating (see below). Datings of the outbreak of plague in
Marseilles to late December or even January 1348 cannot be correct.[10]

A dating of the recognized outbreak in Marseilles to 1 November means that the
city was probably contaminated in the second week of September, a dating that
should be compared to the time of the contamination of Messina, which has been

---

[5] Feroci 1892: 15–16. Michael of Piazza relates that two freight-ships carried the Black Death from Messina
to Pisa, the crews were suffering from plague, and all those in Pisa who spoke to the sailors in the fish market
Piazza dei Pesci immediately contracted the disease. Although this story cannot be dismissed outright, its
anecdotal character is evident, especially the tall story about how everybody who spoke to the sailors was immediately infected.
[6] Del Panta 1980: 111–13.
[7] Mueller 1979a: 71.
[8] Mueller 1979b: 94–5.
[9] Biraben 1975: 91. See also the discussion below of the pace of spread of plague epidemics.
[10] Gasquet 1908: 39; Shrewsbury 1971: 43, asterisked footnote.

estimated at the second week of August. This means that the contamination of Marseilles was caused by a ship that could have sailed on from Messina after only a few days of rest and provisioning, or that could have been cross-infected in the harbour there, or possibly could have been infected in Constantinople and had Marseilles as its final destination.

The surprisingly early invasion of Marseilles by the Black Death may have affected profoundly its pattern of strategic advance in Southern and Western Europe, and also, as we shall see, the invasion of the British Isles. It was another momentous event in the sinister history of the Black Death. Marseilles, a small city with around 15,000 inhabitants on the eve of the arrival of the Black Death,[11] was an important commercial hub of the western Mediterranean. From this commercial centre, communication lines radiated both by sea and by land. This city was an excellent bridgehead for the Black Death's offensive against south-western and Western Europe.

Around the turn of the year 1347–8, the Black Death's deadly armies of bacteria and rat fleas were poised to strike into Europe from several great urban population centres that gave easy access to movement along the main routes of trade and travel both by sea and by land.

[11] Baratier 1961: 66–7.

8

The Southern Balkans: Albania, Macedonia, Southern Yugoslavia, Greece and Bulgaria

The territories constituting present-day Albania, the southern provinces of Yugoslavia and the Republic of Macedonia may quite likely have been invaded from the epicentres that were established on the European side of the straits in the late summer or early autumn of 1347 and in southern Greece in the autumn of 1347. Thus, somewhere in the southern Balkans, conceivably somewhere in Macedonia, the Black Death's Dalmatian army and Greek army met. Possibly its Byzantine European army also reached this region after having engulfed the area of the present-day Republic of Bulgaria. The tentative character of these suggestions must be underlined.

The Venetian ships that carried the infectious forces from Kaffa or Constantinople could also have infected other seaports along the Adriatic Sea. Durres in Albania was, for instance, a Venetian possession at the time; in all likelihood, as many of those ships called at this harbour as in Ragusa (Dubrovnik) or in Spalato (Split). Similarly, Corfu I. (Kérkyra), at the entrance of the Adriatic Sea and facing the coast of both Greece and Albania, belonged to Venice; however, where there are no sources the historian stands defeated.

Arguably, this outline of the probable epidemic movements during the Black Death's conquest of the Balkans suggests that this region of Europe was not only a great crossroads of peoples, cultures, religions and conquerors where human input from Asia, the Near East/Asia Minor and Europe met, but, for the same reason, also a great crossroads of epidemic diseases.

9

The Kingdom of Hungary: Croatia, Bosnia-Herzegovina, Slovakia, Hungary and Western Romania

The spread of the Black Death in the northern Balkans must be discussed within the territorial framework of the Kingdom of Hungary, which comprised a much larger territory at the time of the Black Death than the present-day Republic of Hungary. It stretched down to the Adriatic Sea and comprised much of the area that today constitutes the Republics of Croatia and Bosnia-Herzegovina, and some parts of present-day Yugoslavia including Belgrade; in the north, it included the territories of the present-day Republic of Slovakia, and in the east about the western half of present-day Romania. The fact that all these countries and territories were politically and administratively integrated within the Kingdom of Hungary facilitated the spread of the Black Death.

However, the points of introduction had a different political background. The city state of Venice occupied many islands along the Dalmatian (Croatian) coastline, and had a few bridgeheads in seaports on the mainland, especially Ragusa, present-day Dubrovnik. This highlights the importance of the very early introductions of the Black Death in the form of original epicentres of spread in Spalato (Split), where the outbreak was noticed on 25 December 1347, and in Ragusa, where the outbreak of the Black Death was recognized before 13 January 1348. According to the standard assumption, this implies that they probably became contaminated around 10 November and at the very end of that month, respectively (see also above). Also noteworthy is the early further spread to Sebenico (Šibenik[1]), about 50 km north-west of Spalato.[2]

The army of the Black Death that moved out of Venice along the route eastwards into the Duchy of Carniola, corresponding roughly to the present-day Republic of Slovenia, also played an important part. In August, it was reported to be in Istria,[3] which at the time belonged to the Venetian city state but today is part of the Republic

---

[1] The letter š is pronounced as sh in English and sch in German.
[2] Sticker 1908: 50.
[3] Sticker 1908: 50.

of Croatia, a pattern of spread that implies that it had already ravaged Trieste at the very north-eastern end of the Adriatic Sea, which also constitutes the natural border between Italy and the Balkan Peninsula. The areas that today constitute Slovenia, Croatia, Bosnia-Herzegovina and northern Yugoslavia were conquered either by the Black Death's Dalmatian (Croatian) army or by the Venetian army, or their joined forces.

Within this roughly outlined pattern of spread, the reported outbreak of the Black Death in southern Hungary in January 1349, and the implication that transportation on the R. Danube played an important part in the dissemination of the disease, fits nicely into the picture.[4]

Unfortunately, little more is known except that, in mid-1349, plague ravaged Oradea,[5] on the present-day Romanian border with eastern Hungary. This allows a certain element of speculation to the effect that this invasion was performed by the Byzantine European army, the army of the Black Death that had marched out of the original epicentre on the European side of the straits connecting the Mediterranean and the Black Sea, which was established in the late summer or in the early autumn of 1347. Probably, it is knowledge of this plague movement passed on from the crews on Italian ships that is reflected in the Tuscan city of Lucca's prohibition of all Romanians from entering the city.[6] However, it cannot be entirely ruled out that the Black Death had managed to spread to Oradea from Hungary, where the first outbreak reportedly occurred in the southern areas around the R. Danube in January.

---

[4] Biraben 1975: 81, 83.
[5] Biraben 1975: 83.
[6] Henderson 1992: 144.

10

The Iberian Peninsula:
The Spanish Kingdoms, the Kingdom of Portugal and the Kingdom of Granada[1]

At the time of the Black Death, the Iberian Peninsula contained a number of states. For the sake of convenience, the term Spain is used to denote the territory covered by the modern Spanish state with the exception of the Muslim Kingdom of Granada but including Roussillon, which today belongs to France. There were, accordingly, three Spanish kingdoms, namely the Kingdom of Castile, the Kingdom of Navarre and the Kingdom of Aragon, and two non-Spanish kingdoms, namely the Kingdom of Portugal and the Muslim Kingdom of Granada. After centuries of war against the Muslims, the Kingdom of Castile comprised, in addition to Old Castile, not only the northern provinces Galicia, Asturias and Leon-Castile but also New Castile, Extremadura, Andalucia and the former Kingdom of Murcia. The Kingdom of Aragon also comprised, in addition to Aragon, Catalonia, the former Kingdom of Valencia, Roussillon and the Balearic Islands.

The populations of the Spanish kingdoms taken together have been estimated at about 6 million on the eve of the Black Death (the Kingdom of Granada contained another 1.5 million inhabitants).[2] The Iberian Peninsula comprises about 600,000 sq. km, quite a big chunk of Europe, of which the Spanish kingdoms constituted almost 85 per cent, some 500,000 sq. km. Accordingly, average population density was around 12 persons per sq. km.

The Black Death's conquest of these kingdoms was accomplished with a complex and amazingly efficient strategy and extraordinary impetus and pace. Five separate armies invaded their territory, all of which had their origin in Marseilles, and transport by ship played a pivotal role in the Black Death's grand strategy. The earliest invasion occurred on the Balearic island of Mallorca in December 1347, the second took place in Roussillon in January 1349. Then followed in quick succession in the course of a few months several landings on the Iberian mainland by ship, both from

---

[1]   There are three useful, general papers on the Black Death's introduction and spread in the Iberian Peninsula: López de Meneses 1959: 331–44; Sobrequés Callicó 1966: 67–102; Ubieto Arteta 1975: 47–66.

[2]   Ballesteros Rodriguez 1982: 38.

Rousillon and Mallorca. An army of the Black Death that had reached Bordeaux from Marseilles in forced marches split up in several separate divisions that sailed to a number of destinations in three countries, of which two destinations became bridge-heads for the conquest of north-western Spain and Portugal and of the Kingdom of Navarre in north-eastern Iberia, respectively.

The Black Death's invasion of Spain started with a seemingly fortuitous and unpredictable first attack. What sensible general aiming at conquering Europe and planning an invasion of the Iberian Peninsula would allow the idea to cross his mind that an invasion of Mallorca would be an excellent beginning of the campaign? Mallorca is the main island of the Balearic Islands, situated about 200 km off Spain's south-eastern coast. However, the events would soon prove that it was, actually, an artful strategy, a master stroke based on a dynamic combination of two important facts: firstly, shipping offered by far the speediest and most efficient means of trans-portation in those times; secondly, a fairly large island with around 55,000 inhabit-ants had, of course, a lively commercial exchange by ship with the mainland.[3] This intensive interaction with towns and cities on the coast of the mainland inevitably caused frequent importation of epidemic diseases that would be easily re-exported.[4] These commercial centres would tend to relate to specifically established markets and would often not interact in any intensive way. In short, in this particular case, Mallorca was at the centre of an economic system that would make it easy for the Black Death to enter ships in Mallorcan ports and invade important commercial towns and cities along the south-eastern and southern coasts coasts of Spain; the inva-sion of Mallorca thus facilitated the establishment of important bridgeheads for a multi-pronged invasion of the Peninsula from this quarter.[5]

Consequently, the Black Death entered a ship heading for Mallorca. According to Santamaría Arandéz, there are vague suggestions of the presence of plague in Mallorca in the second half of February,[6] and that on 20 March the information reaching the authorities was so grave that a meeting was convened five days later to 'adopt the measures that the circumstances required'. In order to identify the time of contamination we must take into account that cool winter weather usually slowed down the epidemiological processes,[7] which means that the standard assumption on the time lag between the introduction of contagion and the recognized outbreak should be expanded to 7–8 weeks. These considerations indicate that Mallorca was contaminated at the end of December 1347. The time of invasion shows that Mallorca must have been contaminated by a ship coming directly from the city of Marseilles, which was contaminated in the second week of September (see above) or, possibly, via the city of Montpellier, which, arguably, was contaminated in the first half of December (see below) and had good connections to Mallorca because it belonged likewise to the Kingdom of Aragon (until the following year when it was sold to France).[8]

---

[3] See Durliat and Pons i Marqués 1959: 345–63; Santamaría Arández 1970–1: 165–236.
[4] Cf. Santamaría Arández 1970–1: 180–1.
[5] A large collection of official documentary sources relating to the Black Death in the Kingdom of Aragon was published by López de Meneses in 1956.
[6] Santamaría Arández 1969: 108.
[7] See, e.g., Dubois 1988b: 316.
[8] It cannot be entirely ruled out that desperate people in Sardinia or even Sicily would dare to head out

At the end of March, it was officially reported that the Black Death had broken out in the largish fishing village Allí of Alcudia, and a certain Guillem Brassa is the first documented victim of the Black Death on Spanish soil. The official recognition of the presence of the Black Death came, as so often was the case, when the epidemic had become too obvious and the mortality too frightening to be ignored any more. Soon, the Black Death spread to Palma and further around the island. It appears, therefore, that the epidemic had reached serious proportions no later than the first half of March and that the full brunt of the epidemic was unleashed in the second half of March and in April; at the end of May, it began to subside.[9]

In Mallorca, the Black Death had no difficulty in finding shipping opportunities for reaching the Spanish mainland. On 20 April, King Pedro IV of Aragon declared that the plague had been passed on from Mallorca and now ravaged Roussillon,[10] the south-easternmost part of his kingdom (300 years later, this border area was conquered by France[11]). However, a closer look at the facts does not bear out the king's view. Obviously, the Black Death called first at the harbour of Perpignan, the main urban centre in Roussillon and an important local port. According to the local chroniclers, the plague raged in the months March to June. R. Emery, who has studied the Black Death in Perpignan, is willing to accept that there may have been some cases as early as March, but in his opinion, the evidence suggests that it was only in mid-April that the plague in Perpignan reached 'epidemic proportions'.[12] However, the documentary material used by Emery reflects the epidemiological events as they affected the upper classes and various political and professional élites, which took place with a significant delay in relation to the events in the wards of poor, ordinary people. King Pedro's declaration of 20 April to the effect that Roussillon was being ravaged by the plague must reflect that epidemic developments had been going on for some time and had caused serious mortality among the population, and appears incompatible with Emery's view. The assertions of local chroniclers that the epidemic had acquired serious proportions at the end of March should, therefore, be accepted. According to the standard assumption that has been developed and practised in this book, but with a small addition to take account of the short period of winter weather that presumably slowed down the epidemiological processes somewhat, the chroniclers' statements should be taken to indicate that plague contagion was introduced about seven or perhaps eight weeks earlier, i.e., not later than at the beginning of February. Interestingly, at the beginning of April the Black Death was raging in Cerdaña,[13] a large Pyrenean valley stretching from south-western Roussillon across the border with Spain, which makes it clear that the contagion must have been introduced there in mid-February. Taken together, these pieces of information actually suggests that Perpignan could have been contaminated as early as some time in January.

into the open sea to escape the Black Death and set sail directly for Spain, landing in Mallorca. This is, of course, pure speculation.

[9] López de Meneses 1959: 331–44; Santamaría Arández 1969: 108–9.

[10] López de Meneses 1956: 292; López de Meneses 1965: 533–41.

[11] Because Roussillon and Cerdagne at the time belonged to the Kingdom of Aragon it might be more correct to use the Spanish names Rosellón and Cerdaña.

[12] Emery 1967: 611–23.

[13] López de Meneses 1965: 535–6, 538–9.

An introduction of plague contagion at this date is not compatible with an origin in Mallorca according to the description of the epidemiological developments given by Santamaría Arández, namely that the early epidemic phase that made the developing catastrophe observable and recognizable appears to have started there in the second half of February, which, as mentioned, implies a likely time of contamination at the end of December. Thus, King Pedro was probably mistaken when he asserted that the contagion had come from Mallorca. Contagion from the original epicentre in Marseilles that was established in mid-September 1347 was spreading in a series of metastatic leaps south-westwards towards the Spanish border of Roussillon.[14] It will be shown below that the large French cities of Montpellier and Béziers were probably contaminated in December 1347, the city of Narbonne and the town of Carcassonne, only about 35 and 45 km north of the border, respectively probably around 1 January (see below). Perpignan was therefore probably contaminated from these French sources, which were much closer. This assumption is also strengthened by the early epidemic developments in Perpignan and the time of the expansion out of Roussillon into Spain (see below).[15]

In May, the Black Death emerged with a vengeance in several urban centres on Spain's south-eastern coastline. At the very beginning of May, religious processions against the 'great mortality' were arranged in Barcelona, the greatest city in south-eastern Spain, with a population of around 50,000 inhabitants. The fact that the outbreak had developed quite a broad, deadly presence and had inspired religious countermeasures at the beginning of May shows that the evolving epidemic had already taken on a dramatic character in this large city and indicates that the epidemic presence was recognized at least two or rather three weeks earlier, c. 13–20 April. This implies that Barcelona had been contaminated in the first week of March and that the contamination had arrived by ship from Roussillon, although an origin in Mallorca is also possible.

The determination of the recognizable epidemic outbreak to the third week of April is supported by some specific evidence. A study of the incidence of vacant clerical benefices in the years 1347–9 shows only the quite normal monthly incidence of one vacant position in April 1348. Then, there was an abrupt and dramatic change: there were nine vacancies in May, 25 in June and an astonishing 104 in July. From August on, there was a slowly subsiding development of the epidemic as reflected in the number of vacant priestly benefices until their monthly number reached a quite normal pre-plague level of two vacant positions in June 1349.[16]

In the town of Tarragona, situated about 85 km south-west of Barcelona, the outbreak was recognized on 1 May, which must reflect contamination six to seven weeks earlier, i.e., some time in the second week of March.[17] This indicates that Tarragona was contaminated directly from Mallorca (or, just possibly, by a ship contaminated in the harbour area of Barcelona that then immediately set sail for the city). In Gerona, situated about 90 km north-east of Barcelona, the outbreak must have been recognized roughly at the same time as in Tarragona and the time of

---

[14] Guilleré 1984: 18, 20–1; Biraben 1975: 74.
[15] Guilleré 1984: 21.
[16] Ubieto Arteta 1975: 50–1; Gyug 1983: 378–95.
[17] Ubieto Arteta 1975: 51–2; Trenchs Odena 1969: 45–64; Kern 1969: 71–3.

contamination must be about the same, for the same epidemiological reasons and when taking into account that wills constitute the main type of sources.[18] The time pattern shows that Gerona must have been contaminated by the epidemic forces spreading out of Roussillon. Evidence on ecclesiastical mortality in the diocese of Gerona provides some support for the assumption that this was also the case for the diocese as a whole.[19] The Black Death raged in both cities with extreme intensity in June and July and subsided in August.[20]

The early contamination of Tarragona indicates that the Black Death actually reached Tarrega and Lérida from this city and not from Barcelona, both because the distance is shorter and because the development of the frightening epidemic phase that induced people to flee took longer to develop in Barcelona than in Tarragona.

In the city of Valencia, more than 200 km further south-west, a chronicler asserts that the Black Death broke out in May,[21] and this is supported by the number of wills issued this month. For the eight years 1340–7, there are, on average, slightly less than two wills preserved each year. However, for May 1348 alone there are extant two wills, a fact that clearly indicates an extraordinary situation. In June, when the Black Death blazed up in full ferocity, the number of preserved wills for this month alone amounts to 21, significantly more than in the preceding eight years taken together (15).[22] Wills were made when the will-producing social élites recognized to their horror that the carnage among the poor was spreading and that their own lives would soon be very much at risk; they relate to quite a developed epidemic situation. The small number of wills in May indicates that this situation arose at the end of the month. Presumably, the recognizable epidemic phase set in around mid-May, so that Valencia was contaminated with the Black Death about three weeks later than Barcelona, i.e., at the end of March. Also in this case the contagion probably originated in Mallorca.

It must have been contagion from Mallorca that was the cause of the outbreak of the Black Death in the seaport city of Almería in the small remaining Muslim state in the Iberian Peninsula, the Kingdom of Granada. According to the local physician Ibn Hátima, the Black Death began on 30 May 1348 in a poor ward in Almería, which should be taken to mean that dramatic epidemic developments there came to the attention of the social élites by 30 May. It follows that the outbreak started at least a couple of weeks earlier, which indicates a time of contamination at the end of the first week of April. This does not give any real alternative to an origin in Mallorca, which

---

[18] Guilleré 1984: 23. Alberch i Fugueras and Castells i Calzada 1985: 32. In the case of Gerona, the number of wills began to grow around 10 May, and shot up from about 20 May, which reflects that at this point the will-making upper classes began to feel threatened by the epidemic developments. No doubt, news about a serious epidemic among the poor sections of the population had caught their attention a couple of weeks earlier, which clearly indicates a time of infection around mid-March.

[19] Trenchs Odena has collected evidence of ecclesiastical deaths in the diocese of Gerona, but this evidence provides less accurate information on the progress of the epidemic. However, evidence from other parts of the social scene is welcome, and can in a general way be said to support the outline of the epidemic's progress given here. Trenchs Odena 1980: 183–204.

[20] Guilleré 1984: 23–7; Ubieto Arteta 1975: 51.

[21] Rubio Vela 1979: 24–5.

[22] Trenchs Odena 1978: 27–8. See also Rubio Vela 1979: 25–8. There are small differences in the numbers of wills they have found in the archives and their monthly distribution, but the only significant difference is that Trenchs Odena has identified two issued in May, while Rubio Vela found none; but Rubio Vela found 21 wills issued in June, while Trenchs Odena found only 17.

should be seen in the light of the extensive trade to Morocco from Mallorca that conveniently also took in seaports in the Kingdom of Granada like Almería.[23] Soon, we are told quite credibly, 70 persons died daily. The epidemic in Almería disappeared in February 1349.

Apparently, in the early phase of the epidemic the Black Death did not expand much out of Almería; this appears to have occurred some time in the autumn. This delay of further spread is said to be owing to active precautionary measures to contain the epidemic,[24] although otherwise the Muslim countries in the Middle East and North Africa are known for fatalistic, non-interfering attitudes to epidemics.[25] The first information on further spread in the kingdom is the death of a person in Málaga on 24 April 1349, and it was still taking victims there in the following months, with a well-known poet dying from it on 11 July. In the meantime, another person died from plague in Algeciras, close to Gibraltar, and in Cadiz the bishop died from plague around 1 June or a few days later.[26] One would like to think that this was owing to contamination coming by ship from the Kingdom of Granada, especially from Málaga, or it may possibly have come by ship from Algeria on the other side of Gibraltar, where the Black Death was also raging at the time (see above). Another well-known poet died in Granada on 22 May 1349.[27] Clearly, in 1349 the Black Death was spreading intensively in the Kingdom of Granada, and after having crossed the border with the Kingdom of Spain it would eventually meet other forces pressing on southwards and westwards. In all likelihood Andalucia was mainly or wholly conquered from the south, probably also the southern part of New Castile. In New Castile the Black Death was raging in Toledo in June and July 1349[28] and still had a considerable distance to cover before meeting with the other army of the Black Death that at the time wrought havoc in the Kingdom of Granada and was on its way across the border into Andalucia, undoubtedly passed on by the considerable trade in grain, cattle and olive oil between New Castile and the Muslim state.[29]

It is a misunderstanding that the Black Death also appeared in Sevilla in 1348, as this occurred the following year.[30]

The Black Death's strategic genius made also another masterstroke that greatly increased the pace of its conquest of the Iberian Peninsula. Shortly after its multiple invasions of important urban centres along the coast of the Kingdom of Aragon, it performed a remarkable metastatic leap and emerged triumphantly in the town of Santiago de Compostela in the very opposite, north-westernmost corner of the Iberian Peninsula. The bishop of Santiago is mentioned alive for the last time on 14 June, the circumstances showing quite clearly that he must have died from plague.[31] Bishops were important persons whose actions tended to be reflected in registers and

23 Dufourcq 1970–1: 52–4.
24 Ubieto Arteta 1975: 64.
25 Dols 1977: 56–7.
26 Ubieto Arteta 1975: 60.
27 Ubieto Areta 1975: 64–5.
28 Ubieto Arteta 1975: 65–6.
29 Dufourcq 1970–1: 54; Ubieto Arteta 1975: 54–5; Sobrequés Callicó 1966: 94–6.
30 Ubieto Arteta 1975: 63.
31 Ubieto Arteta 1975: 60.

documents and other sources, and he must therefore be assumed to have died shortly after 14 June. For practical reasons we may realistically assume that he was infected on 14 June or some day in the subsequent week (and died eight days later). The new bishop was instituted by Pope Clemens VI exactly two months later, which, taking into account the normal time for the process of instituting a new bishop, fits very well into the picture.

Santiago was one of the most important goals for pilgrims in the Middle Ages because it was believed that the bones of the Apostle Jacob (Iago) rested under the high altar of the cathedral, which also contained many other precious relics. In the same way as Mecca attracted pilgrims from areas ravaged by the Black Death in the Muslim world and was visited early, the Black Death undoubtedly performed the remarkable feat of leaping to the north-western corner of Spain assisted by pilgrims who were shocked by the Lord's awesome epidemic punishment and wished to temper His wrath by performing a pilgrimage to the shrine of St Jacob. Some of the very same persons who particularly fervently desired to help their fellow men in the time of a terrifying mortality crisis were turned into victims of fate's blackest irony and actually acted as passive carriers and unwitting disseminators of the Black Death. Priests attached to the cathedral in order to serve the spiritual needs of the pilgrims, and help them with problems relating to shelter and food and physical handicaps, would be highly exposed to epidemic diseases that the pilgrims brought with them, not least because pilgrims travelled in groups by land or on overcrowded ships. The priests of the cathedral would therefore be exposed early to the Black Death by pilgrims coming from areas where it raged, and soon the living quarters of these priests would be contaminated by infected rat fleas that they carried with them in their clothing. Deathbeds and deaths of the cathedral's priests and other ecclesiastics would introduce the bishop to their living quarters in order to administer the last rites to them and participate in their funerals. Consequently, it could well be that the bishop contracted the infection in quite an early phase of the epidemic developments, and that the epidemic had surfaced about a fortnight earlier, i.e., 1–7 June. Thus, the time of the bishop's death from the Black Death may be taken to indicate that Santiago was contaminated in the period 20–27 April. This surprisingly early date leaves no doubt that the contagion must have been transported by ship to the seaport of La Coruña, whence the pilgrims would take two days to walk the 50 km to Santiago. The contagion would thus, according to these assumptions, have arrived at La Coruña in the period 18–25 April.

Surprisingly, the bishop of Tuy, a Spanish cathedral city situated about 100 km south of Santiago on the border with Portugal, is correspondingly mentioned alive for the last time on 18 June – in other words, only a few days after the bishop of Santiago was mentioned alive for the last time – and he allegedly also died from plague. According to the same analysis, this implies that the Black Death had reached Tuy at the very end of April. According to Ubieto Arteta, the Spanish historian, there can be no doubt that the Black Death had spread to Tuy from Santiago, because there is no alternative.[32] However, this is an argument that resolves one problem only to create another, namely the contemporaneity of two interdependent epidemiological

---

[32] Ubieto Arteta 1975: 60.

processes in cities situated at a distance of 100 km. Ubieto Arteta's view implies another instance of a metastatic leap by land. Metastatic leaps by land are not usual occurrences, but can be shown to have happened over middle-range distances several times along the road from Arles to Carcassonne via Narbonne, and again somewhere between Carcassonne and Bordeaux (see below); in several instances, the Black Death spread by middle-range metastatic leaps out of Florence and Pisa. In these cases, metastatic leaps by land can be seen to have taken place in some of the most densely populated areas of Europe along heavily trafficked roads, which was not the case with the areas and the roads between Santiago and Tuy. This can be seen also from the fact that plague otherwise spread quite slowly in this region: apparently, the Black Death broke out in the coastal town of Bayona, only 20 km north-west of Tuy, in October[33] and not in the first half of August, as would be expected if the Black Death had spread there out of Tuy after an outbreak starting c. 6–10 June (following contamination in the last days of April). This discussion has uncovered the fact that the alleged death of the bishop of Tuy from the Black Death on Ubieto Arteta's premise is quite problematic and that possible alternatives should be considered. There is, as it seems, only one serious alternative, namely that the Black Death was transported by ship from La Coruña around the coast to the border river Miño and, perhaps via Caminha or some other port along the estuary, further up to Tuy. A new bishop of Tuy was instituted on 18 August, and the process of replacement had taken exactly the same time as in the case of the bishop of Santiago.

One should note that death of bishops in the early phase of an outbreak of the Black Death would tend to be a feature of the early phase of the appearance of the epidemic in a region; as the ferocity of the epidemic became clear and the word spread, precautionary measures would often be employed to protect the bishop from contracting the disease. However, bishops had immensely important tasks to perform in such situations, and the precautions that could be taken would only tend to delay infection and death. This serves to explain why the bishop of Braga, 65 km south of Tuy, and the bishop of Lamego, about 75 km south-east of Braga or 80 km up the R. Douro from Oporto, died at the end of July the following year,[34] presumably at the end of the epidemics in their localities. The bishop of Viseu, about 55 km south of Lamego, died at the beginning of July, presumably in a somewhat earlier phase of the epidemic there. And, of course, bishops were elderly men with quite a high mortality in the best of times, and not all bishops who died during the time of the Black Death would have died from the epidemic. This may have been the case with the bishop of Badajoz on Spain's border with Portugal, roughly 200 km east of Lisboa, whose death on 25 May is difficult to fit into the spatio-temporal pattern of the spread of the Black Death in Iberia.

In the town of Coimbra, about 220 km south of Tuy, the outbreak of the Black Death was recognized on 29 September. Coimbra is situated about 40 km from the coast on the navigable lower stretch of the R. Mondego. Thus, the outbreaks in Tuy and Coimbra probably reflect that, in the summer and autumn, the Black Death was spreading quite widely in the northern half of the Kingdom of Portugal, and that

---

33 Portela Silva 1976: 279.
34 Ubieto Arteta 1975: 60.

metastatic leaps by ship along the coast and up the rivers played a pivotal part in the process of spread.

Contamination of Santiago by 20–27 April rules out the idea that arrival of the Black Death there could have had anything to do with the almost simultaneous outbreaks of the epidemic in south-eastern Spain. This raises an urgent and intriguing question: from where had the contagion come to Santiago? The outbreak in Santiago is so early that there appears to be only one real possibility with respect to origin. As will be argued more comprehensively below (Chapter 12), the amazingly early invasion of Santiago de Compostela should be seen in the light of the surprisingly early invasion of the city of Rouen in north-western France. In both cases, the contagion must have been transported by ships that had set sail from the city of Bordeaux at the end of March. The ship that sailed westwards along the north-western coast of Iberia probably carried the Black Death to La Coruña, a largish seaport from where pilgrims walked to Santiago. No doubt, pilgrims and refugees from the plague streamed to the vital commercial hub of Bordeaux where they could quite easily find shipping opportunities. Pilgrims went aboard ships headed for north-western Spain that could take them as close to Santiago de Compostela as possible: plague refugees entered ships heading for north-western France to get as far away from the Black Death as possible, and brought the contagion with them to Rouen. A ship sailing out of Bordeaux's harbour introduced the Black Death into England in the southern seaport of Melcombe (within present-day Weymouth), but probably put to sea about two weeks later. In Santiago, the Black Death established a new epicentre of spread from which its armies marched southwards and eastwards, eventually to meet armies marching northwards and westwards from other bridgeheads. The Black Death's conquest of the Iberian Peninsula was a brilliant feat of predatory epidemic strategy.

In what follows, the Black Death's Iberian campaign and conquest of the Peninsula will be outlined in quite general terms. The main pattern is clear: the Black Death used ship transport to arrive in important commercial seaports that constituted strategically vital bridgeheads for further expansion and conquest. While moving with particular vigour along the main roads between the main urban population centres, the Black Death continued to spread to all sides along secondary and tertiary lines of communication to local towns and into the countryside.

The early landings on the Spanish mainland in the commercial centres of Perpignan, Barcelona, Tarragona, and Valencia, earliest in Perpignan, shaped the first phase of the Black Death's Iberian campaign as it moved northwards and westwards out of its south-eastern bridgeheads.

Marching out of Perpignan the Black Death soon crossed the southern border with Spain and entered Ripoll(es).[35] As mentioned above, a study of wills in Gerona shows that Gerona was contaminated at a time that implies that it in all likelihood was conquered by epidemic forces coming from the north. These forces of the Black Death pressing on southwards and the forces moving northwards from Barcelona met somewhere south of Gerona and Vich. From Roussillon the Black Death also moved

---

[35] Trenchs Odena 1972–3: 103–15.

early across the Pyrenees into Spain in the west, the bishop of Seo de Urgel apparently dying in the Black Death some time around 1 May.[36] Clearly, south-eastern Spain was conquered in the spring and summer of 1348.

From Valencia the Black Death moved 115 km northwards to Teruel, where the king of Aragon stated that the epidemic raged on 20 July.[37] From Teruel forces of the Black Death sped in the direction of Madrid in the west and towards Calatayud and Zaragoza to the north. Quite likely, Madrid was invaded in the winter or early spring of 1349 by forces of the Black Death marching westwards along the main road from Teruel, while forces coming from Calatayud conquered much of the areas north of Madrid. Toledo, where the Black Death raged in full force in June and July,[38] and therefore quite likely had been contaminated in March or April, was probably also invaded by forces from Teruel, moving along the south-western main road into New Castile.

From Barcelona forces of the Black Death spread out in many directions, but would, as mentioned, on the way northwards meet forces from the early landing in Perpignan that had crossed Roussillon's southern border, then conquer Ripoll, Gerona and Vich and press on southwards. Forces marching westwards would be stopped shortly before reaching Cervera, when they reached areas that had already for some time been ravaged by forces that had marched northwards out of Tarragona towards Tarrega, about 60 km away. Forces from Tarragona moving along a road running north-westwards would then be approaching the important regional city of Lérida,[39] 85 km away (but 135 km west of Barcelona), while forces turning westwards along the road leading from Tarrega to Lérida would cover much of the areas west and north-west of Lérida.

No doubt, it was via the more direct and much shorter route through Lérida and not via Teruel that the Black Death arrived in the city of Zaragoza, about 130 km west of Lérida, where the king of Aragon and the archbishop were resident. In this important royal, religious and commercial centre, it broke out in the second half of September or, possibly, in the early days of October. It appears that the Black Death in Spain moved at quite a fast pace along these main communication lines, covering on average about 2 km a day.

From Zaragoza, the forces of the Black Death took off along main roads in several directions. One division of the Black Death's army corps marched north-westwards and, after having spread about 55 km, it reached Borja, where it was raging on 6 October;[40] about 20 km further down the road it soon reached the cathedral city of Tarazona.[41] From Tarazona it marched on westwards into Old Castile, where it reached the city of Soria at the end of the year.[42]

Shortly before arriving at Borja, another division of the Black Death's army moved off by another road that branched off northwards towards the Kingdom of Navarre, where it could have invaded Tudela,[43] about midway between Zaragoza and

---

36 Ubieto Arteta 1975: 52.
37 Ubieto Arteta 1975: 55–6; López de Meneses 1956: 304–5.
38 Ubieto Arteta 1975: 65–6.
39 Trenchs Odena 1974: 203–10.
40 Gautier-Dalché 1962: 66; Ubieto Arteta 1975: 58.
41 Trenchs Odena 1981: 201–3.
42 Ubieto Arteta 1975: 48; Sobrequés Callicó 1966: 88.
43 Trenchs Odena 1981: 204.

Pamplona, if the town had not already, as seems most likely, been conquered by forces that had crossed into the north-eastern corner of the kingdom either from Biarritz just north of the border with France or from San Sebastian just west of the border with Spain (see below).

From Zaragoza another division of the Black Death's army corps marched south-westwards and soon reached the town of Calatayud, where the epidemic broke out on 25 October;[44] from Calatayud it crossed into New Castile in the direction of Madrid at the turn of the year.

The cathedral city of Huesca was conquered by forces of the Black Death that did not march westwards out of Lérida to Zaragoza, but instead marched north-westwards out of Lérida directly towards Huesca, roughly 110 km away. In Huesca, the Black Death can be seen to have raged in full force from September to November,[45] but must be assumed to have started earlier and continued later. The Black Death had already ravaged the small town of Almudévar, about 20 km south of Huesca, by 27 September,[46] a fact that must be taken to reflect both that the contagion had rapidly been transferred from Huesca and that the epidemiological processes progressed faster in the small town of Almudévar than in the city of Huesca and therefore were observed at an earlier stage of development. Almudévar is situated on the road between Huesca and Zaragoza, but the distances involved and the timing of the outbreaks of the epidemics make it highly likely that Almudévar (and Huesca) was, as mentioned, infected by contagion coming directly via Lérida, and not via Lérida and Zaragoza. The conquest of the important regional ecclesiastical and commercial centre of Huesca heralded the Black Death's final assault on north-western Aragon. From Huesca forces of the Black Death moved also northwards into the mountainous Pyrenean region, and in December there was a plague-related burial in the monastery of San Juan de la Peña, about 50 km to the north, as the crow flies.[47]

The conquest of Huesca also meant that the Black Death approached the Kingdom of Navarre from the west in the direction of Sangüesa. However, the conquest of the Kingdom of Navarre appears to have been wholly or mainly carried out by the armies of the Black Death that originated in Marseilles and by metastatic leaps had moved round the Gulf of Lions to Montpellier (which belonged to the Kingdom of Aragon until 1349 when it was sold to King Philip IV of France) and Béziers, which were, as mentioned, probably contaminated as early as December 1347, while Carcassonne and Narbonne were probably contaminated around 1 January (see below). Roussillon was in all probability invaded from one of these French urban centres not later than 7 February, but quite likely as early as in January (see above), and contagion that was transported out of this town may also have played a part also in the Navarrese campaign, although this must be considered very uncertain. However, from Narbonne the Black Death moved by metastatic leaps rapidly north-westwards in the direction of the Atlantic coast along the main road to Bordeaux, where it arrived not later than late March. At the same time the Black Death moved more slowly into the surrounding regions, crossing into the Spanish areas on the western

44 Trenchs Odena 1981: 203; Ubieto Arteta 1975: 59.
45 Trenchs Odena 1981: 197–200; Ubieto Arteta 1975: 57.
46 Ubieto Arteta 1975: 57.
47 Ubieto Arteta 1975: 57.

slopes of the Pyrenees. In June it was raging in the district of Bigorre in the modern French département of Hautes Pyrénées, and at the end of the month it broke out in the town of Luz, quite close to the border with Spain. However, the Black Death first moved into the north-western corner of Navarre, which means that the contagion had been moved by sea transport either from Bordeaux to Biarritz or from Bordeaux to San Sebastian, and from one or both of these landings marched into the kingdom. In early July, the Black Death was raging in Santesteban, about 15–20 km from the borders with both France and Spain in the north-western corner of Navarre, or about 30 km south-east of San Sebastian and 40 km south of Biarritz. In fact, it had already reached such a violent epidemic intensity that the important iron-works there had to break off their production at this time.[48] Thus, the Black Death appears to have reached Navarre as early as the beginning of May, as it had time to move from the place of invasion by land to Santesteban and unleash its full murderous might by the end of June at the latest. This means that the armies of the Black Death marching into north-western Navarre from Biarritz or San Sebastian in early May would have had time to conquer the whole kingdom before forces moving all the way from Tarragona via Lérida and Zaragoza could cross into the kingdom from the south; although, as pointed out above, it cannot be entirely ruled out that the conquest of Tudela was accomplished by these forces. It also means that the conquest of the kingdom was evidently completed by October 1349.

From the north-western epicentre in Santiago the Black Death conquered large parts of northern Spain, Asturias and Léon Castile, outbreaks being recognized in Lugo in July, and raged in the surrounding districts until December; it arrived in Oviedo some time later, the bishop dying on 13 November, and in Léon not later than in October.[49] It cannot, of course, be ruled out that there were other landings of the Black Death along the northern seaboard. Oviedo could, for instance, have been infected from a landing in Gijon.

Some time in the final months of 1348 the northern and southern plague fronts met in the eastern lands of Old Castile and joined forces for the final and full conquest of the Peninsula.[50]

Individuals or small groups of relatives or friends may be extremely lucky and win the jackpot in national lotteries. During the onslaught of the Black Death the occasional town or village was passed by and, so to speak, won the jackpot in the lottery of life and death. The plain around the coastal town of Costellón, situated about 70 km north of the city of Valencia, appears to have won one of the jackpots of those times and was spared.[51] The Kingdom of Navarra was administratively divided into four regions called 'merindads'; in the 'merindads' of Pamplona and Sangüesa, 15 out of 212 local societies escaped unscathed (7 per cent). As could, perhaps, have been surmised, it was the small hamlets that were spared.[52] However, as time would show,

---

[48] Berthe 1984: 1/307–8 rejects the implications of the sources with respect to the time of invasion of the Kingdom of Navarre, because of mistaken assumptions concerning the origin of contagion and the route and pattern of spread but, according to the present epidemiological analysis, his sources are correct.
[49] Ubieto Arteta 1975: 48, 60, 63.
[50] Ubieto Arteta thinks that this took place in October: 1975: 48.
[51] Doñate Sebastia 1969: 27–43.
[52] Berthe 1984: 1/310.

some years later those communities that counted themselves lucky and assumed that God had intervened and spared them for their good deeds and fervent religious beliefs would learn dearly that, when plague eventually entered their communities, they would be visited with a vengeance.

Generalizing broadly, by the end of 1348, the first year of the Black Death's campaign in the Iberian Peninsula, it had succeeded in conquering most of the territories lying north, west and south of a line drawn slightly north-eastwards from Coimbra in Portugal to Soria in Old Castile, where the line bends sharply southwards and ends south of Valencia, where the Black Death appears not to have made significant progress for some unknown reason (much like what happened in Almería).[53] This suggests that the Black Death had spread into around 35 per cent of the Peninsula in 1348, but many communities within that area remained to be conquered. In 1349, especially after the onset of warmer weather in the spring, the Black Death continued to spread into the remaining regions. This means that it is inaccurate to refer to 1348 as *the* year of the Black Death in Spain, for in all likelihood, the extent of territorial spread was larger in 1349.[54] In less than two years, the Black Death conquered the Iberian Peninsula, around 600,000 sq. km and a sizeable part of Europe.

The grand strategy of the Black Death's Iberian campaign, which can explain the tremendous thrust and dynamics of the conquest, has also been disclosed. It has become clear that Iberia was invaded by five separate armies, which all originated in Marseilles, but only after they had taken new strategic positions for the invasion of Iberia:

(1) The earliest invasion of the mainland was carried out by forces spreading from Marseilles by land or sea transportation and via French south-western Mediterranean cities along the coast of the Gulf of Lions into Roussillon, where they landed in Perpignan, probably in January and not later than 7 February. These forces spread southwards by land and arrived, probably by ship, in Barcelona in February.
(2) A second army sailed from Marseilles to Mallorca, where it apparently went ashore as early as December 1347; this was the earliest invasion of Spanish (Aragonese) territory. From Mallorca these forces were transported to Tarragona, Valencia and Almería. The forces of Tarragona established the most efficient bridgehead for the great march inland, but their campaign was to some extent co-ordinated with forces coming from Barcelona and Valencia. The forces marching north-westwards out of Valencia moved with considerable pace and soon reached the city of Teruel from where these forces of the Black Death turned mainly westwards and south-westwards, marching along the main roads into the heart of New Castile in the direction of Madrid and Toledo, which were invaded some time in the first three or four months of 1349.
(3) The forces arriving in Almería constituted a separate third army, which for some reason did not succeed in making much headway until some time in the autumn, when they began a sustained campaign that in the following year resulted in the

---

[53] See Ubieto Arteta 1975: 47–8.
[54] It cannot be entirely ruled out that there were a few outbreaks in Navarre also in 1350. Berthe 1984: 1/309.

conquest of the Kingdom of Granada, Andalucia and the southern part of New Castile, where they eventually met forces that had marched the long way from Valencia via Teruel, Madrid and Toledo.

(4) An army corps of the Black Death that had advanced with forced marches from Marseilles to Bordeaux and arrived there as early as the end of March split up into several armies for participation in several important campaigns, two of them in Iberia. One army sailed by ship to La Coruña, from where it soon reached Santiago de Compostela and marched southwards into the Kingdom of Portugal, but by further sea transportation also made landings in seaports along the coast of Portugal and sailed up rivers.

(5) The fifth army also employed sea transportation, in this case either to Biarritz or San Sebastian (or both) from where it marched into the north-western corner of the Kingdom of Navarre, reaching Santesteban as early as May.

The Black Death's Iberian campaign showed the artful strategy and violent impetus and irresistible dynamics of its armies, which would be repeated across Europe until the whole continent was conquered in a few years' time.

11

Italy[1]

In the years between 1347 and 1350, and especially in 1348 and 1349, the Black Death wrought havoc on the Italian population. Agnolo di Tura's account of the Black Death in the city of Siena is one of the classic descriptions of its ravages in Italy (it also contains classical rhetorical elements):

> Father abandoned child, wife husband, one brother another; for this illness seemed to strike through the breath and sight. And so they died. And none could be found to bury the dead for money or friendship. Members of a household brought their dead to a ditch as best they could, without priest, without divine offices. Nor did the [death] bell sound. And in many places in Siena great pits were dug and piled deep with the multitude of dead [. . .]
>
> And I, Agnolo di Tura, called the Fat, buried my five children with my own hands. And there were also those who were so sparsely covered with earth that the dogs dragged them forth and devoured many bodies throughout the city.[2]

There was no Italian state in the Middle Ages (and long after). The concept of 'Italy' has mainly geographical/territorial and ethnic meanings and refers to the Italian Peninsula and the northern sub-Alpine and Alpine districts of the modern Italian state, and some other territories. The corresponding territory was divided into a great number of city states in northern and central Italy, the Kingdom of Naples covered southern Italy, and the Papal States were mainly situated in central Italy. In addition, coastal districts on the eastern side of the Adriatic comprising the towns of Spalato (Split) and Ragusa (Dubrovnik) belonged to Venice, the north-western coastline almost all the way to Nice on the present-day French Riviera belonged to Genoa, and there was also a papal territory around Avignon where at the time of the Black Death the popes were actually resident. On the eve of the Black Death, about 11

---

[1]   The only work taking seriously the history of the Black Death in Italy in demographic and epidemiological terms is the quite short account in Del Panta 1980: 111–16. On the introduction of the Black Death into Italy, see also above.
[2]   Cited after Bowsky 1964: 15.

million inhabitants[3] lived within an Italian territory of about 300,000 sq. km, which means that average population density was about 36 persons per sq. km.

In January 1348, the Black Death was poised to strike into mainland Italy from four bridgeheads: Reggio di Calabria, Genoa, Pisa and Venice. Italy's Adriatic coast could also easily be contaminated from Spalato and Ragusa. Southern Italy at the time, as today, was much less economically developed than northern Italy. Northern Italy was then the most advanced industrial and commercial part of Europe, perhaps even in the world; it was the cradle of modern capitalism as well as of the nascent Renaissance. Tuscany and some other parts of northern Italy were the most highly urbanized and most densely settled areas in Europe. While the degree of urbanization of Europe was, on average, 10–12 per cent, 25–30 per cent lived in urban centres in Tuscany. The northern bridgeheads in the important commercial cities of Genoa and Pisa and the famous commercial metropolis of Venice were all situated centrally in the great networks of trade that both bound Italian production centres and commercial centres together, but also linked up with foreign countries. These great networks of trade carried enormous amounts of finished goods for export, and, in the other direction, imported large amounts of raw materials and semi-finished goods for processing and finishing by the advanced Italian manufacturing industries.

The march of the Black Death's armies from Pisa into Tuscany's industrial heartland demonstrates the great importance of bustling commercial activities. After having broken out in Pisa in mid-January, the Black Death presented itself in Lucca in February and, in March, its mighty presence was recognized in the economic and political centre of Tuscany, the city of Florence itself, one of the few metropolises of the time with almost 100,000 inhabitants. According to the standard assumption with the usual addition for the slowing down of the epidemiological processes caused by cool winter weather (see above), Pisa and Lucca had been contaminated about eight weeks earlier, the metropolis of Florence about nine weeks earlier.

Again, the Black Death showed its ability to perform middle-range metastatic leaps along important commercial roads between large commercial and production centres in areas with great population density: the Black Death not only appeared in Florence in March, but also broke out in the cities of Bologna and Modena lying at twice as great a distance from Pisa as Florence.

The unevenness of the Black Death's ability to leap between important urban centres in densely populated areas is conspicuous: the Black Death broke out in the city of Siena in May but, as mentioned, in Bologna and Modena in March and in Perugia in April, all situated at a much greater distance from Florence than Siena. It is hard to explain why Modena, Bologna or Perugia should be attacked earlier than Siena in terms of communication lines and commercial, industrial or demographic factors. This suggests that the early contamination of Modena, Bologna and Perugia probably had to do with fortuitous circumstances with regard to transport of infected rat fleas with people or goods, and with the highly variable luck of infected rat fleas in finding new rat hosts when they were introduced into a new environment. The pattern of spread by metastatic leaps could also have been affected by the preferred

3   Belletini 1973: 497.

destinations of refugees from the Black Death, the movement of refugees from stricken areas affecting the probability that infected rat fleas were introduced into certain communities more than into others. We cannot today identify these streams of people on the run from the Black Death; such studies have, at least, not yet been produced, and the significance of this argument cannot therefore be assessed or considered.

The last great plague epidemic in Europe occurred in southern France as late as 1720–2. The very good source material produced by the far more advanced administrative organizations of the absolutist state shows an interesting sprinkling of places where only one or two plague deaths were registered.[4] This demonstrates the basic process of introduction of plague into new communities, that it was introduced by infected persons or by persons, infected or not, carrying infected fleas in their luggage or clothing. When infected persons were also passive carriers of one or more infected rat fleas, what happened further would depend entirely on whether or not the rat flea(s) succeeded in finding a rat host and unleashed the contagion in the local rat colonies. If not, the community would avoid the plague on this occasion, but the official local register would feature one plague fatality. In other places, this process of introduction led to the outbreak of plague, but the process of introduction was veiled by the high number of casualties.

From Genoa, the Black Death spread both into the northern Italian plains in the direction of the Alpine areas and also westwards, reaching Ventimiglia, close to the present-day French border, by April.

As shown in Table 2, most of northern and central Italy were engulfed by the Black Death by June. In the following months it spread into the valleys and mountain settlements of the Piedmont and other Alpine areas, breaking out in, e.g., Varese near Lago Maggiore in August. The conquest of the Piedmont commenced in October–November, and the outbreak in the city of Turin in the Piedmontese heartland is dated to 11 November.[5] In these Alpine or sub-Alpine areas the Black Death appears to have moved slowly but disastrously from locality to locality, finishing its grisly work only in 1350.[6] Probably it was halted by cold winter weather and resumed its spread in the spring.

The Black Death's spread in the economically far less developed southern and central Italy is less known exactly for this reason, but, for the same reason, it would spread more slowly. In May, the Black Death broke out in the city of Naples and in other places in the Kingdom of Naples. It appears not to have emerged in Rome before August. The reason for this is undoubtedly that Rome was not the religious centre of Christendom at the time. For some decades, the popes had been resident in Avignon. Rome no longer provided services to large numbers of visiting and resident ecclesiastical dignitaries and to multitudes of pilgrims; it had been reduced almost to a local town. This very centre of Catholic Christianity for so many centuries was not at the time crowded with pilgrims from stricken places. This temporary change in Rome's historical role meant that it was not hit early by the Black Death, like Mecca or Santiago de Compostela, and the arrival was instead postponed by some months.

---

4   See the tables rendered by Biraben 1975: 256–79.
5   Comba 1977: 87.
6   Comba 1977: 76, 87; Nada Patrone and Naso 1981: 34.

Table 2. Chronology of the spread of the Black Death in Italy, time of recognized outbreak[a]

Locality	Month, beginning	Year
Messina	end September	1347
Sicily	October	1347
Reggio Calabria	December	1347
Sardinia	December	1347
Corsica	December	1347
Elba	December	1347
Genoa	end December	1347
Pisa	January	1348
Venice	end January	
Lucca	February	
Florence	March	
Bologna	March	
Modena	March	
Pistoia	March–April	
Perugia	April	
Padua	April	
Ventimiglia	April	
Orvieto	end April–May	
Siena	May	
Ancona	May	
Rimini	May	
Naples	May	
Kingd. of Naples	May	
Verona	end May	
Faenza	June	
Cesena	June	
Parma	June	
Reggio Emilia	June	
Trent (Trento)	June	
Piacenza	July	
Ferrara	July	
Friuli	August	
Rome	August (?)	
Varese	August	
Piedmont	Oct.–Nov.	1348–50

[a]   Table 2 is compiled by Del Panta 1980: 112, supplemented with some additional pieces of information on the whereabouts of the Black Death: on Pistoia from Chiapelli 1887: 3–5; on the Piedmont from Comba 1977: 87, cf. map on p. 76; and from Nada Patrone and Naso 1981: 34.

   Information that shows that, e.g., Prato in Tuscany had suffered grave losses by July cannot be introduced in the table, because the information is too inaccurate to be used for retrospective estimates of the beginning of the outbreak or the time of contamination. See Fiumi 1968: 84–5. About Milan, see below.

It is more difficult to pin down the end of the Black Death because, for obvious reasons, chroniclers and authors of related sources were far more interested in and, therefore, more informative about the beginning of the epidemic than about its end. In the places that were hit first, in the autumn of 1347, like Sicily and Sardinia, the Black Death petered out in the early spring of the following year. In areas that were attacked in the winter or the early spring of 1348, such as Florence, Siena, Orvieto and Padua, the epidemic appears to have ended in September or October. However, in the populous Italian country districts many small towns and numerous localities are mentioned as being visited by the Black Death also in 1349 and even in 1350.[7] Valletidone near Piacenza escaped until 1350. Late outbreaks appear to have been most frequent in the Piedmont and other Alpine or sub-Alpine districts.

This lingering circulation of contagion in northern Italy meant that areas or towns or cities that miraculously, as it seemed to contemporaries, had escaped the spread of the Black Death, were eventually visited. Actually, the city of Milan was infected, but appears to have avoided a major outbreak, quite probably by rapid implementation of severe preventive measures. First, the gates to the city were very strictly guarded and only few travellers let in. Nonetheless, according to the well-known contemporary Sienese chronicler Agnolo di Turo, the Black Death managed to penetrate into the city, but only three families died because the authorities immediately walled up the doors and windows of the houses in which they lived in order to isolate them as effectively as possible.[8] This firm and rapid response may, of course, have prevented the Black Death from developing from an incipient endemic phase into the epidemic phase. One would like to know more about the circumstances, where the houses were situated, the environments, and so on. Lorenzo Del Panta, the Italian historical demographer, appears to hold the opinion that Milan escaped entirely, or it could be that he considers the episode of no consequence. However, in the history of the spread of the Black Death it is of significance that the Black Death actually succeeded in getting into Milan, although it did not manage to break out of the isolation imposed on the houses.

Although Italy is less than half the size of the Iberian Peninsula, its population was much larger, the population density three times higher. This may contribute to explain why the Black Death took more time to blanket the Italian Peninsula than the Iberian Peninsula. The numbers of settlements, villages, towns and cities, and the corresponding numbers of rat colonies that could be infected and go through the quite time-consuming epidemiological processes that characterize plague, were much larger: high population density facilitates spread but prolongs the epidemiological processes and expands the time horizon of the epidemic.

The Black Death's conquest of northern Italy paved the way for invasions of Austria and Switzerland along the important communication lines for trade and travel that led across the mountain passes, and into southern France from the plague front that moved westwards from Genoa into the Riviera.

---

[7] Del Panta 1980: 114.
[8] *Cronaca senese* 1934: 553. See also Sticker 1908: 51–2; D'Irsay 1927: 170. In his list of datable outbreaks in Europe, Biraben enters Milan as infected in 1350, but his source is not indicated. Biraben 1975: 76.

12

France[1]

France was Europe's great country and mighty power in the Middle Ages. On the eve of the Black Death, France contained 16–20 million inhabitants,[2] by far the largest population of any European country, e.g., about three times the population of England and Wales. This population inhabited a territory of about 425,000 sq. km,[3] about 75,000 sq. km smaller than today. The average population density was 37–47 persons per sq. km, possibly the highest in Europe.

However, France was politically and administratively fragmented, and dukes and counts and local assemblies of grandees exerted considerable political powers. The English king held a large territory in south-western France in homage of the French king, the Duchy of Guyenne, which also comprised Gascony and the large city and seaport of Bordeaux. At the time of the Black Death, the Hundred Years War had broken out because of conflicting views on the political status of these areas. Even the pope enjoyed possession of French territory, namely Avignon and surrounding districts, situated about 90 km north-west of Marseilles, where at the time of the Black Death, the popes had actually been resident for some decades, and not in Rome.

The Black Death's very early invasion of the city of Marseilles, where the outbreak was recognized 1 November 1347 (see above), had important consequences for its pattern of spread in space and time in France. It meant that contagion had been introduced into the commercial hub of south-eastern Mediterranean France in the second week of September. The pattern of spread was also affected by the early epicentre established in Genoa in December, and soon the Black Death spread westwards along the coast of the Gulf of Genoa. In April, it broke out in the town of Ventimiglia, close to France's present-day border (see above), and shortly afterwards, this army of epidemic death joined the forces of the Black Death that had moved eastwards from Marseilles. This may have taken place in May in the town of Grasse, about 15 km north of Cannes on the Riviera, or in the vicinity. The joint armies of the Black Death formed a plague front that moved northwards in a sharply zigzag-shaped but contin-

[1]   Information on the spread of the Black Death in France will be found in Biraben 1975: 73–83; also useful is Dubois 1988b: 314–21. Dubois is indebted to Biraben but not entirely dependent on him.
[2]   Dubois 1988a: 262; Le Roy Ladurie 1988: 515.
[3]   Dubois 1988a: 261; Le Roy Ladurie 1988: 514.

uous broad movement covering the whole of south-eastern France. In this process of epidemic advance, the Black Death in a characteristic fashion moved relatively quickly to central urban commercial centres from which it radiated into the hinterlands, eventually to blanket the countryside almost completely.

In the discussion of the Black Death's pace and pattern of spread in southern France we must take into consideration Dubois' correct observation on the seasonal pattern of the Black Death's spread in France: 'usually it was stopped or slowed down by the winter'.[4] In the case of southern France, the term winter will be defined as the months November–February. In relation to plague developments in this season in this region, some time must be added to the standard assumption on the time lag from the introduction of contagion to the epidemic presence as recognized by chroniclers; under the circumstances, reasonable additions appear to be roughly eight weeks instead of the usual seven weeks in the case of cities, and seven weeks instead of the usual six weeks in the case of sizeable towns.[5]

From Marseilles, the Black Death moved at quite a brisk pace northwards. Its outbreak was recognized in the largish town of Aix-en-Provence, 30 km to the north, around 1 December (see above), and, in early January, in the papal city of Avignon and in the large town of Arles, both situated at a distance of about 75 km from Aix.[6] The spread of plague contagion was hastened by great population density, a high degree of urbanization with several largish cities and numerous towns, and high traffic density and movement of people and goods along roads and tracks. This implies that plague contagion was being disseminated more widely and rapidly than reflected in the time-pattern of the recognized outbreaks, because, after the arrival of contagion, the epidemiological processes developed more slowly, according to the expanded standard assumption for the winter season. Thus, Aix was probably infected in early October, Avignon and Arles in the second week of November.

The Black Death wrought havoc on Avignon's inhabitants. Pope Clement VI early took on an early active role in organizing religious processions aimed at mitigating the ferocity of the epidemic onslaught by reducing the Lord's anger over their sins, but the processions had no noticeable effect. This opened his mind to the irreligious idea of epidemic causation that the large assemblies of people taking part in the processions rather helped to spread the plague. Pope Clement consulted his personal physician, Gui de Chauliac, who has left us one of the best contemporary descriptions of the Black Death's clinical symptoms and epidemiological characteristics. As a scholarly trained physician he was, of course, a firm believer in the Hippocratic epidemiological theory of miasma (see above). Accordingly, he advised Pope Clement to withdraw to his chamber and not see anyone. The pope spent day and night sheltering between two large fires; the idea was that the fires would destroy pestilen-

---

[4] Dubois 1988b: 316. My translation from French.
[5] Cf. above, pp. 18, 58–60.
[6] In the decades before the Black Death, Arles had about 2,000 registered households and Aix 1,500. Baratier 1961: 65. According to the Italian household structure that has been established as a standard assumption below (see also Baratier 1961: 59), the average urban household size is assumed to be around 4.0 persons, with underregistration estimated at 7.5 per cent. Marseilles had about 15,000 inhabitants. Baratier 1961: 66–7.

tial miasma in the air and prevent infection. The pope also left the city for some time.[7]

In short, Pope Clement behaved as though he did not believe that epidemic disease, in this case the Black Death, was an expression of the Lord's wrath at the abominable sins of his human subjects, but was due to miasma that could be destroyed by fire, and that to go away was not an attempt to avoid God's will. This reflects a tendency towards rational understanding and rational behaviour that later would give rise to anti-epidemic organizations that could muster effective counter-measures against an invisible enemy. It also meant that Pope Clement could reject the popular notions that led to persecution of Jews: (1) the Lord punished the Christians with the Black Death for permitting persons who did not worship him and accept the divinity of Christ to live among them, especially Jews who had taken the initiative to have Christ murdered; (2) the Black Death was caused by poison that Jews had put into the drinking water of Christians because they hated Christians, and so on.

Arles and Avignon were communication nexuses where road systems coming from Languedoc and Provence linked up and connected people and goods with roads running up the Rhône valley and into north-eastern France. At the end of April, the presence of the Black Death was recognized in the city of Lyons,[8] some 200 km north of Avignon, and some 300 km north of the epicentre in Marseilles. Because of the quite chilly season in the preceding months it is likely that plague contagion had been introduced about 7–8 weeks earlier, depending on the particular prevailing weather. One of the exceedingly few surviving parish registers relating to the time of the Black Death is from Lyons, namely the parish of St-Nizier.[9] Unfortunately, it is not complete, evidently because the priest who kept it died from the plague. This register shows an abrupt increase in funerals in May, more specifically a slight increase in the first week of May when the first funeral of a plague victim in the parish is registered on 2 May, and a dramatic increase from the second week.[10] Plague is very distinctly a household disease in the sense that if one member of a household contracted plague from a source of contagion within the house, most members of a household would be likely to be affected. This is because human plague cases normally reflect plague in the house rat colony/colonies in human housing and the release of their infective fleas into the rooms of human habitation when the rats had died off to a degree that made it hard for these fleas to find new rat hosts (see above). This process is easily observed in relation to the first plague cases in the parish of St-Nizier, where the funeral of Stephan Occerius on 2 May was followed by the funeral of his wife on 7 May and one Peter Occerius, probably their son, on 8 May.

In view of the fact that the incubation period and the period of illness taken together lasted, on average, eight days, and that a couple of days would quite likely elapse before the deceased was interred, the time of the first plague funeral indicates

---

[7]   Ziegler 1970: 66–7.
[8]   Dubois 1988b: 315.
[9]   At the time, there was no obligation for parish priests to keep parish registers. The few parochial priests who, nonetheless, did so, acted on a personal initiative and for the purpose of acquiring an overview of their incomes from priestly services, i.e., these registers were not really parish registers but the priests' private account books. Levron 1959: 55. After their death or transfer to another ecclesiastical position none had any interest in preserving them. See more about this in relation to the contemporary parish registers of Givry.
[10] *Inventaire du Trésor de St-Nizier*, introduction by the editor, Guige 1899: xii, xiv, xvii; Drivon 1912: 865–7.

that the endemic phase, when the first persons in this parish was infected, started c. 22 April, and that the first houses in the parish was contaminated about 10–14 days earlier, i.e., around 10 April. Unfortunately, we do not know where in Lyons the plague was first introduced, nor the process of spread that lead to the contamination of St-Nizier. Very likely, Lyons was contaminated several weeks earlier, as indicated by the time the outbreak was recognized.

Lyons was an important industrial and commercial centre and would, therefore, tend to attract epidemic disease. Some illustrations of the Black Death's pace of spread could be useful, and some concrete notions can be formed on the basis of comparison of time of outbreaks and distances. However, it is necessary to adjust for the slowdown in the epidemiological processes according to the assumptions above on the effects of winter weather. As measured in the dating of the recognized outbreaks, the Black Death appears to have taken roughly 170 days to cover the about 300 km from Marseilles northwards to Lyons, i.e., it would have proceeded at an average daily pace of c. 1.75 km. Subtraction of two weeks in order to compensate for the prolongation of the epidemiological processes caused by winter temperatures produces an adjusted average daily pace of c. 2 km. Interestingly, when the same seasonal adjustment is made, this is exactly the same pace that can be estimated for the 105 km from Marseilles to Avignon, which was covered in about 65 days. However, the 30 km from Marseilles to Aix were covered in as many days, i.e., at an average daily pace of 1 km. It is difficult to discern any structural reason for the much slower pace to the large town of Aix than to Arles or Avignon, most of the difference being therefore probably caused by fortuitous circumstances. These data suggest that the Black Death moved along heavily trafficked main roads in densely settled areas at an average pace of around 2 km a day. The pace along secondary and tertiary lines of communication between local towns and in the countryside was much slower. While the Black Death broke out in Lyons, about 200 km north of Avignon, in April, it did not break out in Alés, 65 km north-west of Avignon, until July, in other words after having covered the distance at an average daily pace of roughly 0.7 km.

The Black Death did not only march northwards up the Rhône valley but also moved sideways into the surrounding areas. At the beginning of May, it broke out in the small town of Die,[11] situated about 90 km north of Avignon and 50 km further into the French countryside east of the R. Rhône. Die is situated on the R. Drôme, but since this river is not navigable movement of goods and people must go by land. The Black Death broke out in Die five months after the outbreak in Avignon, meaning that the roughly 140 km from Avignon had been covered at an average daily pace of 1.15 km. Die lies at an altitude of 425 metres, and cool winter weather will last two–three weeks longer than down in the Rhône valley. The contagion could have arrived earlier, and the transport have moved at a faster pace than indicated by the dates of the outbreaks alone.

Die stands at an important route of trade and travel into the French alpine areas that border on the Piedmont. Mountain areas were characterized by a clear tendency to economic specialization in animal husbandry based on extensive use of highland grasslands. This economic specialization presupposed the existence of trade lines that

[11] Biraben 1975: 74.

could handle with regularity the export of excess production of meat, butter, hides, wool and suchlike, and the bringing in to the mountain settlements of necessary products of which there were local deficits, mainly grain and salt. The more special-ized the system of husbandry, the more intensive would the exchange of products and the commercial interaction have to be. Peripheral areas had typically more lively commercial contacts than the anciently settled, and more centrally located, communi-ties on fertile agricultural lands that would be able to meet more of their various needs locally.

At the time, the County of Savoy included the two present-day French départments of Lower and Upper Savoy, large parts of the central and northern areas of the modern Italian province of the Piedmont and the modern province of Valle d'Osta in north-western Italy, and the westernmost districts of the Swiss French-speaking canton of Valais bordering the modern French Savoyard départements. This composite feudal territory was attacked by the Black Death from two or three sides. The mountain valley of Maurienne in the Savoy, an area bordering the Italian Alpine region of the Piedmont, was probably invaded by the Black Death in the first half of April 1348, because the epidemic had caused a considerable diminution of the popu-lation by 19 June. It appears to have reached Upper Maurienne quite late in the year.[12] The Black Death must have come from the west, i.e., from the Rhône valley. Although our knowledge on the temporal pattern of the Black Death's spread across the Piedmont is frustratingly small, the northern parts of the Piedmont apparently were invaded from the original Italian epicentre of contamination and spread in Genoa later than the outbreak in Maurienne. The distance between the Rhône valley and Maurienne is almost 150 km as the crow flies, but considerably farther on the ground. On the other hand, the R. Isère is a large tributary to the R. Rhône that flows south-eastwards through Lower Savoy and across Dauphiné before it meets the Rhône north of Valence (see Map 6). The Isère is navigable for 150 km upstream from the Rhône, and a little way north of Montmélian in south-western Lower Savoy the large tributary R. Arc flows into it after having traversed Maurienne. These geographical facts may serve to explain why the Black Death could reach the Maurienne in the first half of April, roughly at the same time that it reached Die, although the area was situated both farther north and farther inland than Die. Trans-port by boat could have taken place as a metastatic leap, e.g., to Grenoble, or even farther upstream. Some of the forces of the Black Death that entered the Savoy marched north-eastwards into Upper Savoy where, for instance, Ugine was ravaged.[13] Probably the westernmost areas of the canton of Valais were invaded by these forces of the Black Death as they continued to move eastwards. However, it cannot be excluded that the forces of the Black Death that had marched out of Lyons north-eastwards towards Geneva and Lausanne, where they turned southwards, can have reached these westernmost parts of Valais at about the same time and have conquered some of these areas.

Movement westwards out of the Rhône valley was much slower; the Black Death

12 Gelting 1991: 21–2.
13 Demotz 1975: 93–5.

did not break out, e.g., on the plains of Forez until July–August,[14] despite being situated at a considerably shorter distance from the R. Rhône than Maurienne.

From Marseilles, the Black Death moved also westwards and, then, south-westwards along the coast of the Gulf of Lions in the direction of the Spanish border at Roussillon. Interestingly, the main thrust of spread appears to have occurred by a series of middle-range metastatic leaps starting in the small city of Arles where the epidemic presence of the Black Death was, as mentioned, recognized at the beginning of January,[15] via the large cities of Montpellier and Béziers to the smallish town of Carcassonne, roughly 270 km away, where, in all three cases, the presence of the Black Death was recognized as early as February. In the large city of Narbonne, between Béziers and Carcassonne, the outbreak was recognized around 1 March.[16] According to the seasonally adjusted standard assumption, Arles was contaminated in the second week of November, while the dating of the recognized outbreaks in Montpellier and Béziers indicates that they were contaminated in the first half of December, and not later than around mid-December. Both Narbonne and Carcassonne were probably contaminated around 1 January when we pay heed to both the epidemiological structural difference owing to size and the effects of winter climate. Although the sailing season did not really include these months because of fear of winter storms, the early infection of Mallorca shows that desperate people fleeing from the ravages of the Black Death dared to take to sea in order to escape, and, thus, may have caused metastatic spread by ship. What happened next points, as we shall see, to the importance of pilgrims moving along the roads.

Thus, the Black Death had entered Carcassonne with a metastatic leap around 1 January, and was now moving along the important commercial road that led from the seaport city of Narbonne on the Mediterranean to the great seaport city of Bordeaux on southern France's Atlantic coast (which, as mentioned, at the time was in the possession of the king of England as part of the Duchy of Guyenne). Bordeaux is estimated to have had at least 30,000 inhabitants on the eve of the Black Death.[17] The time of the outbreak in Bordeaux is both problematic and important, and will be subject to some quite lengthy discussion. There is no usable information provided by chroniclers or documentary sources.[18] The only way to determine an approximate dating of the Black Death's arrival in Bordeaux is to use the time of outbreaks elsewhere owing to importation of contagion from Bordeaux as bases for a process of retrospective epidemiological analysis. There are three such outbreaks that can serve as bases for this analysis, namely the outbreaks in Santiago de Compostela in north-western Spain, in the city of Rouen in north-western France and in the town of Weymouth in southern England. As can readily be seen, these outbreaks represent three very important metastatic leaps by sea leading to the establishment of new northern plague fronts in the Iberian Peninsula and in France, and introducing the

---

[14] Neveux 1975: 43.

[15] Biraben 1975: 74.

[16] Guilleré 1984: 18, 20–1; Biraben 1975: 74. The information on the size of urban centres is taken from Higounet-Nadal 1988: 303–4.

[17] Higounet-Nadal 1988: 304.

[18] The datings given by Dubois 1988b: 315, and by Biraben 1975: 74, 97, namely June/July, are untenable.

Black Death into England, events that greatly hastened the spread of the Black Death and the pace of its conquest of Europe.

The Norman chronicle *Normanniae nova Chronica* contains a notice to the effect that the plague had broken out in the countryside around Rouen and in the city of Rouen around the Feast of St John the Baptist, i.e., around 24 June.[19] According to the epidemiological standard assumption, an outbreak on 24 June implies that this large city was probably contaminated around 7 May. However, in this case, the contamination occurred probably somewhat earlier, because it is stated that the plague broke out in the surrounding countryside at the same time as in the city. This does not appear likely because plague in the countryside must have originated in the city, and because the reference to the countryside must be assumed to refer to a number of local outbreaks that constituted an epidemic, not to outbreaks in one or two villages. These considerations make it likely that the epidemic in the countryside at the time had been spreading in the form of frightening severe outbreaks for at least a couple of weeks. The greater transparency and observability of the epidemic developments in the countryside than in the big city meant that they caught the attention of contemporaries at an earlier stage of development. The chronicler has unwittingly provided a piece of information indicating that the epidemiological processes in this large city took longer than presumed by the standard assumption, before the Black Death's presence became obvious and was recognized by the chronicle-writing social élites. In other words, the contemporaneity of recognition conceals a significant difference in the pace of epidemiological events leading to recognition in the great city and in the countryside respectively, and that, in this case, a couple of weeks should be added to the period of time contained in the standard assumption. The outcome of this discussion is, then, that the Black Death more likely reached Rouen at the end of April.

Ship transportation in those times was dependent on the vicissitudes of wind and weather, and the time taken to cover the same distance varied greatly. At the time, sailing ships were poorly developed to sail against the wind and brave inclement or foul weather. Ships following the coastline in order to avoid the dangers of sailing in open sea would usually not sail at night to avoid the dangers caused by darkness. Assuming a normal incidence of inclement weather and adverse winds, an average pace at sea of 40 km per day over long distances seems reasonable and can be substantiated.[20] This means that a ship from Bordeaux with plague on board that arrived in

---

[19] Fournée 1978: 6; Jouet 1972: 267. The sources on the arrival of plague in Rouen is discussed below and related to the outbreak in Paris according to the same retrospective methodological approach.

[20] It appears that little research has so far been carried out on the average or usual pace of sailing of commercial ships in the Middle Ages. A couple of scholars have presented some data relating to Norway and Hanseatic trading with Norway, and the present author can add some data from the end of the Late Middle Ages.

In the century preceding the Black Death, the usual duration of the voyage of about 550 km from Bergen further northwards to Nidaros (Trondheim) by Norwegian ships was two weeks, corresponding to an average daily rate of c. 40 km. At the beginning of the fourteenth century, it is said that the usual time needed by a (commercial) ship to sail the distance of roughly 1,100 km between Nidaros and Tønsberg in the inner Oslo fjord area was a month, which indicates a normal or average pace of sailing of 37 km a day. Steen 1934: 227.

In 1485, the East German (Wendish) Hanseatic towns and cities proposed to the merchants in Lübeck who traded with Bergen that their ships should sail in convoy and that they should assemble on 24 June outside Lübeck in order to arrive in Bergen one month later. Consequently, they expected that the average daily pace of sailing would be roughly 37 km. Because this indication of duration appears to reflect a general-

Rouen, roughly 1,200 km away, at the end of April would have set sail at the end of March.

The bishop of Santiago de Compostela died from the Black Death c. 22 June, and it has been argued above that this reflects that Santiago was contaminated 20–27 April. On the same assumptions as to the usual pace of sailing, a ship would take about 25 days to sail the roughly 1,000 km from Bordeaux to La Coruña. Adding a couple of days for pilgrims to walk the 50 km from La Coruña to Santiago, this indicates that, also in this case, the contaminated ship left Bordeaux at the very end of March. Under the circumstances, and in view of the rough-hewn assumptions upon which the analysis is based, the retrospective discussions of the outbreaks in Rouen and Santiago de Compostela both indicate that the Black Death was present, at least in Bordeaux's harbour area, at the end of March at the latest.

The conclusion that the Black Death was present in Bordeaux's harbour area at the end of March has consequences for the discussion of the spread of the Black Death along the road from Narbonne to Bordeaux. It has been shown above that the Black Death probably arrived in Carcassonne c. 1 January. In order to cover the c. 320 km from Carcassonne to Bordeaux as a plague front within the indicated time span, the Black Death would have to spread by an average daily pace of 3.5 km, which exceeds all certain registrations of pace at a distance, and seems particularly unlikely in winter. Instead, we will have to assume that the series of metastatic middle-range leaps that have been identified on the stretch from Arles to Carcassonne included at least one additional leap somewhere along this road. In the large city of Toulouse, 90 km north-west of Carcassonne, and in the small city of Monteauban, 140 km down the road, the presence of the Black Death was recognized at the end of April; and in the town of Agen, 70 km farther down the road, only a few days later, at the very beginning of May. All these outbreaks should be seen in the light that their respective urban centres were contaminated in cool winter weather that caused a pronounced slowdown of the epidemiological developments. The fact that the outbreaks were recognized almost at the same time in these three urban centres indicates that plague contagion had been widely distributed along this road in metastatic leaps in cool winter weather that produce a marked contemporaneity of recognized outbreaks,

ized notion of the usual time required for Hanseatic merchant ships to cover the distance of roughly 1,100 km from Lübeck to Bergen, it must be given more weight than the few, and, perhaps, unrepresentative reflections in the extant sources of the duration of voyages that also comprise instances of substantially shorter and longer durations, which are mentioned precisely because they are unusual. All the three individually known durations of this voyage from the second half of the fifteenth century, one in 1455 and two in 1483, lasted much longer, namely eight weeks.

In the first half of the sixteenth century, the usual or normal average daily rate for ships sailing from Lübeck to Bergen still appears to have been 40 km; although it is usually assumed that ships at the time tended to be more developed than two centuries earlier, the roughly 1,100 km were usually covered in three to four weeks. Bruns 1900: page C.

In 1529, Crown Prince Christian (III) sailed the about 540 km along the sea lanes from Copenhagen to Oslo with a following of Danish councillors of state. After having waited for suitable wind and weather for some time, they put out of the harbour of Copenhagen on 30 June and called at the harbour of Oslo on 13 July; thus, the average daily rate was slightly below 40 km. *Diplomatarium Norvegicum* XI, No. 530; *Diplomatarium Norvegicum* X, No. 580; *Norske Regnskaber og Jordebøger*, Vol. 4, p. 351. They put out of the harbour of Oslo on 8 September and called at the harbour of Varberg, about 360 km farther south, nine days later, having sailed at about the same average daily rate. *Diplomatarium Norvegicum* VIII, No. 607; *Diplomatarium Norvegicum* XI, No. IX, No. 644.

much as the metastatic leaps from Arles to Carcassonne produced recognized contemporaneous outbreaks in February over the long distance from Montpellier via Béziers to Carcassonne.

In this perspective, it does not seem unlikely or far-fetched that Bordeaux was also involved in this process, and could have been contaminated at the end of March, the distance from Carcassonne to Bordeaux being only about 50 km longer than the distance from Arles to Carcassonne that was covered in about two months. This dating can also be co-ordinated with a recognized outbreak in June in this large city, especially, if we, like Biraben,[21] assume that the contagion was introduced first into the harbour area by goods or pilgrims, and that it would take some time before contagion was spread from this area into the city itself.

Crowds of pilgrims, awed and inspired by the ravages of the Black Death, and hoping fervently that they could mollify the Good Lord and do their suffering fellow men good by going to Santiago de Compostela could, of course, easily have occasioned metastatic leaps by land along the roads leading from Arles to Bordeaux. In Bordeaux, they would seek shipping opportunities for Santiago. Other crowds of people gathering in Bordeaux's harbour area looking for the chance to sail away may simply have been refugees from the horrors of the Black Death. Before these people, pilgrims or refugees, had entered ships carrying the Black Death in their few belongings, they could have contaminated the quarters around the harbour, and, thus, unwittingly, have made it easier for the Black Death to enter ships headed for La Coruña (in northern Spain from where the pilgrims would walk to Santiago on foot), Rouen, or Weymouth, or other destinations. Moreover, large quantities of goods were exported from Bordeaux, which in turn means that large quantities of goods were transported to the city's harbour area, making infection by goods or people the more likely.

This scenario outlines a pattern of events that may serve to explain several important developments in the history of the Black Death, namely the metastatic leaps to Santiago de Compostela, Rouen and Weymouth that significantly hastened the Black Death's conquest of Europe. One should keep in mind that the three metastatic leaps by ship are empirical facts independent of the theory of a common origin in Bordeaux that has been argued here. It is also certain that they must have taken place considerably earlier than formerly recognized. This means that it is also certain that the city of Bordeaux must have been contaminated significantly earlier than assumed until now.[22]

The Black Death had now covered the whole of south-western France from the Mediterranean to the Atlantic coast in a band that was at least 200 km in territorial depth and could move on northwards along a front that, despite a sharp zigzag-shape, was continuous from the Mediterranean coast to the Atlantic coast.

---

[21] Biraben 1975: 97.

[22] Both Dubois and Biraben hold in effect that the Black Death broke out at the same time or earlier in Rouen and Weymouth (Melcombe) than in Bordeaux, although they also hold that Rouen and Weymouth were contaminated by ships from Bordeaux. Dubois 1988b: 315; Biraben 1975: 74. Biraben appears to have recognized the contradiction on pp. 96–7 and attempts to resolve it by hypothesizing that plague contagion could have been present in Bordeaux's harbour area at the beginning of June, and have moved into the city itself in July. However, this will not do, because it only allows time for transport by a ship that must have been quite lucky with wind and weather, especially in relation to Rouen, but allows no time for the epidemiological processes from the time of contamination to the time of a recognized outbreak, which add another six and seven weeks in the cases of Weymouth and Rouen, respectively. There are also other objections.

*

The Black Death also sent its armies into the remaining parts of France from several other quarters. It continued to move up the Rhône valley and beyond. One should note that, at the time, Lyons was situated on the border with the County of Savoy,[23] which was part of a loosely organized constellations of principalities and countries pompously called the Holy Roman Empire of the German Nation (see below), which was also the case with the Duchy of Burgundy, which was not formally incorporated into France until 1482. Thus, when the Black Death moved on northwards and north-eastwards from Lyons it remained within the present-day borders of France but, at the time, it entered the system of principalities joined under the auspices of the German emperor.

Having entered the Savoy, the Black Death immediately started to penetrate deep into the Savoyan region, while it also marched north-eastwards towards Geneva and Lausanne, from where it turned southwards eventually to approach the westernmost cantons of present-day Switzerland, which at the time belonged to the County of Savoy. These movements will be discussed below.

In mid-July, the Black Death broke out in Givry, a small town situated 12 km west of the city of Chalon (on the R. Saône) in Burgundy, about 120 km north of Lyons. The vicar of Givry at the time has blessed research on the Black Death with a set of almost complete parish registers that record funerals and marriages from 1334 throughout the period of the Black Death, but there are lacunae for a few years in the preceding 13–14 years.[24] At the time, parish priests were not obliged to keep parish registers, the few extant specimens being really the priests' private account books where they recorded the income from priestly services. In the funeral register of Givry the names of the deceased are followed by the price paid per family and the payment. However, because the parish priest has also entered the names of the poor people who could not afford to pay anything, it can be considered a real parish register.[25]

According to these funeral registers, in the years 1334–41 and 1345–7, on average, 23 people a year died in this small urban community, or some two funerals a month. In the period of the Black Death, according to the burial register, 626 persons were interred in the cemetery. This means that in the four months of the epidemic, fifteen times more persons were entered in the burial register than the annual average for the preceding eleven years, and 2.5 times more persons than in these eleven years taken together (256).

The beginning of the Black Death is reflected in the register by a small sprinkling of burials beginning on 17 July and adding up to a total of nine interments in the last fifteen days of July. This sprinkling of cases reflects clearly the endemic phase and indicates that the contagion was introduced into Givry almost four weeks earlier,[26]

---

[23] The continental use of the term county must not be confused with the English use of the word. It has been suggested that the corresponding European title of count is more related to the English title of earl, in that case a continental county or countship would tend to correspond to the English term earldom.

[24] Gras 1939: 295–308. The funeral register breaks off at the end of November 1348, but at that time the epidemic is clearly subsiding rapidly and approaching its end.

[25] Levron 1959: 55.

[26] Epizootic phase 10–14 days + 3 days of starvation before the rat fleas begin to attack human beings + 3–5 days of incubation period + 3–5 days of course of mortal illness. About 23 days after the introduction of

under ordinary epidemiological circumstances around 23 June (probably passed on from Chalon). If we assume that the outbreak in Lyons was recognized at the end of April and in Givry around 1 August, this difference in time indicates that the Black Death took about 95 days to cover the c. 110 km to Givry. This shows within wide margins of error a sudden, sharp diminution of the average pace of progression, down from about 2 km a day to about 1.2 km a day.

The city of Chalon contained an important crossroads where important roads ran north-westwards in the direction of Paris, northwards in the direction of Dijon and Rheims or Nancy, and north-eastwards in the direction of the cities of Besançon in Burgundy and Strasbourg in northern Alsace on the border with Germany on the R. Rhine. Presumably, the Black Death began to spread from Chalon north-eastwards towards Besançon at about the same time as it began to spread westwards towards Givry, which indicates that the spread started around 13 June. A sudden rise in the number of wills registered at Besançon's 'Officialité', i.e., the Ecclesiastical Court, shows that the Black Death must have begun to ravage this city in Burgundy in the last months of 1348. In the years 1340–7, there were, on average, 44 wills registered at the Court annually, but in 1348 the number increased to 77, and then, in 1349, it reached the sky-high number of 312 wills.[27] In this case, a retrospective analysis can be usefully employed: Allowing time for a substantial rise in the number of registered wills before the end of the year as well as the standard time horizon for psychological developments, and taking into account the time demanded by the epidemiological processes leading to the subsequent recognition of the presence of the Black Death in mid-November, Besançon was probably contaminated at the end of September, corresponding to a will-producing recognition of the presence of the Black Death in mid-November, according to the standard time horizon for the epidemiological and psychological developments. This implies that the Black Death had moved the about 120 km from Chalon to Besançon in roughly 108 days, corresponding to an average daily pace of c. 1.1 km.

From Besançon, the Black Death marched 220 km farther north-eastwards via Montbéliard, Mulhouse and Colmar to Strasbourg, where its outbreak was noted on 8 July 1349.[28] Our assumption that the recognized outbreak in Besançon started almost eight months earlier implies that the Black Death had covered the 220 km in about 240 days and had moved at a daily pace of 0.9 km or, as it would seem, slightly slower than the pace from Chalon to Besançon.[29] Thus, a developmental pattern emerges in which the pace of spread diminishes strongly north of Lyons. The main reason must be a sharply reduced density of traffic on the highways north of Lyons compared with that on the highways south of Lyons. Cool winter weather caused a further sharp seasonal decrease in pace; it took almost six months from the time the

---

contagion the first plague death will occur. See the discussion of the time horizon of these epidemiological processes above in the introduction to the plague in Constantinople and below under England.

[27] Andenmatten and Morerod 1987: 22. Consequently, Biraben's assertion that the Black Death broke out in May 1349 cannot be correct. Biraben 1975: 76.

[28] Fößel 1987: 9–10. The outbreak lasted until October.

[29] According to Biraben, the presence of the Black Death was observed in Colmar, 60 km south of Strasbourg, in June, which could be taken to indicate that along this stretch plague had moved at a daily pace of 2 km. However, while Biraben can point out the time of the outbreak in Strasbourg was recognized, it is not clear whether he means that it broke out in Colmar in June or that it was raging in June but could have started earlier.

outbreak in Besançon was recognized in mid-November to the time of the outbreak in Montbéliard, about 70 km down the road, was recognized in May, corresponding to an average daily pace of c. 0.4 km. From Montbéliard the Black Death marched on in warm spring weather at the same pace as before the winter set in.

By now, the Black Death was positioned to move rapidly on Paris, by far the largest urban centre in Europe, a metropolis containing about 200,000 inhabitants,[30] and the commercial centre for a vast hinterland. Its political and administrative centre functions should not be overrated in a historical period when the kings were constantly journeying about the country accompanied by most of their administration as a part of the royal household and entourage. There was as yet no real political capital in France or in any other European country and only the faint beginnings of what would become central bureaucracies and administrations in the Early Modern period.

The first cases in Paris were reported on the outskirts of the metropolis, in the village Roissy-en-France, which today is a suburb, and it is assumed that either Saint Denis[31] or Pointoise,[32] two nearby towns, served as the link between Roissy and Paris.[33] The presence of the Black Death in Paris was noted on 20 August. The standard assumption for the time lag between contamination of a metropolis and the recognition of its presence, namely about 8 weeks, indicates that the Black Death had invaded Paris at the end of June.

A study of wills registered in the account books of the churchwarden of the parish of Saint-Germain-l'Auxerrois shows an abrupt increase in the last days of August.[34] Because we do not know where the plague contagion was originally introduced and the pattern of spread until its effects surfaced in the account books of the churchwarden of this parish, the real significance of this information is to underscore that Paris can hardly have been contaminated later than the end of June, and that it could have occurred significantly earlier.

Clearly, Paris seems to have been invaded from the north-west, by the army of the Black Death that had invaded the city of Rouen at the end of April by a metastatic leap from Bordeaux (see above), based on the recognition of its presence both in Rouen and in the surrounding countryside on 24 June by *Normanniae nova Cronica* ('The New Chronicle of Normandy'). However, there is also a different dating of the recognized outbreak to 25 July.[35] In the latter case, importation of infection by ship from southern England cannot be ruled out. The question of the time Rouen was invaded by the Black Death relative to the time of the recognized outbreak can be discussed in relation to the time of the outbreak in Paris. The distance from Rouen to Paris by land is roughly 120 km, a distance that, assuming an average daily pace by land of 2 km, would be covered in 60 days, which corresponds very well with the reported time of the observed outbreak in Rouen and surrounding districts on

---

[30] Higounet-Nadal 1988: 305–6.
[31] Fourquin 1964: 227.
[32] Dubois 1988b: 316.
[33] Fourquin 1964: 227–8.
[34] Mollat 1963: 510.
[35] Porquet 1898: 22.

24 June. Possibly, the Black Death could also have moved by boat up the R. Seine, which could have sped up the arrival in Paris considerably.

On the other hand, it seems impossible to reconcile a dating of the recognized outbreak in Rouen to 25 July with a recognized outbreak in Paris less than four weeks later, since the latter reflects a likely time of contamination there at the end of June or in early July at the latest. The time span from the time of contamination to an early epidemic phase that would be observed and recognized in villages and, perhaps, small towns is, as noted above, 5.4 weeks, but in a great metropolis with frequent visitations of dangerous epidemic diseases this would hardly be noticed at all; only a more developed epidemic phase involving many cases and conspicuous mortality would catch the attention of chroniclers. Time is also needed for transport from Rouen to Paris. Therefore, the only dating of the outbreak to appear tenable and realistic is that of 24 June in the *Normanniae nova Cronica*. This is in accord with the rule stated above: when chronicles contain disparate assertions on the time of outbreak in the same community that can be tested with independent material, the earliest dating can be systematically shown to be correct or most likely.

It should be expected that transport of contagion by land from Rouen along the busy road to Paris would take a somewhat shorter time than along the less busy road from Rouen to smaller cities. This reasonable assumption can be put in perspective by the fact that the Black Death's outbreak in the Norman city of Caen, situated south-west of Rouen, at a somewhat shorter distance than Paris, started at the end of September and was in October reflected in an abrupt increase in donations from the upper classes to the parish churches for attractive burial places; in November the full onslaught set in.[36]

The outbreak in Caen represents an instance of the Black Death's progression south- and south-westwards from Rouen, eventually to meet the forces of the Black Death that expanded by land northwards from Guyenne and Languedoc. On 30 November, the Black Death's presence was noted in the city of Angers, almost 200 km south of Caen, having thus invaded Anjou, an area bordering on Brittany.

The Black Death also conquered new territory further north, breaking out in Calais on the north-western coast in December. Calais was a French town, but had been conquered by the English in 1346 in the first phase of the Hundred Years War both because it was an important harbour for the export of English quality raw wool for the Flemish cloth industry (and for the English Crown's export taxes), and for the safeguarding of the transports of English troops across the Channel to the Continent. Obviously, the English conquest increased Calais' exposure to contamination, and the time of the outbreak can easily be co-ordinated with the spread of the Black Death in south-eastern England in the autumn of 1348. However, in this case, dissemination could have taken place also by land from Rouen, or in the form of a metastatic leap by ship along the French coast. The number of possible routes and means of communication that the Black Death could choose for its invasion of Calais in time to produce a recognized outbreak in December show that it had spread widely and could approach most destinations from several quarters, and that it was only a question of months before the whole of France was conquered by its armies of death.

The following month, in January 1349, the Black Death broke out in the city of

[36] Jouet 1972: 272–3.

Amiens on the R. Somme's northern riverside, about 130 km north of Paris.[37] In the prevailing winter weather, the Black Death managed only to move slowly in a northerly direction along a broad, sharply zigzagged, front. It must have crossed France's contemporary northern border into the Low Countries, but not its present-day border, in the late spring and summer, breaking out in the city of Valencienne in the County of Hainault in June and in the city of Lille in Artois, the southern region of the County of Flanders in August.[38] It had also invaded the territory of the present-day Kingdom of Belgium (see below).[39] The focus appears to be on the urban centres. This is, however, a reflection of the sources. They provide only a few incidental glimpses of the ravages of the Black Death in the countryside, e.g., in the villages of Izel and Esquerchin, east of Arras in eastern Artois.[40]

Although the Black Death was approaching France's borders both in the north and the east at the end of 1348, France was such a large and populous country that the epidemic also continued to expand inland in 1349. This was the case, for instance, with Brittany, which was invaded from Angers, and Auvergne, which was invaded by the plague front moving up from the south,[41] and it continued to spread in Normandy.

As in Italy, the Black Death reached the last and most peripheral areas in 1351, and even, perhaps, in 1352, when its presence is mentioned in Tonnerre in Burgundy.

Also in France there were lucky places where people won the jackpot in the great lottery of life and death managed by the Black Death. This appears to have been the case with, e.g., Béarn in the south-western corner of France,[42] and with Carpentras,[43] situated only about 20 km north-east of Avignon that was ravaged so cruelly, and with the surrounding Comtat Venaissain; it may also have been the case in a small part of Flanders and, perhaps, in a part of central France. Inexplicably, Carpentras does not appear to have been invaded by any of the following waves of plague epidemics before in 1395, and, then again not until 1468.

---

[37] Biraben 1975: 76.
[38] Biraben 1975: 76; Aubry 1983: 338.
[39] Dubois 1988b: 316; Blockmans 1980: 836.
[40] Bocquet 1969: 38.
[41] No local chronicles are preserved in Auvergne; the dating of the Black Death in this area to 1349 is an inference based on knowledge of the movements and whereabouts of the plague fronts, and on the demographic facts, which show that the population of this area suffered grave losses. Audisio 1968: 259–61; Boudet and Grand 1902: 138.
[42] Tucco Chala 1951: 80–5.
[43] Dubled 1969: 19–20.

13

Belgium[1]

Historically, the terms the Low Countries and the Netherlands used to refer to both the country that today is called Belgium and the country that is still called the Netherlands, and some adjacent areas.[2] The Black Death invaded Belgium from France and in a couple of cases also evidently from England, and it is generally assumed that the Netherlands was invaded from Germany. However, as we shall see, the Netherlands was invaded both from the north and east with an even more complicated pattern of invasion and spread, and with a significant delay in time. The Black Death's conquests of these two countries reflect different phases in the history of the Black Death and the progression of different plague fronts. For this reason, the presentation of the history of the Black Death in these two countries has been divided: its Belgian history is discussed here in what is a continuation of the chapter on its French history, while its 'Netherlandish' history is discussed in the continuation of the chapter on its German history (see Chapters 20 and 21 below).

At the time of the Black Death, the territory of Belgium was divided into a number of principalities; the countship of Flanders was held by the French king, while the countships of Hainault and Limbourg, the duchies of Brabant and Luxembourg,[3] and the diocese of Liège were held by the German emperor.[4] One should note that the present-day territory of Belgium is not conterminous or identical with these principalities at the time of the Black Death, and that this makes for some artificiality in the handling of geographical and political concepts. For instance, in the south, Flanders also included Artois in present-day France and, in the north, some areas that today belong to the Netherlands on the southern shores of the R. Western Schelde's long

---

[1] The best presentation of the Black Death in the Low Countries is Blockmans 1980.

[2] The term Holland, which, especially in American English, is much used in the meaning of the country properly called The Netherlands must be considered unfortunate, because Holland is the name of one of The Netherlands' provinces.

[3] The larger part of the medieval Duchy of Luxembourg is today a province in Belgium adjacent to the remaining part that today constitutes the independent principality of the Duchy of Luxembourg. For various reasons, it has been impossible to separate these two areas in this context.

[4] This means that the diocese was held by the bishop both in the capacity of the leader of an ecclesiastical division of the Catholic Church and in the capacity of tenant-in-chief of the German emperor. The diocese thus also had the formal status of a principality within the Holy Roman Empire of the German Nation (see under Austria and Germany).

estuary. Hainault stretched further southwards. The Duchy of Brabant is today divided between Belgium and the Netherlands so that northern Brabant is a Dutch province, while the Belgian part is divided into the provinces of Antwerp and Brabant, and so on.[5]

Belgium's present-day territory comprises about 29,500 sq. km. On the eve of the Black Death, the southern part of the Low Countries also comprised the present-day Duchy of Luxembourg with about 4,500 sq. km and Artois with about 5,100 sq. km; Hainault comprised roughly another 2,500 sq. km of territory that today belongs to France, and the Duchy of Brabant contained also the part that today belongs to the Netherlands, northern Brabant, which covers 5,100 sq. km. In all, the southern part of the Low Countries, here inaccurately called Belgium, may have comprised about 47,000 sq. km at the time.

The size of Belgium's pre-plague population can only be guestimated. The population of the Low Countries in 1469 is estimated at slightly above 2,600,000 persons, with an average population density of 34 persons per sq. km. Flanders, Brabant, Hainault, Luxembourg and Limbourg, which constitute most of present-day Belgium, contained almost exactly one-half of this population, but there was also Artois with 180,000 inhabitants and some additional areas, so that, in 1469, there may have been about 1,600,000 inhabitants within what we may, perhaps, call Belgium's historical borders.[6]

It has further been shown that the number of hearths, i.e., households, in the County of Hainault declined by 28 per cent from 1365 to 1479. In the preceding sixteen years, Hainault had been ravaged by the Black Death in 1349–50, by another major plague epidemic in 1360–1, and by a relatively smaller one in 1364[7] that must have caused considerable net reduction of the population.[8]

For a few areas in Hainault, it is has been possible to estimate the development in the number of heads of households, corresponding quite closely to the concept of hearth, in three bailiwicks[9] between 1286 and 1365. In these three areas, the number of heads of households or hearths declined from 562 to 289, i.e., a decline of 48.5 per cent.[10] In the ensuing 63 years from 1286 up to the time of the Black Death, the population may first have continued to grow significantly for three decades. This period was followed by a dramatic year of starvation, dearth and a hunger epidemic in 1315 that may have caused significant population reduction, but there is no substantial reason to assume that the size of the population would have fallen below the level of 1286. Moreover, the population would have had time to recuperate before it again was struck by a major calamity when, in 1340, the southern parts of the county was ravaged both by French and English military forces. Although the diminution of the bailiwicks' populations as reflected in the fall in the of number of households cannot with confidence be ascribed to plague alone, most of it seems to be owing to the Black Death and the ensuing two plague epidemics.

5   See maps in Prevenier 1980: 272, 274.
6   Prevenier 1983: 271–2.
7   Blockmans 1980: 844.
8   Blockmans 1980: 858–9.
9   'Prévoté'.
10 Sivéry 1965: 433.

If we assume, quite hypothetically, that these data are representative of the development of Hainault's population, and that the development of Hainault's population is representative of that of the territory of Belgium, the population reduction caused by plague in the period 1349–1469 cannot have been smaller than about 50 per cent, and the area's population at the time of the Black Death would have been of the order of magnitude of 3.2 million persons. Expressed in rounded figures to take some account of the formidable margins of uncertainty, this population size corresponds to an average population density of 40 persons in 1469, 50 persons in 1365, and, possibly, 75–80 persons per sq. km on the eve of the Black Death's arrival in 1349, twice as high as the average for France, Italy or England, and tremendously higher than for a country like Norway with about one person per sq. km.

These averages veil great variety, for the population density in Flanders must at least have been of the order of magnitude of 150 persons per sq. km. This demonstrates within substantial margins of uncertainty that the Low Countries were demographically different from other countries, although some Italian city states, especially Florence, may have had significant structural similarity. This part of Europe had an exceptional degree of urbanization together with extreme population density in the countryside, where villages would tend to contain more than 1,000 persons per sq. km and take on the character of small towns. In 1469, when the Low Countries' population may have been reduced by at least 50 per cent by recurrent plague epidemics, almost all of Belgium's constituent dukedoms and countships had urban population levels between 36 and 29 per cent.[11] It has been shown above that urbanization for special reasons of plague epidemiology tends to have a negative effect on morbidity rates, and consequently also on mortality rates in plague epidemics.[12] For this structural reason it should be expected that the Black Death did not perform up to its best murderous capabilities in the Low Countries.

In 1950, H. Van Werveke published a paper in which he maintained that the Low Countries largely avoided the ravages of the Black Death: the epidemic would only have raged in fringe areas, especially in some cities in the south of Artois, Flanders and Hainault; within the Netherlands' territory of today in the cities of Deventer and Groningen; and in the province of Friesland. Thus, he concluded, 'the wide swathe through the North and the South remained largely saved'. According to this territorial incidence of the Black Death, the cities in Artois, Flanders and Hainault had obviously been contaminated from the French epidemic, while it was assumed that Deventer, Groningen and Friesland were offshoots from the German epidemic.[13] If these observations were correct and exhaustive, Van Werveke's conclusion to the effect that the Low Countries were only marginally affected would also be valid.

This position presented itself immediately as an epidemiological conundrum that simply defied explanation. First, it was well known that plague ravaged the Low Countries many times in the following centuries. This fact demonstrated that there were no structural obstacles to the effective spread of plague within the territory, and

---

[11] Prevenier 1983: 270–3.
[12] See above, pp. 31–34, 'Can it really be true that plague spreads more effectively in the countryside than in towns and cities?'
[13] Van Werveke 1950. My translation from Dutch.

that an area typified by very intensive economic exchange with other countries had a high degree of exposure to importation of contagion. Consequently, it appears impossible to explain in epidemiological terms what could have prevented the Black Death from spreading efficiently across the territory of the Low Countries when it actually had succeeded in crossing the borders. Unsurprisingly, this position was immediately challenged, albeit indecisively at first.[14] However, in the following decades, there appeared a number of papers on the Black Death in the Low Countries that increasingly undermined Van Werveke's position.

The arrival of warm weather heralded the coming of the Black Death: the outbreak in the city of Valenciennes (medieval Hainault) took place in June 1349, which means that the epizootic phase probably had started in early May, and there were then outbreaks in the cities of Tournai (Flanders), Mons (Hainault) and Lille (Artois) in early July.[15] It has also been shown that it raged in the countryside, e.g., in the villages of Izel and Esquerchin, east of the city of Arras in eastern Artois.[16]

Interestingly, the epidemic can be seen to have an unusually strong tendency to linger on in the same areas. The district of Ath, for instance, where the Black Death broke out in the summer of 1349, can be seen to be still suffering high mortality in the tax register running from April 1351 to 1 May 1352. This tendency of prolonged epidemic duration can also be shown to manifest itself at the regional level of the duchy: southern Hainault was severely attacked by the Black Death in the second half of 1349, and in the north-eastern parts of the county the mortality was still strong in 1351–2.[17] This phenomenon is explicable in view of the extreme population density: Hainault's population is estimated at 209,000 in 1469,[18] which means that it hardly can have been smaller than about 420,000 persons on the eve of the Black Death, and while this proportional relationship is considered a quite hypothetical guestimate in relation to the Low Countries as a whole, it can be considered a conservative real estimate for Hainault. This population was distributed in an area that at the time comprised 5,000 sq. km,[19] which means an average density of at least 112 persons per sq. km, three times higher than average population density in England, Italy or France. In order to blanket the district of Ath, the Black Death was required to enter, in relation to the size of the territory, an extraordinary number of houses and trigger an extraordinary number of rat epizootics that must have run their course before the rat fleas, for lack of rat hosts, turned on human beings in their immediate vicinity, an obviously time-consuming process.

Mons was the countship's largest city. Interestingly, there are clear indications that there was a sudden increase in Mons's population at the time of the Black Death, and that this increment was caused by an influx of peasants fleeing there from the

---

[14] Rogghe 1952; Van Werveke 1953–4.

[15] Biraben 1975: 76–7; Dubois 1988b: 316. According to Aubry 1983: 338, the Black Death broke out in Lille and Tournai in August–September. However, this delay is probably a factor of the special character of the material she has used, namely the development in the annual number of deaths of purchasers of annuities for life, a social class that, presumably, would be hit with a delay in relation to the poor classes. In addition, one should keep in mind the time that would elapse from the introduction of the contagion in the rat colonies to the transition into an epidemic phase.

[16] Bocquet 1969: 38.

[17] Sivéry 1965: 438.

[18] Prevenier 1983: 271.

[19] The present-day province of Hainault comprises 3,700 sq. km.

countryside.[20] The influx of peasants is another reflection of the fact that the country-side was badly ravaged by the plague. The mortality in Mons was relatively moderate for a plague epidemic, which agrees with the special epidemiological characteristics of plague that, according to some studies presented above, include a strong tendency towards lower mortality in towns and cities than in the countryside.

There are also clear economic indications of an epidemic catastrophe that affected normal economic relationships, the county's administrative capabilities and the demographic relationships. The reduced supply of labour pushed up wages.[21] The count's domainal revenues were, however, severely affected only temporarily. The reason for this is clear. The enormous population pressure that had built up in this extremely densely populated area had created large landless or all-but-landless agricultural proletarian classes, consisting of sub-tenants, cottars and other social categories of poor and indigent people who mostly had to work for wages as day labourers in order to keep body and soul together. This agricultural proletariat was now reduced twice over, both by plague, as with other people, and by social mobility as the survivors moved into the great number of good tenancies vacated by the Black Death.

Medieval people had no economic theory that would explain the consequences of a dramatic and lasting reduction in the population on rents and wages and on public or manorial incomes. Princes, landlords and ordinary people alike just assumed that everything would soon revert to normal. The new tenants who before the plague could only dream of getting hold of a good tenement considered themselves very fortunate to become tenants on the terms prevailing in pre-plague society. Only grad-ually did the new social and economic realities dawn upon princes, landlords and poor people alike. Rents and fines fell precipitously and real wages reached record heights. Concomitantly, the manorial and domainal revenues declined strongly, producing a social and economic crisis for the manorial classes of nobility, gentry, prelates and ecclesiastical institutions, and for the rulers, in this case the count himself.

The Black Death was also in action far deeper into Belgian territory. In 1980, Griet Maréchal proved that also the great seaport and trading city of Bruges, with 40,000 inhabitants, had been severely attacked by the Black Death, although nothing is said in chronicles.[22] He used three categories of sources that reflect a dramatic increase in mortality. A deed issued by the Chapter of St Donatus in the autumn of 1350 comments on the annual output of the Chapter's estates and describes the present situation in this way: 'The tithes of our church yield less rents nowadays than usual due to the very high mortality and to the inconvenience of wars and rain.'

An *obituary* is a register in which a religious institution entered notices on the date of death of brothers, sisters, other spiritual staff, dignitaries and donors. *The Obituary of the Hospital of Our Lady of the Potterie* in Bruges records 60 deaths in the hundred years 1301–1400. If the deaths due to plague around 1350 are subtracted, the mortality in the Black Death in 1349 was eighteen times higher than the annual average for the period. Moreover, the relatively high number of deaths in 1351, representing the second highest

---

[20] Sivéry 1965: 438, n. 1.
[21] Sivéry 1965: 439–43.
[22] Maréchal 1980. My translation from Flemish.

annual level recorded in a hundred years, show that the Black Death was still around. The reason that no death is recorded in 1350 could quite likely be that the administrative functions had broken down under the impact of the onslaught, which indicates that the real increase in mortality was substantially higher (see below).

Stone buildings were inconvenient ecological niches for rats, and it has been repeatedly observed that social institutions in stone buildings – hospitals, orphanages and the like – have avoided epidemics that were raging all around them.[23] Plague deaths among hospital staff would, therefore, quite likely be due to a special variant of epidemiological causation: one might reasonably assume that the hospital staff would have been infected by rat fleas carried in the clothing of patients brought in from infected houses; and one might therefore also reasonably assume that hospital staff could be affected quite early in the epidemic. The first death of a member of the staff was recorded on 12 July 1349, to be followed by a succession of deaths in the ensuing months until October. Obviously, the epidemic had first developed somewhere else; a number of patients would quite likely be admitted before a blocked rat flea was introduced that attacked a member of the staff; this member would go through an incubation period and a period of illness before a death could be registered in the obituary. For these reasons, it appears unlikely that Bruges could have been contaminated later than 1 June.

This dating should be seen in the light of the fact that already by 15 August the Count of Flanders had to respond to a request by the magistracy of Bruges to lay out two new graveyards. This suggests that the mortality in Bruges as early as at the end of July had reached such extraordinary and disastrous proportions that the magistracy realized the need for extreme and unprecedented measures. This also suggests that the time of contamination was earlier than 1 June. The early dating of the outbreak means that Bruges was quite likely contaminated from England, although a metastatic leap by ship along the coast from Rouen or Calais or some other town on the north-western coast of France cannot be ruled out.

The city of Ghent lies 40 km east of Bruges; it was the largest medieval city in Western Europe after Paris and possibly London, containing in the years 1356–8, i.e., after the onslaught of the Black Death, around 64,000 persons.[24] It is puzzling to modern historians that no chronicler in this great city with so many educated persons found it worthwhile or useful to comment on the ravages of the Black Death.[25] Instead, historians have to rely on economic reflections of a sudden dramatic increase in mortality. The first reflection is an increase in the number of registrations of tutelage, i.e., guardianship for orphaned children. The registration of tutelage contracts before the aldermen began in August 1349, and may be seen as a reflection of dramatic mortality and a corresponding dramatic increase in the need for tutelage contracts. Disastrous mortality may explain why there are almost no tutelage deeds from the autumn of 1349, in the same way as it may explain why there are no preserved account books or registers for any institution in the city of Ghent for the time of the Black Death. Nonetheless, it can be shown that even in 1350–2 there was

---

[23] Sticker 1908: 264; Alexander 1980: 263–4.
[24] Prevenier 1980: 255.
[25] This point, i.e., the subjects chroniclers addressed, is commented on below in relation to the history of the Black Death in Germany. See also above pp. 70–71.

an appreciable increase in tutelage deeds compared with the number for subsequent years, although much smaller than in the following plague epidemics of 1360–1 and 1368–9.

The city collected a so-called *exue*-duty when property that had been put under its jurisdiction, mainly in cases of guardianship, was transferred to the ownership of another person. The incidence of this event would obviously be affected by changes in mortality. There is a conspicuous doubling of the revenue from *exue*-duties in (the accounting year) 1349–50.

Although it cannot be proven in an indisputable way that the Black Death wrought havoc on the inhabitants of Ghent as early as in the summer and autumn of 1349 according to the same pattern as in Bruges only 40 km away, there are indications to this effect. There is also clear evidence of a substantial increase in mortality in 1350–2. Ghent could have been contaminated from Tournai via intensive shipping of grain on the R. Scheldt to cover the needs of its large population, and certainly also from the nearby city of Bruges.[26]

Farther to the east, it has been shown that the Black Death raged at least in some parts of Brabant, more accurately in the so-called Walloon-Brabant, the southern part of the province of Brabant (including Brussels) that was inhabited predominantly by French-speaking people (in contrast to areas inhabited by Flemish-speaking people). Very unusually indeed, G. Despy has succeeded in using a work of religious literature to demonstrate the presence of the Black Death in a large area of Walloon-Brabant situated south-east of Brussels. That is a booklet entitled *Miracula Beate Marie* (the Miracles of St Mary) written by the prior of the Benedictine monastery in Basse-Wavre. The monastery was in the possession of a holy shrine with widely recognized anti-epidemic effects that in the course of three years was paraded through many localities in order to persuade the Lord to temper the threatening epidemic storm for his sinful but profoundly contrite human lambs; actually almost a hundred localities are mentioned. The area in question stretches from Wavre, situated 20 km southeast of Brussels via Jodoigne, to Hannut, about 50 km from Brussels.

As usual, no contemporary chronicle is preserved that comments on the Black Death. However, a much later chronicler writing at a time when it had become more appropriate to mention serious epidemic events cites or at least renders quite closely, a contemporary chronicler whose work has since been lost to the effect that the Duchy of Brabant was ravaged by an epidemic that caused depopulation in 1349–50.[27] This piece of information expands the territorial horizon from Walloon-Brabant to the Duchy of Brabant.

Again, the almost fortuitous nature of the extant sources that reflect the ravages of the Black Death is striking.

Other sources show that the city of Ypres, and the towns of Luxembourg and Bavay (between Valenciennes and Maubeuge) were visited by the Black Death in 1349, but the date is not known.

There is clear evidence that the Black Death was present in the diocese of Liège in 1351, first in the small town of Amay (near Huy) on the R. Meuse about 25 km

---

[26] Blockmans 1980: 839–43.
[27] Despy 1977.

upstream from the city of Liège. Later, it broke out in the cathedral city itself.[28] This structure of the epidemic events indicates that the contagion had been transported downstream by ship, and could be connected with the provisioning of the city, especially with cereals.

Summing up, it is no longer possible to maintain that the southern or Belgian part of the Low Countries escaped the Black Death largely unharmed, only being affected in the fringe areas. Slowly, new small pieces of evidence have been adduced showing that it actually raged over most of the territory.

---

[28] According to Biraben, the Black Death was present in the city of Liège in 1349, but his source is not indicated, and this early dating is not mentioned by Blockmans. Biraben 1975: 76–7, 415.

14

Switzerland[1]

At the time of the Black Death, the state of Switzerland was still in the making. The core territory of the present-day state of Switzerland had quite recently emerged as a loose confederation of a few areas, called 'cantons'. The territory and composition of the cantons that constitute Switzerland today are the results of a long historical process. For instance, at the time of the Black Death the easternmost areas of the canton of Valais belonged to the County of Savoy, some of the eastern cantons belonged to the Austrian Habsburg dynasty,[2] and St Gallen to the east was an episcopal fief of the Holy Roman Empire.[3] Such cantons were therefore organized and run according to feudal principles.

Little is known about the history of the Black Death in the small cluster of cantons that on the eve of the Black Death constituted the Swiss confederation. Arguably, the Black Death's history in those areas that have joined Switzerland later ought to be discussed in relation to the countries to which they belonged at the time. For some reasons, this is also an unsatisfactory approach. First, the modern people of Switzerland would like to consider this dramatic event in the history of the present-day territory of their country in its national perspective, and this is the way Swiss historians approach the issue. Secondly, the emergence and development of the state of Switzerland is not a fortuitous historical process, but reflects the fact that these territories/cantons were drawn into the same political sphere because they interacted in ways that made political unification advantageous for profound economic and political reasons. In short, they constituted an economically and socially comprehensively integrated territory at a time when many of the present-day constituent parts belonged to other states. In epidemiological terms, this is the overriding argument because this means that the dissemination of the contagion within this territory would tend to be a strong function of interaction by people living within it. As we shall see, the pattern of the spread of the Black Death confirms the comprehensive territorial integration of the cantons that today constitute the state of Switzerland.

---

[1] The most useful paper on the history of the Black Death in Switzerland, from which some of the data and perspectives in this chapter have been drawn, is Andenmatten and Morerod 1987: 19–49. It relates, however, mostly to western Switzerland. For some additional information, see Dubuis 1979 and 1980b.
[2] See under Austria.
[3] This means that it was at the same time an administrative division of the Catholic Church led by the bishop and a fief of the Holy Roman Empire held by the bishop as tenant-in-chief directly of the emperor.

The present-day territory of Switzerland covers about 41,000 sq. km, but the medieval population is not known, and hence no estimate of population density can be offered.

The Black Death's conquest of (the area that today constitutes) Switzerland was mostly carried out by epidemic forces that had marched out of Marseilles and moved up the Rhône valley, while some parts in the east and the south-east were invaded by epidemic forces coming from Italy. In March 1348, the Black Death invaded the city of Lyons, about 110 km from the present-day Swiss border, and moved on relentlessly. Thus, the history of the Black Death in Switzerland began right across the western border, in the city of Geneva. In the *Chronicle of Berne*, Justinger states that, in Switzerland, the Black Death moved from the sunset to the sunrise.[4]

The most important category of historical sources used to uncover the pattern and time of spread of the Black Death in Switzerland is wills, which have been shown to reflect quite accurately the period of the full outbreak when the upper social classes realized that their own lives were also at risk. Thus, the making of plague-related wills started presumably shortly after the growing epidemic in the poor sections of the city alerted the chroniclers. The response to the presence of the Black Death in the form of wills started in Geneva on 10 August 1348, indicating mid-June as the probable time of contamination.

From Geneva, the Black Death moved north-eastwards on the main road to the largish town of Lausanne, provoking the same reflection in wills in Nyon, about 20 km down the road, on 20 September, and in Lausanne, about 60 km from Geneva, on 10 November 1348. The 60 km between these two quite large towns were covered in ninety days, giving an average daily speed of spread of 0.66 km.

At the same time, Switzerland was also invaded across the north-western, Lombardian border of Italy. Varese, situated about 60 km north of Milan and close to the Italian border, is reported to have been ravaged from August. Varese must be the source of infection for the town of Bellinzona in the canton of Ticino, situated 50 km north of Varese near the end of L. Maggiore, where the epidemic broke out in October or November.[5] It appears that the Black Death did not succeed in breaking out of this canton over the St Gotthard pass or the St Bernard pass; this outbreak would, therefore, not develop into a significant factor in the history of the Black Death in Switzerland.

From Lausanne the Black Death marched on in two main directions, along the two main roads that ran north-eastwards all the way to the city of Zurich and along the main road that ran south-eastwards to the cathedral city of Sion. Moving

---

[4] Hoeniger 1881: 17.

[5] Biraben 1975: 75. According to Biraben, at the same time the Black Death also broke out in the town of Disentis up in the mountains south-east of Altdorf at the southern end of L. Vierwaldstätter. It would have taken months for the Black Death to move from Bellinzona to Disentis even if it had managed to cross the St Gotthard pass or the St Bernard pass, and there is no source for such an early outbreak from the north or the east. Actually, it would fit in quite nicely if the outbreak in Disentis has been misdated by one year, and occurred in October or November 1349. Disentis would then have been contaminated by the army of the Black Death that marched southwards from Luzern, and on the way sent an expeditionary force up the valley to Engelberg. The army marched on via Altdorf and Andermatt, where it turned eastwards up into the mountains to Disentis, which is situated at a crossroads for the routes over the Upper Alps and the Lukman pass.

north-eastwards, the Black Death arrived first in the town of Berne, where it broke out in February 1349.[6] In Olten, in the canton of Solothurn, about 60 km north-east of Berne, there is an important crossroads with roads leading northwards to Basle, where the Black Death broke out at the beginning of May,[7] and southwards to Lucerne. In the annals of the parochial church of Rusweil near Lucerne, it is stated that the Black Death broke out on 29 July.[8] It raged in the town of Engelberg, roughly 30 km south of Lucerne, almost exactly in the territorial centre of Switzerland, from 8 September 1849 to 6 January 1350.[9] However, situated at the foot of insurmountable mountains, Engelberg, was a dead-end road. The Black Death also marched further eastwards on the road to Zurich where the plague is said to have broken out on 11 October.[10] In the city of Constance, in the north-eastern corner of Switzerland, it broke out at some time in the last months of 1349.[11]

Interestingly, in May the Black Death was raging in and around Pfäfers in the south-eastern corner of the canton of St Gallen, near the border with Austria.[12] It is impossible to reconcile the time of this epidemic with the other datings on the spread of the Black Death across Switzerland from the west to the (north-)east. However, it is easily reconcilable with an invasion from the east, from Austria: the inner mountain areas of the province of the Tyrol were already ravaged in September 1348, and were, therefore, probably contaminated at the end of July (see below). The distance from the Brenner pass northwards to the town of Innsbruck, and from Innsbruck west-wards to Feldkirch, on the borders of the canton of St Gallen and Liechtenstein, is about 180 km. Altogether, the Black Death would have to travel roughly 200 km from the Brenner pass and the Austrian Tyrolese mountains to arrive in Pfäfers, which means that the distance could be covered in time to cause the outbreak in May (or in late April) with an average daily pace of c. 0.8 km.[13]

From Lausanne, where the Black Death broke out at the beginning of November 1348, it also marched south-eastwards towards the canton of Valais and its urban centre, the cathedral city of Sion. In December, it broke out in Chillon, about 30 km down the road, a few kilometres south of Montreux at the eastern end of L. Léman.[14] About 50 km down the road from Lausanne, it reached the parish of Saint Maurice d'Agaune in the castellany[15] of Monthey. Extraordinarily, a burial register is preserved that reflects the ravages of the Black Death in the parish. Only four parish registers are preserved from the mid-fourteenth century that reflect the effects of the Black Death, all of them relating to French-speaking areas. Two of these parish regis-ters have been mentioned, the burial registers of St-Nizier in Lyons and of Givry, and

---

[6] Biraben 1975: 76–7.
[7] Biraben 1975: 76–7, 90.
[8] Hoeniger 1881: 17.
[9] Fößel 1987: 9, n. 38. Engelberg is situated in the canton of Uri.
[10] Biraben 1975: 76–7.
[11] Hoeniger 1881: 17–18.
[12] Bucher 1979: 14–15; Sticker 1908: 56.
[13] Theoretically, the Black Death could also have spread north-westwards from Trent in north-eastern Italy (province of Trentino-Alto Adige), where the outbreak reportedly started on 2 June 1348. The distance from Trent to Pfäfers is 170 km as the crow flies. For topographical reasons and because no important commercial roads ran in that direction, this scenario appears quite unlikely.
[14] Biraben 1975: 75.
[15] The term castellany refers to the lordship of a castle and its district.

in Givry a marriage register is also preserved. The fourth parish register is the burial register of St Maurice.

Unfortunately, like the burial register of St-Nizier, this burial register is also incomplete, starting on 9 April, when the Black Death had reached the height of its intensity, and continuing until 8 June, i.e., roughly from Easter to Whitsun, when it breaks off. The reason the register is incomplete is probably that the church's priest at the onset of the epidemic died from plague and was replaced by a new priest who started to keep a register. The rarity of medieval parish registers reflects the fact that there was no ecclesiastical obligation to keep parish registers of any sort, and medieval registers of priestly services are really account books kept voluntarily by priests who wished to record their incomes from performing burials, baptisms and marriages. Because these registers were private account books, their successors would normally not have any substantial interest in preserving them, and thus almost all such registers perished.

Observation of the presence of the Black Death is reflected in the wills from 22 January. Because the epidemic developments must be assumed to have been slowed down by cold winter weather, the contagion was probably introduced into the little community at the beginning of December. This relatively long duration of the plague epidemic within a parish community reflects its large territory and the diversity of its socio-economic make-up, comprising the small town of St Maurice, a surrounding fertile plain and quite extensive mountain areas.

As should be expected, the Black Death started in the little town and radiated out from this local epicentre. The central economic nexus of the town was to provide the mountain settlements with additional grain in exchange for excess production of animal products in these areas, much like the economic system described below in the case of Norway. As reiterated already several times, grain was a product that was particularly well suited for the dissemination of dangerous rat fleas that carried the Black Death with them in their ventricular system.

The fact that the parish register breaks off on 8 June, while the epidemic continued until the autumn, suggests that also the new priest succumbed to the Black Death.

The arrival of the Black Death in the cathedral city of Sion is reflected in the wills from 3 March. The Black Death had covered the 150 km from Geneva to Sion in slightly less than 200 days, corresponding to an average daily pace of 0.75 km, which presumably was slowed down by cool or cold winter weather for about half the time on the road. According to the evidence in the number of wills, the Black Death petered out in Sion around 1 October 1349. Thus, in general, the Black Death appears to have completed its conquest of Switzerland in the late autumn of 1349, although sporadic cases continued to occur into January 1350 as the killer epidemic was finishing its deadly course.

Switzerland was invaded at least twice by epidemic forces coming from Italy. It was first invaded by one of the armies of the Black Death that moved out of the original epicentres in Florence or Genoa, or, perhaps, they joined forces somewhere on their way into the mountain areas of north-western Italy whence these forces of epidemic death crossed into the canton of Ticino and attacked the town of Bellinzona. The eastern canton of St Gallen was invaded by the army of the Black Death that moved northwards out of the epicentre in Venice and crossed into the Austrian province of the Tyrol over the Brenner pass, which probably took place at the end of July (see below). The early invasion of the Tyrol gave the Black Death good time to reach eastern St Gallen in time to unleash an outbreak in May. Thus, the Black Death conquered Switzerland in a three-pronged attack: three armies marched out of three original epicentres, one from Marseilles up the Rhône valley in the west; the second marched out of one or both epicentres in north-western Italy; a third army came from Venice. Because the army that attacked the canton of Ticino failed to cross the St Gotthard pass, the conquest of Switzerland took on the strategic character of a mighty pincer movement. Most of the conquest was carried out by the western arm(y) of the pincer.

15

The British Isles[1]

The British Isles comprise Ireland, England, Wales and Scotland. At the time, the Shetland Islands and the Orkney Islands were Norse settlements that belonged territorially to the Kingdom of Norway and were invaded by the Black Death by ship from Bergen on Norway's western coast. England contains by far the largest part of the territory and the population of the British Isles. On the eve of the Black Death, England and Wales contained about 6 million inhabitants[2] distributed in a territory of 150,000 sq. km, and, thus, living at an average density of 40 persons per sq. km, much the same as in Italy and France.

Several categories of English sources yield valuable information on the history of the Black Death:

First, *registers of institutions*: in each diocese, the Bishop's Registrar kept a list of all the institutions made to vacant benefices in the parishes by the bishop in which the time of institution of a new incumbent in a specified cure was carefully noted down. Benefices became vacant because of resignations, but most vacancies were caused by the incumbent's death. The *registers of institutions* provide, therefore, information on the incidence of deaths and the resignations of the beneficed clergy in a diocese in normal years that can be compared with the entries in the years of the Black Death. The number of vacant benefices distributed according to various divisions of time and according to territorial incidence provides information on the Black Death's pattern of spread in time and space, and on the ecclesiastical mortality it caused.[3]

---

[1] There are four works in which the history of the Black Death in the British Isles is dealt with at some length: Creighton 1891; Gasquet 1908; Ziegler 1969/1970, and Shrewsbury 1971. In my opinion, Ziegler's account is still by far the best. Gasquet's book is an impressive pioneering work, although much research in many relevant fields of study has been produced since his book appeared. Unfortunately, to some extent this is now also true with respect to Ziegler's book, which was published a generation ago. Shrewsbury's book is based on untenable epidemiological assumptions but contains much valuable concrete information. John Hatcher has written (1977) a small but excellent book on *Plague, Population and the English Economy 1348–1530*, which contains also a valuable discussion of the Black Death.

[2] Hallam 1988: 536–7; Smith 1988: 191; Smith 1991: 48–9.

[3] A related type of information is found in the *Patent Rolls*: on these royal rolls were entered, among other things, royal presentations to vacant ecclesiastical livings that were in the King's gift, and presentations to livings, which the king performed on behalf of lay and ecclesiastical lords, in the first case as guardian for sons during their minority, in the second case when their offices were vacant.

As sources for the study of the spread of the Black Death in time and space institutions provide two valuable, but in themselves insufficient, pieces of information that can be used in a retrospective method of subtraction from the time of an institution to the time when the Black Death entered local society. First, an institution provides the starting point for the subtraction. Secondly, it is a valuable piece of information that it would usually take four to six weeks from the death of a parish priest to the institution of his successor.[4] When this time lag is deducted, the probable time of the death of the incumbent from the Black Death will be indicated.

In order to determine the time the Black Death invaded a parish it is necessary to take into account and subtract the time consumed by the epidemiological processes up to the time of the death of the parish priest. The ordinary pattern, causation and duration of these epidemiological events are well known and were discussed in some detail above. To summarize, after plague infection has been introduced into a house by an infective rat flea, the first human cases of plague illness will usually occur after 16–23 days, the first plague deaths after about 20–28 days, and within this range most often after about 23–24 days. When the parish priest for the first time was called upon to administer the last rites in a plague case and for the first time entered a house containing numerous dangerous rat fleas, about three weeks would, on average, have elapsed since the first rat was infected in his parish.

Although, the parish priest would be at risk from the first case, it cannot be assumed that he would normally be personally involved in the epidemiological process at once, in the sense that he either would be bitten or would carry one or more rat fleas in his clothing to his own house in connection with the first plague case in his parish. His stays in plague-infected houses to administer the last rites would be quite brief. However, the chances of becoming involved increased rapidly as the endemic phase gradually developed into an early epidemic phase. Thus, it can be assumed that parish priests would tend to become personally involved quite early in the epidemic, as shown, among other things, by the substantial incidence of two or more institutions to the same parish benefice[5] despite the fact that the time from the death of an incumbent to the institution of his successor normally took between four to six weeks, which reduced substantially the clerical population at risk and the period of exposure.[6] Slightly arbitrarily, it will be assumed that the parish priest would usually become embroiled with the Black Death in the early epidemic phase, about the time that a wider spread manifested itself in a rapidly growing number of cases.

Next, one must clarify the composition and usual duration of the ordinary chain of events in the epidemiological processes until the death of the parish priest. The priest could, as mentioned, become personally embroiled in the epidemic process either by being bitten by a blocked rat flea in the house of a dying parishioner, or one or more rat fleas could have jumped onto his clothing and ridden with him to his house.

4   Thompson 1911: 316–17; Ziegler 1970: 148. Cf. Gasquet 1908: 165. This standard time lag of four to six weeks is not a rule without exception: Davies found that, in the diocese of Coventry and Lichfield, the time lag between the death of the beneficed priest and the institution of his successor was, on average, only eighteen days. R.A. Davis 1989: 88.
5   See, e.g., Jessopp 1922: 205; Thompson 1911: 316.
6   Cf. Hatcher 1977: 23.

Because of the long and quite thick clothing that priests wore, and because of the brief duration of the stays at deathbeds, and because many of the rat fleas would be infected but not yet have developed the blockage that made them infective,[7] the second alternative would occur more often than the first.

These alternatives make for two scenarios with markedly different time horizons. In the first case, the priest would usually die in about eight days (incubation period plus duration of mortal illness). This means that a small but significant proportion of the parish priests died around six weeks after the first rat was infected by plague, namely (on average) 12 days (epizootic phase) + 3–4 days (before first infective transmission by starved fleas), + 7 days (endemic phase) + 5 days (early epidemic phase) + 8 days incubation and illness for the early epidemic cases that triggered his involvement, + 8 days (incubation and illness for the priest) – 43–44 days in all, or 6.2 weeks.

In the second case, the rat fleas would need some time to find a rat host in the priest's house, and if they were not blocked it would, in any case, probably take a few days before they could trigger the epizootic process. Then, the basic processes would be repeated, the epizootic phase followed by the phase when the rat colony was so decimated that the rat fleas began to be attracted to human beings in their immediate surroundings as sources for nourishment for want of their natural hosts. In this phase, the priest would quite likely be infected within a few days because he now shared the same environment with the dangerous rat fleas for a much longer period of day and night. This second and usual alternative implies a significantly longer time horizon from when the first rat was infected in the parish to the death of the parish priest, namely 12 (epizootic phase) + 3–4 days (before infective transmission by starved fleas), + 7 days (endemic phase) + 5 days (early epidemic phase) + 8 days (incubation and illness of the early epidemic cases that triggered his involvement), + 2 days (before the infected flea(s) brought to the priest's house found a rat host), + 12 days (epizootic), + 3–4 days (before infective transmission), + 8 days (incubation and illness) – in all 60–61 days, or 8.6 weeks.

When the time that normally elapsed from the death of the parish priest to the institution of his successor, namely four to six weeks, on average five weeks, is added on to the outlined epidemiological processes we find, according to the two scenarios, either a usual minimum duration of 11 weeks or a usual maximum duration of 15 weeks from the introduction of plague contagion into a parish until the death of the parish priest from the disease led to the institution of his successor. An average of thirteen weeks is obviously the practical solution to obtain an operational standard assumption, but it is, then, important to keep in mind that this figure more often than not will be short, and that in real life there would have been considerable variation in the individual cases owing to fortuitous circumstances and individual variation in behaviour and health. The standard assumption is a generalized gauge based

---

[7] As to the difference between infected and infective fleas, see above, pp. 15–17. Readers ought, perhaps, also to be reminded that the usual fleas of the black rat are fur fleas, which are evolutionarily adapted to riding with their hosts and for this reason also tolerate light well, while human fleas are typical nest fleas that stay near beds and other sleeping arrangements to emerge during the night to feed, and for this reason have great aversion to light, and ride with their hosts only accidentally.

on a statistical average and represents the usual or ordinary course of epidemiolog-ical, physiological and ecclesiastical events under the circumstances.[8]

Hollingsworth has suggested that the use of auxiliary priests in the richer benefices meant that 'much of the visitation of the sick to perform the last rites would probably have been done by the non-beneficed'.[9] He refers to an important paper by Thompson on the institution of priests in the diocese of York during the Black Death, but Thompson does not mention that the non-beneficed auxiliary priests should have performed these duties. It appears that the beneficed parish priests died quite early in the epidemic in their local communities, as reflected, for instance, in the quite signifi-cant incidence of two (or more) institutions in the same parish.[10] This must be taken as an indication that the parishioners had a strong wish to have the last rites adminis-tered by their parish priest, and that such serious business was considered among the duties he should perform personally. When the number of parishioners in their death throes began to increase substantially, both the parish priest and his auxiliary priest would become busily engaged in administering to the parishioners the sacramental prerequisites for salvation.

Institutions to benefices can be summarized according to counties and dioceses on a monthly basis. Applying the deductions established on the preceding pages, this approach produces quite good data on the onset and duration of the Black Death, which can be used to reconstruct the Black Death's pattern of spread in time and space throughout England.[11]

Secondly, *manorial court rolls*: on these rolls were entered the business of the manorial courts, and this would include death of householders since the previous court, and whether there were inheriting relatives or the holding was escheated to the lord of the manor. These sources exist in great numbers in England. In the best cases, they provide a usable basis for demographic analysis. Occasionally they will make it possible to establish the number of tenants in a manor and the number of plague victims among them, and thus the mortality rate of tenants; more often they will indicate the incidence, time and duration of a mortality crisis, and thus, in the present context, the whereabouts and pattern of spread of the Black Death. The value of the manorial court rolls as historical sources is often substantially increased when they can be used together with *manorial account rolls*.[12]

The studies that are based on these sources provide a more detailed picture of the Black Death's spread and demographic effects in England than is available for any other country.

The Black Death entered the British Isles in the town of Weymouth, a seaport in the county of Dorset on the southern coastline of England that was of considerable importance at the time. This infamous event is described in the *Grey Friars' Chronicle*:

---

[8] This standard assumption must not be confused with the standard assumption on the time elapsing from the contamination of a community until its presence was recognized by the upper classes and became reflected in chronicles (see above).

[9] For some interesting points, see Hollingworth 1969: 232–5.

[10] See., e.g., Wood-Legh 1948: 158.

[11] Further comments on the use of institutions to benefices will be given in Part 4 below on mortality.

[12] Gasquet 1908: 86–7; Ziegler 1970: 126–7.

> In this year, in Melcombe [= 'Weymouth'[13]], in the county of Dorset, a little before the Feast of St John the Baptist, two ships, one of them from Bristol, came alongside. One of the sailors had brought with him from Gascony the seeds of the terrible pestilence and through him the men of the town of Melcombe were the first in England to be infected.[14]

The chroniclers give various dates for the time when the presence of the Black Death was first recognized. The earliest date is given in the cited *Grey Friars' Chronicle*, a few days before 24 June; Ranulphus Higden asserts in his *Polychronicon* that it occurred on 24 June;[15] Robert of Avesbury dates the event to 'about St Peter's Day', i.e., around 29 June; the so-called monk of Malmesbury says in his chronicle *Eulogium Historiarum* that it took place on 7 July; one chronicler indicates 25 July, two others 1 August and others mention August or the autumn.[16] Summing up, there is a certain tendency of clustering in the chroniclers' assertions that indicate either the period c. 21 June–7 July or the couple of weeks around 1 August as the time that the presence of the Black Death became apparent.[17]

As shown in the discussion of the time horizon of the epidemiological process, one should as a rule of thumb, what is here called a standard assumption, assume a time lag of 6–7 weeks before the introduction of plague into towns took on epidemic proportions that would make its presence recognized by the chronicle-producing upper classes; in cities this would be seven weeks, in the larger cities approaching eight weeks. This means that an assertion to the effect that the presence of the Black Death was recognized, even on the basis of hindsight, to a few days before 24 June, implies that the plague probably entered Weymouth around 8 May.

The pivotal question, of course, is which of these contemporary assertions with respect to the time of the Black Death's arrival in Weymouth can be corroborated by independent empirical evidence? In other words, which of them is compatible with the data on the first phase of spread in England, with the facts on the ground? One should keep in mind that dissemination of plague contagion with goods could start at once in the harbour as illustrated by the ship that, according to the *Grey Friar's Chronicle*, was contaminated in Weymouth's harbour immediately after the arrival of the ship that carried the contagion from Gascony. In fact, early contamination of ships in Weymouth's harbour happened at least twice. The Irish friar John Clyn states in his chronicle that in Ireland the Black Death broke out first in Dalkey (Howth) and Drogheda, two small towns on the coast of the Pale, and that people next started to die from it in Dublin at the beginning of August 1348 (his account is discussed below and found credible). In itself this piece of information excludes dating of the outbreak of the Black Death in Weymouth to around 1 August. That the Black Death was recognized earlier in Dalkey and Drogheda than in Dublin does not necessarily mean that contagion was introduced later in Dublin, since the epidemiological processes leading to recogni-

---

[13] Melcombe was situated within the area covered by Weymouth today. It is therefore usual to refer to Weymouth as the name of the seaport where the Black Death entered England.

[14] Grandson 1957: 274.

[15] Higden 1865: 355.

[16] Creighton 1891: 115–16; Ziegler 1970: 122–4.

[17] Chroniclers like dating to the best-known feasts of saints, e.g., as in this case, to the Nativity of St John the Baptist, and they were certainly not pedants. Typically, the two dates given for the beginning of the Black Death in London are Michaelmas and All Saints' Day.

tion of the presence of the epidemic would take some days longer in a fairly large town like Dublin than in quite small towns. In this case all three towns could have been contaminated on the same day or with a difference of only a few days earlier in Dalkey or Drogheda. According to the standard assumption on this point, 6–7 weeks would normally elapse from the date when a town was contaminated until the presence of a plague epidemic was recognized. This implies that Dublin was contaminated no later than c. 30 June, probably a few days earlier, around 27 June, and not unlikely as early as 23 June, i.e., at about the same time as earliest recognition of the presence of the Black Death in Weymouth. However, the transport of the Black Death by ship from Weymouth to the Pale must also be taken into account. If we assume that the contaminated ship made a usual type of voyage at the time, following the coast quite closely, sailing only in daylight and at an average pace of 40 km per day, that it crossed over to Wexford harbour in Ireland form the western tip of Wales, and then followed the coast to Dublin, this was a voyage of roughly 1,000 km that would take about 26 days. Consequently, according to this discussion, under normal circumstances the ship that contaminated towns in the Pale would have left Weymouth around 1 June. This shows that the earliest dating of the recognized outbreak in Weymouth must be accepted; it also confirms that the indicated time of contamination of Weymouth is realistic.

William Rees of University College in Cardiff has presented evidence to the effect that 'by the beginning of August, most of the tenants of Frome Braunch in Somerset were dead and there were other deaths in North and South Cadbury'.[18] This means that, by early August, the Black Death would have had time to spread from Weymouth on the coast of Dorset overland northwards to the vicinity of the small town of Frome in the easternmost part of central Somerset, a distance of about 70 km as the crow flies; and the Black Death would, in addition, have had time to kill off most of the tenants of the manor of Frome Braunch. This indicates, of course, the earliest possible date of introduction of the contagion and early effective spread of the contagion into the surrounding region. It actually indicates quite strongly that contaminated goods were transported out of Weymouth before the earliest recognition of the presence of the Black Death.

According to Geoffrey le Baker, a cleric of the abbey of Osney near Oxford who wrote one of the most used contemporary chronicles, the Black Death broke out in Bristol on 15 August, a date that appears to be widely accepted.[19] This indicates that the Black Death was introduced into this small city about seven weeks earlier, i.e., at the end of June. Assuming ship transport of the usual type along the coast from Weymouth around Cornwall and into the Bristol Channel up to Bristol, a voyage of about 700 km that would normally take about 17 days, this indicates 10 June as the time when the ship that contaminated Bristol left Weymouth. The importance of ship transport in this case is also signified by the fact that the Black Death did not penetrate into Cornwall until the end of 1348, as demonstrated by a small but significant rise in institutions of parish priests from January 1349; and the epidemic spread overland from Devon, causing the death of the reeve of Rillaton manor on 12 March.[20] Also the date of the outbreak in Bristol must be taken to support the earliest dating of

[18] Rees 1923: 29.
[19] Creighton 1891: 116; Boucher 1938: 34; Shrewsbury 1971: 40.
[20] Hatcher 1970: 103.

the Black Death's outbreak in Weymouth, and provides another case of a ship that had left Weymouth with contamination on board before the Black Death reached a phase that led to recognition of its presence. In general terms, this fits well with the account of the *Grey Friars' Chronicle* in which it is actually stated that a ship from Bristol was involved in the introduction of the Black Death in Weymouth, although it is not clear whether or not it was the ship from Bristol that had carried the contagion from Gascony or it was the ship lying next to her. Whatever the case, the ship of Bristol in question could not have been the ship that contaminated the city, since a date for the recognized outbreak in Bristol of 15 August is too late.

An interesting piece of evidence for this discussion of the time of arrival is that the parish priest of West Chickerell in the immediate vicinity of Weymouth appears to have been the first incumbent to die from the Black Death. The institution of the new incumbent is dated to 30 September,[21] which means that after the deduction of 13 weeks according to the established standard assumption, the death of the preceding incumbent quite likely occurred around 1 July. If we allow time for the outbreak in Weymouth to develop and time for the spread of plague by chance of transport with persons or goods the short distance from Weymouth to West Chickerell, and some time for the epidemic to develop there, this incidence also supports the earliest dating of the introduction of the Black Death into Weymouth.[22] Shortly afterwards, other parish priests died in parishes some kilometres west of Weymouth, and institutions are recorded on 9 and 19 October,[23] corresponding, according to the standard assumption, to contamination of the parishes on 10 July and 18 July, respectively. In November, institutions were recorded in parishes at a distance of some 30–40 km north and north-east of Weymouth.[24]

In August, two ecclesiastical institutions situated on the R. Otter in the south-eastern corner of Devon suffered great losses from the Black Death: many of the canons of the collegiate church of Ottery St Mary, roughly 70 km northwest of Weymouth, died; in Honiton, c. 10 km north-east of Ottery, it killed 23 of the 26 brethren in the Cistercian house of Newenham.[25] Both these institutions must have been contaminated in the first half of July, in order to have developed full-blown epidemic situations in the second half of August. Their fates support the earliest dating of the Black Death's arrival in Weymouth.[26] This early dating suggests that the contamination was spread by ship from Weymouth to the small town of Budleigh Salterton on the estuary of the R. Otter, and was then transported by boat or barge some way upstream. It does not appear possible to construct a realistic scenario for

---

[21] Fletcher 1922: 7.

[22] The normal time lag of 13 weeks between the institution of a new incumbent and the presence of the Black Death in a parish makes it unlikely that the institution on 17 July to the vacant rectory of Wareham St Michael on Portland I. outside Weymouth was owing to the Black Death. Shrewsbury 1971: 57.

[23] Fletcher 1922: 7. 'From then on, the deaths of Dorset clergy followed one another in quick succession.'

[24] See also Watts 1998: 23–6.

[25] Shrewsbury 1971: 60.

[26] The time of the outbreak of the Black Death in the town of Exeter appears not to be known. Pickard 1947: 22–7. The early presence of the Black Death 15 and 25 km from Exeter could, therefore, hypothetically be explained by an early leap to Exeter by ship. However, this hypothetical alternative implies a quite similar time perspective comprising ship transport, introduction into Exeter, outbreak in this town, and further spread into the surrounding districts.

movement by land in these two distances in time to produce full-blown epidemic situations with high mortality in the second half of August.

Finally, the earliest dating of the recognized outbreak of the Black Death in England (a few days before 24 June) is supported by the fact that the Bishop of Lincoln and the Bishop of York on 25 July and 28 July, respectively, issued mandates in which they proclaimed the imminence of the great pestilence and gave orders for religious processions and intercessory prayers in order to temper the wrath of the Lord and induce Him to spare them. In this case, a time horizon of a month must be the absolute minimum: this episcopal action was triggered by a chain of events starting with the outbreak, recognition of its significance, the spread of the news all the way to these two bishops in the opposite corner of England, and the production of a decision by them to issue mandates on the matter.[27]

Summing up, the early facts on the ground that reflect the early phase of the spread of the Black Death in southern England support the earliest dating of the recognized outbreak of the Black Death in Weymouth in the chronicles, i.e., a few days before 24 June. According to the standard assumption, the contamination will have occurred about 6–7 weeks earlier, around 8 May. Assuming again that ships moving along the coast would at the time cover, on average, about 40 km a day, it is indicated that the contaminated ship would have left Bordeaux's harbour about 24 days earlier, around mid-April.[28] This dating is easily compatible with the redating of the contamination of the city of Bordeaux (see above).

Although the standard assumptions offer rather coarse analytical tools that include significant uncertainty, they appear to have provided a consistent and credible scenario that combines both standard knowledge of plague epidemiology as uncovered by physicians, bacteriologists and entomologists and the facts on the ground as uncovered by historians in relation to the history of the Black Death.

From Weymouth, the Black Death spread by leaps and bounds along the coast westwards and eastwards. It soon rounded the Cornish peninsula, moved into the Bristol Channel and spread to places along the coasts of Devon and Somerset, sailed up the R. Avon, and in an amazingly short time reached the city of Bristol where its presence, as mentioned above, was recognized as early as 15 August, implying contamination around 1 July. The Black Death also sailed up the last stretch of the Bristol Channel, into the R. Severn, and reached the town of Gloucester, roughly 50 km north of Bristol.

The inhabitants of Gloucester attempted to defend themselves against invasion of the forces of the Black Death by shutting their gates, not allowing any alien person to enter the town. However, it was all to no avail, because, as in the case of Kaffa, such measures could not prevent the Black Death from entering the town through crevices in the town wall or between the gate and the gateway, riding triumphantly and invisibly in the bodies of rodents or their consort of fleas. Furthermore, the townsmen needed food to survive and would have to open the gates to let grain and other foodstuffs be brought in. Nonetheless, shutting the gates and screening entrants as meticulously as possible was, of course, the only rational action that offered any hope of

---

[27] Thompson 1914: 102–3; Gasquet 1908: 175
[28] Cf. above pp. 85, 101–104; Contamine 1976: 75.

avoiding the plague, however small the chances. Actually, Milan appears to have succeeded by adopting similar measures (see above).

Bristol and Gloucester were situated on navigable rivers at some distance inland. The Black Death's easy conquest of these urban centres was part of a broader pattern of its movement along coastal waterways, while seizing the opportunities to send expeditionary forces inland up rivers, making early appearances along navigable waterways.[29] The fact that the British Isles are typified by much precipitation and many rivers and waterways affected significantly the Black Death's pattern and pace of spread. All British scholars who have studied the spread of the Black Death agree that transport by fishing boats and ships along the coast and up the estuaries and navigable rivers played a major role in the process of dissemination, especially in the first phase.[30]

This is, of course, as should be expected: all students of pre-industrial economic history observe that the prevailing technological level of old-time society made transport by boat or ship both in terms of pace and capacity by far the most efficient way of moving people and goods. The pattern of spread of the Black Death confirms the vitality and substantial volume of trade and travel by ship in pre-plague society, and that this type of transport must have comprised a large number of vessels. In addition, the fishing industry was much developed in coastal waters, comprising a great number of small fishing boats that would enter various seaports to sell their catch and purchase grain and other necessities in exchange. Thus, the assumption that fishing boats played a significant role in the dissemination of the Black Death is justified.

Studies of the diocesan registers of institutions show that the incidence of institutions to vacant benefices began to increase substantially in the diocese of Salisbury (comprising the counties of Dorset, Wiltshire and Berkshire) from October,[31] presumably in the second half of the month, which means that, according to the standard assumption, the Black Death was spreading rapidly in the diocese in the second half of July, producing epidemic situations in contaminated rural parishes and in local towns with a standard time lag of about of 5.5–6 weeks. Conversely, the time parish priests were beginning to die from plague is indicated by deducting the standard time required to have a new parish priest installed, i.e., on average, five weeks, which takes us to the second week of September. As should be expected, this epidemic process began in southern Dorset where Weymouth is situated, reflecting the original epicentre of spread. The spread by land westwards into the neighbouring diocese of Exeter comprising Devon and the Duchy of Cornwall, England's two south-western-most counties, is reflected in an abrupt rise in the incidence of institutions in Devon in November. Cornwall was invaded overland from Devon at the end of 1348, the presence of the epidemic being disclosed, as mentioned, by a significant rise in the institutions of parish priests from January 1349; the reeve of Ralliston manor, quite close to the border, died on 12 March.[32] In Cornwall, the Black Death raged with full

---

[29] Gasquet 1908: 97; Coulton 1947: 496–7. For East Anglia, see Jessopp 1898: 210.
[30] See, e.g., Gasquet 1908: 89–90; Ziegler 1970: 138.
[31] Gasquet 1908: 90–1; Shrewsbury 1971: 59.
[32] Hatcher 1970: 103.

force from Easter to Michaelmas.[33] This pattern shows that, generally speaking, in the south-westernmost counties the Black Death began to spread effectively in Devon in August and in Cornwall a couple of months later. The distribution of institutions in these two dioceses according to months shows that the Black Death could have lasted for a year in this region,[34] although the institutions performed in the last months could quite likely reflect not the time of the incumbent's death, but late replacements reflecting the difficulties in finding suitable candidates in the last part of the epidemic when the pool of auxiliary priests was severely depleted. As the Black Death moved on, the pattern of time and space shifted month by month through 1348 and 1349.

From Bristol and Gloucester the Black Death marched on further northwards and north-westwards into the Midland counties and the counties bordering on Wales, and westwards into Oxfordshire and along the main road in the direction of London. However, it is clear that this movement overland was quite slow.[35] It broke out on the manor of Cuxham in southern Oxfordshire in March, or possibly in February.[36] Taking into account the slowness of epidemic process in cool winter climate and the time needed for the epidemic to spread over the south-western borders of Oxfordshire to Cuxham, it becomes clear that the invasion of the county must have taken place in late 1348. The same goes for south-eastern Buckinghamshire where epidemics also broke out in early 1349, reaching the height of their intensity in May and the following months.[37] The same was the case for Cornwall in the extreme south-west. This slowdown reflects the generally dampening effects of cool winter weather on plague's powers of spread that, in the case of the Black Death, have also been observed in Italy, Spain and France and will again be shown to be the case in Germany, the Nordic countries and Russia, where the Black Death stopped spreading in the winter. The plague history of Norway from the Black Death to the last epidemics in 1654 has recently been published, and shows there was not a single instance of a winter epidemic of plague in any of the over thirty waves of plague epidemics that hit this country in the course of 300 years.[38]

The Black Death leapt also along the coast eastwards from Weymouth, and soon crossed from Dorset into the county of Hampshire in the diocese of Winchester. One could have assumed that Southampton had been attacked early because one of the most quoted chroniclers believed that this was the town where the Black Death first went ashore.[39] However, the first probable reflections of the epidemic relate to other places, including a somewhat suspicious institution to a vacancy at the living of Stratfield Turgis on 23 September. More decisive evidence has been found that shows that, at the end of October, the epidemic was raging in the village of Titchfield, which also functioned as a small port on the Meon where the estuary reaches the Solent and Spithead, the straits between the mainland and the northern shores of the Isle of

---

[33] Hatcher 1970: 102–3.
[34] Hatcher 1970: 103; Shrewsbury 1971: 59–64. Readers who would like to consult Shrewsbury's book are warned that his views on plague epidemiology and mortality are not accepted by any other scholar; he has, however, collected a great amount of useful data.
[35] Page 1934: 120, 123.
[36] P.D.A. Harvey 1965: 135.
[37] P.D.A. Harvey 1965: 135; Shrewsbury 1971: 103.
[38] Benedictow 2002.
[39] Ziegler 1970: 123.

Wight. At the court held on 31 October, the number of recorded deaths of villeins, namely eight, was significantly above the average, and a week later, unusually, an additional court was held, obviously prompted by the onset of catastrophic mortality, when now the deaths of 25 villeins were recorded.[40] This means that the phase characterized by a sprinkling of endemic deaths started c. 20–25 October followed by the usual explosive epidemic development. Presumably, the village was contaminated in the second week of September. It is not clear that the Black Death in Hampshire had its first epidemic outbreak at Titchfield, only that the study of the manor of Titchfield has established the earliest evidence so far. It would not be surprising if similar studies of settlements or communities along the Solent or in the New Forest would yield earlier evidence indicating contamination at the end of August.

Again this accords well with the fact that Bishop Edyngton of Winchester was already distraught in October because of the ravages of the Black Death in his diocese. This corresponds well with the fact that there was a significant increase in institutions in this diocese in December, followed by an abrupt surge in January. The standard assumption that has been established for retrospective analysis on the basis of institutions can also be tested: when institutions to vacant benefices in the diocese show a marked increase from the month of December, a deduction of an average of five weeks for the time elapsing from the death of a parish priest until the institution of his successor in the cure indicates again October as the month the Black Death made itself felt.[41]

The Black Death also marched into the heartlands of England from bridgeheads established along the eastern coast, which can be seen from the fact that it invaded Cambridgeshire several months earlier than Oxfordshire and Buckingham- shire: on the manors of Crowland Abbey, a few kilometres north of Cambridge, the onslaught began in October 1348,[42] while it broke out on the manor of Cuxham in southern Oxfordshire in March, or quite possibly in February.[43] Thus, the Black Death again made its conquest with a large strategic pincer movement.

The time pattern of the epidemic's spread and intensity in Cambridgeshire can be seen from Table 3 when two factors are taken into account: (1) the average delay between the death of a parish priest and the institution of his successor was 4–6 weeks, (2) the pre-plague annual average of institutions in the diocese of Ely (comprising Cambridgeshire and the Isle of Ely) was 3.5 institutions[44] (= monthly average of 0.3). The institution of February and possibly also the institution of March 1349 thus reflect clerical deaths at the end of 1348.

The onset of the rise in the incidence of institutions seems to start somewhat late to really accord with a start of the onslaught of the Black Death in Cambridgeshire in October. This could be taken to suggest that the scholar who has provided the monthly figures for 1349 may have neglected to include institutions in late 1348 that reflected the epidemic process in October and early November, and that the epidemic subsided with the advent of cold or cool winter weather. Table 3 read in the skewed

---

[40] Watts 1998: 23–4. See also James 1999.
[41] Shrewsbury 1971: 91.
[42] Page 1934: 120, 123.
[43] P.D.A. Harvey 1965: 135.
[44] Aberth 1995: 278–9. See also under mortality in England, below, Ch. 32, pp. 354–358.

Table 3: Institutions of new parish priests in Cambridgeshire in 1349

J	F	M	A	M	J	J	A	S	O	N	D
0	1	1	6	6	18	24	12	9	6	3	4

Source: Wood-Legh 1949: 158. See also Aberth 1995: 280.

time perspective of institutions indicates that the epidemic accelerated in the second half of February, reached its peak in May and June and began subsiding in the summer, in late June or, possibly, in early July. One should, however, note that there are about twenty institutions in 1350–1 in excess of the normal incidence, which must reflect clerical deaths in the epidemic for which it had been difficult to find successors, and which are sufficiently numerous to potentially affect the shape of Table 3 when distributed according to various hypothetical alternatives.

By the early autumn, the Black Death was closing in on London in a three-pronged attack, moving by land fastest along two important roads: the road that ran south-eastwards from Gloucester, and the road that ran north-eastwards from Weymouth by way of the towns of Salisbury and Winchester. These two roads met near Reading in a pivotal crossroads where they joined the main road to London. The third prong advanced by ship transport along the coast, allowing a sudden metastatic leap that with remarkable speed could carry the Black Death into the harbour of the great city of London. The Black Death's amazingly rapid movement by ship westwards and north-eastwards up the Bristol Channel may have been exceptionally fast because a ship from Bristol reportedly was involved in the original introduction of plague in England in Weymouth harbour. Otherwise, there is no reason why the Black Death should not move eastwards along the coast from Weymouth by ship as quickly as it had moved westwards. The fact that at the end of September the prior of Christ Church, Canterbury, wrote an alarmed letter to the Bishop of London informing him about various invasions of the Black Death in the diocese,[45] which also comprised the eastern county of Essex with busy seaports like Colchester and Harwich, fits well into this picture. Also the outbreak of the Black Death in the manors of Crowland Abbey just north of Cambridge in October fits into the pattern.[46] This means that under otherwise equal circumstances, the Black Death would be expected to reach London by sea with quite a moderate time lag in relation to its invasion of Bristol, keeping in mind that the coastal distance from Weymouth to Bristol is longer than to London.

Two disparate dates are given by chroniclers with respect to the time of the Black Death's outbreak in London, Michaelmas and All Saints',[47] i.e., 29 September and 1 November, respectively. This represents not only a problem relating to the time-structure of the epidemic's progression but also a problem as regards the route and means of transport used by the Black Death's army of lethal bacteria and fleas in

[45] Ziegler 1970: 161.
[46] Page 1934; 120, 123.
[47] Gasquet 1908: 107.

order to invade this great city. An important clue to the effect that plague was carried to London by ship is the fact pointed out by Ziegler, that the Black Death broke out in London earlier than in the surrounding countryside.[48] Another clue is afforded by the fact that the first clerical death from plague in Winchester occurred on 1 January 1349, because Winchester is situated on the highway from Weymouth to London, and at the time the Black Death had ravaged London for at least two months.[49] At the time, London was approaching the sociological status of a metropolis, and a recognized outbreak on 29 September implies, according to the standard assumption, that London was contaminated nearly or about eight weeks earlier, i.e., around 4 August.

At the time, with out-parishes, London contained probably about 80,000 inhabitants, possibly even 100,000, according to recent research,[50] corresponding to around 1.5 per cent of the population of England and Wales, quite a high percentage for an urban centre in the medieval period. This would reflect the economic dynamism of the city and an extraordinary vitality in the economic interaction with large parts of south-eastern England and even beyond. From the second half of the thirteenth century, the general economic and demographic situation in England was characterized by extreme population pressure on land and other resources for making a living and scraping together the wages and production that would enable people to keep body and soul together. The serious situation for the lower classes manifested itself also in a significant diminution of the English population in the first half of the fourteenth century, even before the arrival of the Black Death.[51] The population pressure on the resources for agricultural production tended to force the population to give up self-sufficiency in economic production in favour of economic specialization in order to produce as efficiently as possible. Instead, they would acquire needed products by barter or sale and purchase that had likewise been produced efficiently and at competitive prices by specialized producers elsewhere. In short, from the end of the thirteenth century until the advent of the Black Death a substantial economic modernization of the English economy would have taken place with a considerably increased emphasis on a market economy. This societal change, which implied greatly increased movement of people and goods and exchange of products, strengthened correspondingly the Black Death's power of spread throughout England and ensured that London would be invaded quite early.

The great size of London measured in number of houses, numbers of people and extension of territory also ensured that the number of rat colonies and their territorial distribution were such as to keep the epidemic going considerably longer than in other communities; there were a substantial number of cases far into 1350.

London's ecclesiastical registers have been lost, and for this reason the Black Death's spread across the city and its out-parishes, and the time pattern of the intensity of the onslaught cannot be identified on the basis of institutions. Instead, as Gasquet discovered, the wills proved in the Court of Hustings provide useful information. These wills have recently been studied more thoroughly by B.E. Megson than Gasquet had the opportunity to do in his pioneering general study of the Black Death

---

[48] Ziegler 1970: 161.
[49] Shrewsbury 1971: 88.
[50] Smith 1991: 50–1.
[51] See, e.g., Smith 1991; Astill and Grant 1991: 226–9.

in England. Wills were legal instruments used by affluent members of society, who in London usually lived in stone or half-timbered houses. They were accustomed to frequent epidemics among the poor masses, and would not be much induced to make their wills in a hurry because some malign epidemic was spreading in the more typical working-class areas and among the poor and destitute. There would be a considerable time lag between the introduction of the Black Death in the environments of the lower classes and when its epidemic manifestations became so clear, near and frightening that the affluent hurried to make wills in the face of an all too likely sudden death. In this great city where the Black Death would need quite some time to develop a more generally threatening epidemic character, the time lag would probably be much the same as for institutions.

The distribution of the wills proved at the Court of Hustings at the time of the Black Death can be seen from Table 4. The court was in recess in August and September, which explains the systematic absence of data for these months. In view of the fact that the annual average of registered wills in the years 1346–8 was twenty-two, important insights emerge from the table. There is an abrupt dramatic surge in the number of wills proved in the court in January 1349, almost equal to the annual average in the preceding three years, which heralds the beginning of the epidemic as reflected in wills. This accords with other events. At the beginning of January, the king prorogued the Parliament that was summoned to assemble in London in that month because '. . . the plague of deadly pestilence had suddenly broken out' in London and its neighbourhood, and 'daily increased in severity so that grave fears were entertained for the safety of those coming there at that time'.[52]

Table 4: Wills proved in the Court of Hustings in London 1348–50

Month	1348	1349	1350
January	3	19	5
February	2	42	19
March	3	39	6
April	–	82	6
May	2	38	4
June	–	29	4
July	8	51	2
August	–	–	–
September	–	–	–
October	2	34	2
November	3	11	3
December	–	7	–
Totals	23	352	51

[52] Gasquet 1908: 107.

One should keep in mind that wills used to be enrolled several months after they had been drawn up, but that this changed abruptly with the Black Death, when the interval between dating and probate decreased sharply. From February 1349 nearly all wills were brought to court within weeks, and sometimes within days after they had been written. The exceptions are the wills proved in January that in several cases bear dates from the previous autumn. Thus, the wills proved in January 1349 indicate that the upper classes began to feel threatened by the epidemic developments in the late autumn, certainly in December, and quite likely also in November. Since the beginning of the epidemic among the poor classes presumably started earlier, the wills tend to confirm the time pattern of the early epidemic developments in London that was outlined above on the basis of other sources: introduction of the contagion at the beginning of August; the first epidemic manifestations emerging in the second half of September, followed by increasing spread and mortality among the poor classes in an early phase that was drawn out by the advent of cool and cold weather in the late autumn; the beginning of the epidemic scare among the affluent classes starting in November or December at the latest; and the epidemic exploding, as it were, with the arrival of warm spring weather. The wills indicate that the Black Death began to abate in the autumn. The wills that could not be proved under the court's recess were presumably proved in the following months, which indicates such a sharply reduced monthly incidence that the process of abatement may quite likely have started in August. It can be seen to have lasted until spring 1350, with many of the wills proved in February still dated from 1349 – so this quite high figure does not suggest any late upsurge of the epidemic. Among the poor, the plague still continued to produce casualties for a number of months.

There were over hundred burial places in London and the suburbs, but nonetheless two emergency cemeteries were established on the outskirts of the City for victims of the Black Death in 1348.[53] This fact further indicates that the early date of the introduction of the plague into London should be preferred. From November on, cool weather slowed down the pace of the epidemiological developments.

At the end of 1348, the Black Death had reached all around the southern coast and northwards along the eastern coast so far that it had been carried up the R. Stour, the border river between Essex and Suffolk/East Anglia. After sailing up the roughly 15 km-long estuary and farther up the river for about another 30 km, the Black Death would have reached the small town of Sudbury. Certainly, its presence is recorded a few kilometres south of this town, in the court of the manor of Cornard Parva (= Little) that was held on 31 March 1349: although there can have been no more than fifty tenants on the manor, six women and three men were registered as having died since the previous court two months earlier, and this, of course, was only the beginning of the epidemic.[54]

Although this is the earliest episode of the Black Death in East Anglia to be found so far, one would like to assume on elementary grounds of epidemiology that this inland manor was not really the first place in the area to be attacked by the Black

[53] Hawkins 1990: 637–8.
[54] Jessopp 1898: 201. It is unfortunate that so little has been done to uncover the spread and mortality of the Black Death in East Anglia since Jessopp published his pioneering work over a hundred years ago.

Death. It is more likely that the Black Death had first landed at Harwich, at the mouth of the estuary,[55] and had been carried up the river by boat or barge. In normal circumstances, it would take some time for the Black Death to move up the river all the way to Sudbury, which quite likely was the local epicentre of dissemination. In addition, it would take some time for the Black Death to develop endemic and epidemic character there, extended by cold or at least cool winter weather, before it was in some way carried on to the manor of Cornard Parva where, for the same seasonal reason, at least five weeks would elapse before the Black Death began to harvest human victims in a distinct epidemic form. These elementary epidemiological considerations suggest that the Black Death was introduced into these southernmost districts of East Anglia at the end of 1348.

It is easy to imagine that the further development of the Black Death in this part of England eventually took on the character of inundation: plague contagion now flowed out of London in all directions and was closing in on the floods of contamination that were flowing south-eastwards from the early epicentres in western England, and northwards and eastwards from landings on the coasts of Hampshire and Sussex in the south, and northwards and westwards from landings on the coasts of Kent and Essex.

From this part of England, the Black Death moved further northwards and inland according to the same main strategy and the locally specialized types of tactics that it had employed with such outstanding success: finding transportation along the coast by ship, slipping contagion ashore in seaports and sending expeditionary forces up estuaries and navigable rivers; moving at a slower and more erratic pace along highways and roads; fanning out into the countryside along tracks and other local lines of communication, penetrating villages and manors; continuously recruiting fresh local forces of rats and fleas.

From the conquered areas in south-eastern England the Black Death struck into the dioceses of Lincoln and York, which for reasons of the pattern of spread of the Black Death in central and northern England must be discussed together. The large diocese of Lincoln comprised eight counties running from Oxfordshire in the south to the southern shores of the Humber in the north. The number of institutions began to increase noticeably from April 1349, but other sources conspicuously and surprisingly disclose that the Black Death had clearly begun its ravages earlier, not only in the south of the diocese, but also in the north. It broke out on the manor of Cuxham in southern Oxfordshire in March or quite possibly as early as in February; if we take into account the characteristic slowdown of the epidemic process by cool winter weather, the contamination of the manor in all likelihood took place in January.[56] In the cathedral city of Lincoln, which is situated about 190 km north-east of Cuxham as the crow flies and about 55 km south of the Humber, the outbreak of the Black Death was recognized on 5 April (Palm Sunday).[57] If we also take into account the slowdown of the epidemic process caused by cool weather, this dating implies, according to the standard assumption, that the contagion had been introduced around mid-February.

[55] Shrewsbury 1971: 85, n. 4.
[56] P.D.A. Harvey 1965: 135–6.
[57] Ziegler 1970: 185.

When we also take into account that some time would elapse before the spread of the Black Death in southern Oxfordshire and in northern Lincolnshire reached Cuxham and Lincoln, it becomes clear that both southern Oxfordshire and Lincolnshire must have been invaded in the last months of 1348. The invasion of the southern parts of the diocese must be seen in the context of the part of the south-western plague front that moved eastwards from Gloucestershire and Wiltshire. The outbreak in Lincoln must have a very different background: the close contemporaneity of the outbreaks of the Black Death in the south of Oxfordshire and in northern Lincolnshire 190 km away shows with great clarity that, in the autumn of 1348, the Black Death must have made at least one metastatic leap from the contaminated towns on the coast of south-eastern England to a seaport town that cannot have been situated far from Lincoln. Grimsby immediately comes to mind, and possibly also Hull if we assume rapid and widespread dissemination out of Hull by ship along both sides of the Humber. If it is justified on the basis of this indirect evidence to assume that the Black Death landed in Grimsby in late 1348, the Black Death would have had time to spread by land the distance of about 50 km to Lincoln by February.

However, there is also an alternative way the Black Death could have used to reach Lincoln at that time. This point can be made in the light of the epidemic events in the diocese of York. In addition to Yorkshire, which at the time stretched down to the northern shores of the Humber, the diocese of York included in the west the medieval county of Lancashire north of the R. Ribble and in the south Nottinghamshire, which (also at that time) was conterminous with Lincolnshire along its eastern border. The earliest concrete reference to the Black Death is a licence issued by the archbishop on 15 May 1349 that permitted the consecration of a new cemetery for the town of Newark, because of the alarming growth of the 'pestilence'. Newark is situated on the R. Trent in east-central Nottinghamshire, about 70 km upstream from the inner area of the Humber. Quite some time would elapse from the introduction of plague contagion into Newark until such a licence would be produced: it would comprise the time from the contamination until epidemic mortality reached such levels that it became urgent to address the archbishop in order to obtain such a licence, and, in addition the time needed to identify his whereabouts and to reach him with this plea. February may appear to be a likely time for the beginning of these developments. In this case, plague contagion must have been transported by ship from Grimsby (or possibly Hull) to the mouth of the R. Trent and 70 km upstream to Newark. Quite likely, this did not take place in a single metastatic leap by a ship sailing directly to Newark, but in one or two intermediary steps, which implies quite a time-consuming process and again indicates that plague contagion arrived in Grimsby (or possibly Hull) in late 1348. Newark is situated only about 25 km south-west of Lincoln, so it becomes perhaps at least as likely that the contamination of the cathedral city was occasioned by contagion passed on by land from Newark than by land from Grimsby. The early outbreak of Newark discloses also that the Black Death was now spreading rapidly by boat down the R. Trent to mid-England where it would meet the plague front that was moving northwards from southern England, which it had conquered in 1348.

A local chronicler dates the outbreak in the cathedral city of York to around Ascension Day, which that year was 21 May. According to the standard assumption on the time-structure of the epidemiological processes from the time of contamination of an urban centre of this size to the recognition of the epidemic outbreak of plague, this

implies that the city was probably contaminated around 1 April. Again it is a conspicuous fact that York, like Newark, is situated on a large river flowing into the Humber,
namely the R. Ouse. Although the time of the recognized outbreak in York was 1.5
months later than in Lincoln, it must be probable that the source of contagion in the
region was the same as for Newark and Lincoln.

The long coastlines of Lincolnshire and Yorkshire made these counties vulnerable
to the naval tactics employed so successfully by the Black Death. Plague contagion
was transported by ship from a contaminated seaport town in south-eastern England
to a port on the Humberside in the autumn of 1348, probably to Grimsby, or possibly
Hull, or both; in the following months it was spread further upstream along the large
rivers that flow into the Humber, most importantly the R. Trent and the R. Ouse and
this river's extensive ramifications of tributaries. These large rivers are navigable by
ship over large or largish distances, further upstream for quite some distances with
boats and barges, the Trent all the way from the river mouth to Burton-upon-Trent in
Staffordshire in the very heartland of England. Only this pattern can explain the
spread of the Black Death to Newark in Nottinghamshire (upstream on the R. Trent)
and to the cathedral city of York (upstream on the R. Ouse) in early 1349. However,
inevitably plague must also have been disseminated quite rapidly up the large tributaries that flow into the Ouse at various places along its course: the R. Derwent from
the north-west, but more importantly from the north-east the R. Swale, the R. Ure,
the R. Nidd and the R. Wharfe. In addition, the substantial R. Aire flows into the
Humber close to the mouth of R. Ouse after having been joined by the R. Calder
from the west. about 15 km south-east of Leeds. Along this great river system plague
contagion fanned out with great intensity north-westwards, westwards, southwards
and south-westwards.

In the first half of 1349, a great plague front was established in north-eastern
England on the basis of at least one landing of contagion on Humberside in late 1348,
quite probably in Grimsby. Its rapidly growing forces soon split up into two plague
fronts. One front spread southwards and south-westwards, the other westwards
through Yorkshire into Lancashire, where it reached the Irish Sea, and also moved
northwards into the diocese of Durham. Thus, from the first half of 1349 three plague
fronts were expanding through England: one front moved northwards out of
southern England, another moved south-westwards and southwards out of Humberside and a third moved north-westwards and northwards, also out of Humberside.
Only this pattern of spread can explain that the Black Death in 1349 succeeded in
covering the remaining main bulk of England's territory from the frontier it had
established in southern England in 1348, and even make significant conquests in
southern Scotland.

This is a general description of the process of the final conquest of England in
1349, but there were, of course, a great number of smaller but significant epidemic
events. When the sailing season reopened in March or early April the Black Death
again leapt along the coast to seaport towns.

On the western side of England, the Black Death spread also northwards out of
Gloucestershire. In the diocese of Coventry and Lichfield, the archdeaconry of
Coventry, which covered roughly the north-eastern half of the county of Warwick,
lost its first parish priest in the beginning of April. Arguably, this priest's death was
probably not due to plague. According to the standard assumption relating to institu-

tions, the time of contamination of this parish should ordinarily have occurred 11 or 15 weeks earlier. However, it has been shown that in the case of the diocese of Coventry and Lichfield the time lag between the death of the beneficed priest and the institution of his successor was, on average, only 18 days, and not the ordinary average of five weeks. Consequently, in this special case, the standard assumption should be reduced to 8.5 or 12.5 weeks.[58] Thus the time of contamination of this priest's parish appears to have been around 7 February, according to the first alternative of this standard assumption, or around 20 January. This does not fit well with what we otherwise know about the spread of the Black Death, and it therefore appears likely that this parish priest's death was not caused by the Black Death.

In the archdeaconry of Stafford, the first priest died from plague at the very end of April, but the whereabouts of his parish is not known, which makes it problematic to identify the direction whence the Black Death first moved into Staffordshire. According to the standard assumption, the parish of this priest could have been contaminated by plague in early March or, alternatively, a month earlier. Since the Black Death did not break out in the manor of Halesowen in northern Worcestershire until May,[59] indicating a time of contamination about six weeks earlier in this case, the death of this priest appears to have been occasioned by plague contagion on the move by boat south-westwards upstream on the R. Trent: Newark had probably been contaminated as early as in February and the Trent is, as mentioned, navigable all the way to Burton in east-central Staffordshire. No doubt, soon afterwards the plague crossed also the northern borders of Worcestershire and Warwickshire into southern Staffordshire.

This process of epidemic territorial conquest developed with decreasing pace as the northern plague front was expanding southwards and approaching the western English counties on the border with Wales and made its way through districts that at the time were increasingly peripheral to the main lines of commercial activity, transport of goods and travel in England. In Derbyshire and Cheshire, the mortality of the parish clergy took on serious proportions in mid-June. Shropshire was not noticeably affected until the end of the month.[60] Spread by land across Hereford and Cheshire from the north and south, and across Staffordshire and Worcestershire was also a fairly slow process.

Thus, it is possible to discern a pattern where the southern plague front that was moving northwards from the positions conquered in 1348 and the northern front that was moving southwards from north-eastern England met in central England along an obviously sharply zigzagged line, but probably somewhere in Shropshire, Staffordshire, Leicestershire and Northamptonshire.

The registers of institutions for the diocese of Durham and the diocese of Carlisle in northern England bordering on the Kingdom of Scotland appear to have been lost or to be only partially extant and cannot, therefore, be of much use for the history of the Black Death. It is known that it was present in the county of Durham in the summer.[61] Almost nothing is known about the progression of the Black Death in

---

[58] R.A. Davis 1989: 88.
[59] Razi 1980: 102. Cf. Dyer 1980: 237.
[60] R.A. Davis 1989: 86.
[61] R. Lomas 1989: 128.

these dioceses, although they were clearly ravaged by plague in the second half of 1349.[62]

The English sources for the history of the Black Death do not lend themselves well to analysis of the pace of its spread. Apparently, the Black Death started its spread out of Weymouth around 1 June and its conquest of England was completed in 1349 at a time when the remainder of that year permitted it to make significant territorial gains in southern Scotland. It took roughly 500 days to cover the full length of the English land area, a distance of roughly 500 km as the crow flies. The resultant average pace of 1 km per day in a crow-flying perspective provides some sense of proportion to the question of pace, but has, obviously, considerable weaknesses. One must, for instance, take into account that England was conquered by three plague fronts, one established in the summer of 1348 in southern England and two others were formed in north-eastern England in the first half of 1349. This fact suggests that each plague front moved at considerably slower pace, perhaps much like in Switzerland. Admittedly, as the crow flies is an artificial gauge of distance for those times, although not quite so much with respect to transportation by ship along the coast as by land. It makes it quite likely that, on the ground, even when spurred on by ship transport along coastal sea lanes or navigable waterways, it is probable that the thrust in a specific direction usually did not take place at a higher average pace than something in the order of magnitude of 2 km per day, and that the normal average daily pace along roads and tracks with their bends and curves and shifting directions may have been something in the order of magnitude of 1–1.5 km. However, one is sorely missing more information on the spread of plague upstream along the numerous navigable English rivers.

Wales, Ireland and Scotland

In the middle of the fourteenth century, Wales was in practice divided into the lowland 'Englishry' and the upland 'Welshry'. The Englishry was largely controlled by colonizers from England. It was run on a manorial basis similar to that of England, and, thus, the preserved records are similar in type and volume to those that obtain in England. In the Welshry, the native Welsh population still retained control of their country, and precisely because the writ of the English hardly ran, the few surviving records provide scant information on the Black Death.[63]

The Black Death's early leap to Bristol and Gloucester ensured that Wales would be invaded quite early. By March 1349 at the latest, the lordship of Abergavenny in the county of Monmouth was in the merciless grip of the Black Death. Rees considers that it probably had been introduced by ship from England, and that this also was the case with the outbreak in Carmarthen. Two of the officials of the Staple in Carmarthen were among the early victims, and since they were in regular contact with the vessels calling at the harbour, they would have a particularly high risk of

---

[62] Gasquet 1908: 183–7; Ziegler 1970: 191–3; Shrewsbury 1971: 115, 117–19.
[63] Ziegler 1970: 198–9.

exposure to plague contagion. The incomes of the Lord of Carmarthen fell disastrously.

It appears that the Black Death also entered Wales in the north-west after having made its way through the English border counties (Herefordshire, Shropshire and Cheshire). Its ravages in the Lordship of Ruthin in the county of Denbigh have been studied by Rees, who has succeeded in demonstrating how mortality suddenly shot up from early June and abated in the late autumn. The Black Death caused severe if not consistently high mortality also in the mountain region of Snowdonia and in the Isle of Anglesey farther west.[64]

What little is known about the Black Death's arrival and ravages in Ireland comes mostly from a longish contemporary account by John Clyn, a Minorite friar of the convent of Kilkenny in south-eastern Ireland.[65] He writes:

> It first commenced near Dublin, at Howth and at Drogheda. These cities – Dublin and Drogheda – it almost destroyed and emptied of inhabitants, so that from the beginning of August to the Nativity of our Lord, in Dublin alone 14,000 people died.

Ignoring the mortality statistic, which must have been taken out of thin air, John Clyn provides some important information on the early phase of the Black Death: it broke out in epidemic form in the towns Drogheda, almost 50 km north of Dublin, and Howth (= Dalkey) on the southern tip of Dublin Bay just outside Dublin at the beginning of August; the outbreak in Dublin is also dated to August, and must, consequently, have started only a week or two later than the original outbreaks.

The epidemic was apparently quite widespread in September and October 1348, when people and ecclesiastics streamed to the pilgrimage centre of Teach Molinge (on the R. Burrow) 'some through devotion, others, and indeed most, through fear of the pestilence which then was very prevalent'.

According to this information, the Black Death must have been shipped from south-western England to Ireland without much delay. In order to have had time to develop epidemic form by the beginning of August, the contagion must have been introduced into Drogheda and Howth directly from Weymouth by a ship contaminated shortly before the recognized outbreak, c. 21 June. An introduction from Bristol, as often assumed, appears almost impossible.

Not much is known about the further spread of the Black Death in Ireland, but John Clyn notes that eight friars had died between Christmas and 6 March in his own convent of Kilkenny:

> And I, Brother John Clyn, of the order of Minorites, and the convent of Kilkenny, have written these noteworthy things which have happened in my time and which I have learned as worthy of belief. And lest notable acts should perish with time and pass out of the memory of future generations, seeing these many ills, and that the world is placed in the midst of evils, I, as

---

[64] Rees 1923: 30–1.
[65] His account is rendered by Gasquet 1908: 138–40. The best accounts of the Black Death in Ireland is Gwynn 1935 and Ziegler 1970: 202–5.

if amongst the dead, waiting till death do come, have put into writing truth-
fully what I have heard and verified. And that the writing may not perish
with the scribe, and the work fail with the labourer, I add parchment to continue it, if by chance anyone may be left in the future and any child of Adam
may escape this pestilence and continue the work thus commenced.

Here follows a single paragraph written in 1349, and the copyist's brief entry: '*Videtur
quod Author hic obiit*' = 'It seems that the author died here.'

Although there is nothing unrealistic in John Clyn's emphatic statement to the effect
that the Black Death broke out in Ireland in August 1348, considerable doubt has been
expressed on this point, especially by Ziegler. He points out that, in a sermon preached
before Pope Clemens in Avignon in August 1349, Archbishop Richard Fitzralph of
Armagh states that the pestilence had killed two-thirds of the English but had not yet
done conspicuous harm to the Irish or to the Scots. Ziegler infers from this that the Black
Death could not have broken out by the time the archbishop had left Ireland, or, just
possibly, that John Clyn could have observed some endemic cases in 1348. Ziegler
supports his doubts by pointing out that the Archbishop of Dublin died on 14 July 1349
and the Bishop of Meath in the same month.[66]

There is no way that John Clyn's account can be reconciled with a sprinkling of
endemic cases. Probably, another part of the archbishop's sermon should be underlined, in which he states that few Irishmen would be able to make a certain
pilgrimage because there were few ships in Ireland, and now there was also a shortage
of seamen 'for the plague has fallen most heavily on those who lived near the sea, and
has found more victims among fisherfolk and sailors than among any other class of
men'. This shows that the archbishop was aware that serious mortality caused by the
Black Death had already taken place in Ireland, which highlights a different interpretation from Ziegler's, namely that the archbishop referred to the English within the
Pale. The Pale was at the time a band of land on the eastern coast that was in the
hands of the English Crown, stretching from Dundalk near the border of present-day
Northern Ireland to Dalkey (= Howth) at the end of Dublin Bay. This area had seen
intensive colonization and settlement by English peasants within a familiar
socio-economic manorial context since it was established at the end of the twelfth
century.[67] In other words, Archbishop Fitzralph's statement should quite likely be
taken to mean that the English both in England and within the Pale in Ireland had
suffered immensely from the Black Death and that the epidemic by the summer of
1349 had not yet spread much in the Irish-dominated part of Ireland or in Scotland.

It appears quite unlikely that John Clyn should misdate by a year the time of the
most dramatic event, which he relates with such intensity. Importantly, his dating
does not stand alone. In the Annals of Clonmacnoise it is stated under 1348: 'There
was a general plague in Moylurg and all Ireland in general, whereof the earl of
Ulster's grandchild died.'[68] John Clyn states that several of his brothers in the
convent died of plague in the period stretching from Christmas 1348 until 6 March
1349, and it appears that he himself died shortly afterwards, according to the terse

---

[66] Ziegler 1970: 203.
[67] Otway-Ruthven 1968: 109.
[68] Shrewsbury 1971: 48.

statement added by another hand. It appears difficult to reconcile these facts with the implication of Ziegler's doubts, that the Black Death ravaged the convent of Kilkenny in 1350.

There is such a severe paucity of source material for the history of the Black Death in Scotland that it is virtually impossible to discuss the matter at all. Southern parts of Scotland were apparently invaded by the Black Death in the second half of 1349, but 1350 was the year when most of Scotland was affected.[69]

---

[69] Ziegler 1970: 205–8.

16

Norway[1]

From England, the Black Death sailed north-westwards to Norway. It arrived later in Denmark, and quite likely not directly from England. The Black Death was poised to strike Iceland from Bergen in the autumn of 1349, probably in mid-August. It had entered an Icelandic ship that was preparing to leave for Iceland, but the epidemic broke out on board before it was ready to sail and the voyage had to be cancelled. This story is tersely related in one of the Icelandic chronicles cited below. No ship arrived in Iceland from Norway in 1349, and this prevented the Black Death from ending its series of metastatic leaps by ship northwards along Europe's western coasts with a triumphant landing in Iceland. Iceland was not attacked by plague until the fifteenth century.[2]

However, the Black Death succeeded in reaching the other Norse settlements in the Atlantic Ocean, namely the Shetland Islands, the Orkney Islands and the Faroe Islands by metastatic leaps by ship from western Norway. The Faroe Islands were to be the final north-western destination of the Black Death's spread by metastatic leaps by ship in Europe. In the north of Europe, the Black Death's use of metastatic leaps scored its final triumph, as far as we are able to know, in the cathedral city of Nidaros (Trondheim) in central Norway.

There is no evidence that the Black Death reached Greenland, and all notions to this effect are pure speculation. The desolation of the Norse settlement there in the course of the fifteenth century is explained on entirely independent grounds.

There is a severe paucity of sources for the history of the Black Death in the Nordic countries.

One should note that the Nordic countries, Norway, Iceland, Denmark, Sweden and Finland, together cover roughly 1.3 million sq. km and thus constitute a large

---

[1] The central works on the Black Death's history in Norway are Benedictow 1993/1996a and Benedictow 2002, which gives the complete plague history of Norway from 1348 to 1654 and also contains some new material on the Black Death and develops some points further, but which is available only in Norwegian.

[2] I must, unfortunately, warn readers interested in the history of plague in Northern Europe against a paper on the two Icelandic plague epidemics in the fifteenth century that was published a few years ago: G. Karlsson, 'Plague without rats: the case of fifteenth-century Iceland', *Journal of Medieval History*, 22, 1996: 263–84. The special nature of this paper provoked strong reactions among Icelandic scholars. After a heated conference where this paper was very much in a critical focus, nine papers were published in the Icelandic historical journal *Sagnir. Tímarit um söguleg efni*, 18, 1997: 73–114.

part of Europe, a territory almost as large as that of Spain, Italy, France and England and Wales added together (c. 1.4 million sq. km).

The social systems of the Nordic countries differed in important respects from those of contemporary Europe. They were only partly feudalized, Norway (and Iceland) the least. Agricultural land was privately owned and not, in principle, in the king's gift, being distributed on the basis of homage and feudal service. The peasantry was personally free and owned probably around one-half of the agricultural land in Sweden and possibly around one-third of the agricultural land in Norway,[3] but only about 10–15 per cent in Denmark.[4] Manors and estates consisted mostly of quite widely dispersed tenements. Also for this reason, manors and estates did not function as a level of the administrative and judicial system of the respective countries. Instead, there was a national administrative system based on territorially integrated and continuous areas that were all held directly on a personal contractual basis from the king by noblemen (including gentry), and occasionally also by bishops, on condition of performing various essential administrative services. In Norway, such an administrative district was called 'sysle', or as in the other Nordic countries, 'len'; for practical considerations of language the English territorial synonymous terms county and shire will be used. The main administrative subdivision was 'herred', which corresponds quite closely to the English term hundred.

Around the middle of the seventeenth century Sweden made substantial and permanent territorial gains, especially from Denmark, but also from Norway, which lost about 10 per cent of its population. Thus, the modern territories of the Nordic countries differ from the medieval, as does the relative size of the populations, Sweden's being much enlarged, while especially Denmark's is much diminished. At the time of the Black Death, the counties of Bohuslän, Jämtland and Härjedalen, comprising c. 55,000 sq. km, belonged to the state of Norway. Bohuslän was the quite densely populated south-easternmost county in Norway, reaching all the way to the R. Göta Älv, the old-time border river between southern Norway and Sweden that runs past present-day Gothenburg. Jämtland and Härjedalen constituted the eastern-most parts of central Norway. They comprised large territories but contained only tiny populations. Jämtland comprised, for instance, an area of 37,500 sq. km, corresponding to the size of present-day Denmark or twice the size of Wales, but contained only 1,130 peasant holdings or about 5,600 inhabitants, giving a population density of only 0.15 persons per sq. km. The medieval Norwegian national territory constituted about 350,000 sq. km,[5] which was inhabited by about 350,000 persons of whom

---

[3] Rosén 1962: 661. The empirical basis of the Norwegian figure has still not been published several decades after it was first forwarded, and must by now be considered quite uncertain, or rather, unfortunately, unusable.

[4] Rasmussen 1994: 70.

[5] The northernmost region of Finmark comprises 47,500 sq. km, a much larger territory than modern Denmark (39,000 sq. km), Belgium, the Netherlands or Switzerland, but still contained only a few thousand inhabitants in 1567, and may have had a population density of the order of magnitude of 0.06 persons per sq. km, considerably smaller than the county of Jämtland. However, almost all inhabitants, whether Norwegians or Saami, lived along the coast. For these reasons, the terrritory of Finmark is largely subtracted because the borders were obscure and the tiny population lived along the coast. Including Finmark, Norway's medieval territory would be 380,000 sq. km; subtracting most of Finmark for the mentioned reasons gives a rough estimate of Norway's functional state territory of around 350,000 sq. km.

about 15,000 lived in urban centres.[6] Consequently, population density was only one person per sq. km. This is, of course, a somewhat artificial estimate, because most of the country consisted of enormous tracts of almost uncolonized mountains, forests, moors and lakes, with vast regions like Jämtland, Härjedalen and Finmark almost uninhabited. The population was strongly concentrated in the more or less fertile agricultural areas that were suitable for arable and animal husbandry.

In the High Middle Ages, Norway's population grew considerably, producing an increasing population pressure of a distinctly Malthusian kind that led to considerable colonization also in mountain areas. In the mountain settlements, the peasants had to concentrate on animal husbandry based on extensive use of vast grazing lands, but they also endeavoured to grow as much grain as possible, which often meant a substantial deficit. The mountain settlements were, therefore, based on a more specialized type of production and, as a consequence, were more dependent on exchange of goods in a market-oriented type of economy than the more self-sufficient anciently settled communities in the lowlands. They were dependent on exchange of goods for their survival and had to sell or barter excess production from animal husbandry and products from exploitation of the more specific resources of the mountain areas in order to obtain products that were essential for their survival, especially salt and grain.

The epidemiological point is that this type of specialized economy was dependent on regular trade through stable trade and communication lines stretching all the way from coast to mountains.[7] These communication lines strengthened the territorial integration of the country, but were also suitable for the transport and dissemination of the Black Death. Furthermore, the vital transport of grain up to the mountain settlements was a product of particular epidemiological importance. As emphasized above, the black rat much prefers grain for nourishment, which is why it is a typical house rat and ship rat. As a result its ordinary type of flea has developed the ability to live off grain and grain debris (because this is a usual nutritional element in the environments where they fall off or are scratched off by the self-cleansing activities of rats), and are dependent on blood only for reproduction. Plague infection is, therefore, easily transported at a distance in the gut of fleas in shipments of grain both by sea and by land, which is the usual basis for plague's metastatic leaps (above, p. 20). Thus, in the centuries preceding the arrival of the Black Death, demographic and economic circumstances had developed that were highly suited to the dissemination of disease in general and of the Black Death in particular.

Ship transport had, of course, always been important, and played a major role in the Norwegian economic system. In the High Middle Ages, a substantial trade developed with other countries, especially with England, and towards the end of the thir-

---

[6]   Benedictow 1996b: 179–80; Benedictow 1996c: 177–81; Benedictow 2000: 84–89. The estimate of the size of Norway's population is based mainly on an estimate of the total number of free holdings and of tenements in operation in Norway in the first decades of the fourteenth century. Recently, this estimate has on persuasive grounds been revised upwards from 60,000 to somewhat above 64,000 within the present borders of Norway. The territorial losses of the seventeenth century caused a decrease in the number of agricultural holdings of c. 12.5 per cent, thus, the number within Norway's medieval borders amounted to around 73,250, containing, on average, 4.5 persons. The non-farming population can be roughly estimated at about 5 per cent of the total population.
[7]   Martens 1989: 73–91; Martens 1990: 70–80.

teenth century increasingly with the Hanseatic cities along the German coasts of the North Sea and the Baltic Sea. In this trade, the Hansards primarily brought grain to Norway, to some extent also the English merchants.[8] In connection with the Black Death, the lively economic exchange with England was to decide the time and place of the plague's arrival. The ominous importance of the English–Norwegian trading connections in this case can be illustrated with a concrete instance: on 8 May 1349, King Edward III issued an export licence for Thomas and William de Melchebourn, giving them the right to export 1,000 quarters of grain in order to do business with Norway.[9]

The Black Death invaded Norway with two separate metastatic leaps by ship from England, the first one in all likelihood to Oslo, by far the largest town in southern Norway, the other to Bergen on the western coast.

What induced the townsmen of Oslo to take the initiative to found an altar to St Sebastian in the cathedral of Oslo in the late autumn of 1348?[10] Before the arrival of the Black Death in Europe, altars to this saint were not usual, and this was the first time an altar for this saint had been founded in Norway. His reputation as a protector saint against plague dated back to the first identified pandemic of plague that ravaged large parts of Europe from 541 to 767.[11] After plague returned with the Black Death, there was a spontaneous tremendous increase in his popularity. Interestingly, the new altar for St Sebastian in Oslo is one of the very earliest to be mentioned in Europe.

The lively commercial contacts between seaports in south-eastern England and Norway, particularly Oslo and Bergen, makes it technically possible that the Black Death could have been introduced into Oslo by a ship (returning) from England at the end of the shipping season and had demonstrated its presence by at least a sprinkling of endemic cases before winter cold suppressed the incipient epidemic. Observations and accounts by returned merchants and crew members with some knowledge of the epidemic disaster that ravaged southern England could have spurred the townsmen into action. On the basis of the usual religious understanding of the cause of epidemic disease they would seek protection through religious precautionary action. They could possibly have learned what the English had done to halt the plague epidemic or they could, of course, have consulted some of the learned ecclesiastics at the cathedral on the advisable religious action.[12] Because the foundation of the altar for St Sebastian can be explained independently as a precautionary preventive measure inspired by the grisly catastrophe that unfolded in England, it does not constitute proof to the effect that the Black Death had invaded Oslo in the autumn of 1348.

---

[8] Bruns 1900; Hansen 1912; Rafto 1958.

[9] *Regesta Norvegica*, Vol. 5, No. 1158a; Calendar of Patent Rolls Edward III, 1348–50, p. 287.

[10] The altar is mentioned for the first time in a document issued 20 February in Oslo, and is referred to as 'newly built'. As the funding and making of such an altar would take some time, it is reasonable to assume that the initiative was taken some time in the late autumn.

[11] Biraben and Goff 1969: 1484–1510. These authors are wrong in their assumption that the first plague pandemic did not reach the British Isles. See also above, p. 39.

[12] Benedictow 1993/1996a: 93–4.

Several sources show that the Black Death was already raging in south-eastern Norway in the summer of 1349. It is stated quite concretely in a document issued in the hundred of Upper Eiker, about 60–80 km south-west of Oslo, where the dating formula refers to 'the summer of the great mortality'.[13] In this part of the country, the outbreak of the epidemic must have started in the late spring or early in the summer, in May or around 1 June at the latest, in order to have spread sufficiently to warrant the use of this dating. The plague in this area must have originated in Oslo, and considering the normal spread rate of plague, this must be taken to indicate that the Black Death had started to spread out of Oslo in April, i.e., roughly at the same time that an English merchant vessel with plague on board and bound for Oslo theoretically could have left a south-eastern port in England at the start of the shipping season for a voyage that normally would take more than a month. Even so, we have not yet taken into account the time for the epidemic processes to develop in Oslo to the point that would start the process of spread out of the city. This highlights the other interesting alternative, that the Black Death went ashore in Oslo from a ship coming from England in late 1348, was prevented by the onset of winter from developing into a full-blown epidemic and, instead, smouldered on in the rat colonies until spring brought warmer weather

Hamar was a small cathedral city lying on the eastern shore of L. Mjøsa, Norway's largest lake, about 130 km north of Oslo. The road to the cathedral city of Nidaros (present-day Trondheim), where the Norwegian archbishop was resident and the cult of St Olav had its international centre, ran through Hamar and was, therefore, much used by pilgrims. *The Chronicle of Hamar* contains a very sentimental, but also to a large extent factually oriented history of this small town. It was written in the mid-sixteenth century,[14] but is still valuable because the anonymous author used the episcopal archives quite extensively, archives that were lost a few decades later. He states that the Black Death ravaged Hamar between *Nativitatis Mariae* and continued to *All Saints'*, i.e., that it started on 8 September and continued to 1 November.[15] The editor has shown that the author generally produced his specifications of time on the basis of dating formulae in relevant case documents or account books and registers, in this specific case using sources that contained references to the Black Death in the text or in dating formulae. This implies that the epidemic quite likely started earlier and ended later than indicated by the author. Certainly, it would take some time for the epidemic process to reach the catastrophic level of mortality that would increase the likelihood that the dramatic events would be reflected in written sources.

The Icelandic annals include Bishop Hallvard of Hamar among the Norwegian bishops who died in the Black Death. The time of the death of Bishop Hallvard of Hamar must be seen in the light of the normal time elapsing in the consequent eccle-

---

13 Benedictow 1993/1996a: 81.

14 The original version of *The Chronicle of Hamar* disappeared long ago. The Chronicle is handed down to posterity in a number of much later transcripts that are themselves transcripts of earlier transcripts, and they have in the process of transcription accumulated a substantial number of so-called scribe's errors that must be taken into account and considered according to the ordinary rules of source criticism. These problems are extensively discussed by Benedictow 1993/1996a on the basis of a very valuable introduction to the original edition by Professor Gustav Storm and later papers by Storm and other Norwegian scholars. See also Ulsig 1994: 97.

15 Hamarkrøniken 1895: 136.

siastical process that comprised the time needed to summon an electoral council of canons at the cathedral church, and the time needed for the bishop elect to prepare for and travel the 415 km to Nidaros with an entourage of elderly ecclesiastics in time to be consecrated by Archbishop Arne before his death on 17 October,[16] or more accurately, before the archbishop fell ill from plague 3–5 days earlier. The journey would have taken about a fortnight, which implies that the new bishop started his journey in the very last days of September or on 1 October at the very latest, if we assume that the consecration was performed on the last day before the archbishop fell ill. More moderate assumptions on this point, including time for the electoral process and preparation for the journey to Nidaros, indicate that Bishop Hallvard probably died in the first half of September. The time he was infected emerges when the normal time for incubation and illness, 6–10 days, is subtracted, which means that he probably was infected around 1 September. Most Norwegian bishops died quite early in the epidemic process, which suggests that the Black Death began to take on an epidemic character in Hamar in mid-August, and hardly later than in the third week of the month. Because it would take almost six weeks from the time plague contagion was introduced into rat colonies in Hamar until the epidemic phase began to develop among the human inhabitants, it appears that the Black Death entered Hamar in the first half of July, and probably early within this time frame.[17]

However, the Black Death in Norway cannot have started in Hamar 130 km inland: it must have spread there from Oslo. As mentioned above, the pace of spread at a distance by land in Western and Northern Europe was usually in the range of 0.66–1.5 km per day, but in a sparsely settled country like Norway one would expect a spread rate in the lower reaches of that range. However, this does not agree with the facts on the ground, which includes a distance of 130 km from Oslo to Hamar and a climate that makes it unlikely that temperatures would reach a level that would allow an epidemic to develop in time to start spreading out of Oslo before the first half of April. The spread rate must have been at or close to the indicated maximum level in order to make it possible for the Black Death to cover the distance from Oslo to Hamar in about 90 days, which would take us back to the first half of April. This conclusion strengthens further the assumption that the Black Death was introduced into Oslo late in the autumn of 1348, because the spread out of Oslo must have started before a ship from England with plague contagion on board could have sailed into the harbour in the following spring; nor have we taken into account the time required for the development of the epidemic from the introduction of contagion to an epidemic phase.

The reason for the high spread rate must have been that Hamar was situated on the main road to Nidaros and that in those dramatic days there was a stream of pilgrims along this road to Nidaros and the shrine of St Olav, the national patron saint.

There is also quite a good indication that the Black Death was raging in the hundred of Idd at the end of August, an area situated about 100 km south of Oslo on the eastern side of the Oslofjord.[18] This indication probably reflects that plague,

---

[16] *Monumenta historica Norvegiæ* 1880: 190; see also the comments by the editor, Gustav Storm.

[17] Benedictow 1993/1996a: 82–7.

[18] Benedictow 1993/1996a: 81–2.

following the main road southwards from Oslo on the eastern side of Oslofjord and sending continuously small expeditionary epidemic forces into the countryside, had also reached this district in the first half of July. This fits well into a pattern in which the Black Death had its epicentre in Oslo, radiating from here along the main roads in various directions, reaching Hamar, 130 km to the north, and the hundred of Idd, about 100 km to the south, at much the same time, while arriving in the hundred of Eiker, 60–80 km from Oslo on the western side of the Oslofjord, correspondingly earlier. This coincidence of events probably reflects that the intensity of movement by people and goods along the road to Hamar and Nidaros was higher than along the roads that ran southwards along the Oslofjord, and that this differentiated the pace of spread of plague correspondingly.

This piece of somewhat uncertain evidence should be seen in the light of a so-called 'open letter' (*litteræ apertæ*) from King Magnus Eriksson of Norway and Sweden to the population of the Swedish diocese of Linköping that was issued some time in September 1349, probably in the first half of September, and within this time frame quite likely around 10 September.[19] In this 'open letter', he informs them, among other things, of the terrible epidemic events that were taking place in countries to the west of them, and that he had summoned the bishops of Linköping and Skara and a number of lay members of the Council of the Realm to a meeting in the town of Lödöse, the precursor of Gothenburg, lying about 10 km upstream on the R. Göta Älv, the border river between medieval south-eastern Norway and Sweden. The purpose of the meeting was to discuss the religious countermeasures that should be taken to prevent the grisly epidemic that at the time was raging 'all over' his Kingdom of Norway, and in Halland,[20] from coming to Sweden. The likely visitation of the Black Death in the hundred of Idd at the end of August fits well into this pattern and may serve to explain the consternation with which King Magnus considered the epidemic developments in Norway at the time. The king's assertion that the Black Death raged over all Norway must be taken to mean that he also had received news of the outbreak in Bergen on the western coast.

There is also evidence to the effect that the Black Death was rife in Toten, a fertile lowland district situated on the western side of L. Mjøsa, at the end of September.[21] In this case, the Black Death would have spread from Oslo northwards along the main road to Vestlandet (the 'West Country') and Bergen, and have sent an arm of contamination along secondary country tracks to Toten, which explains why the Black Death broke out later in Toten than in Hamar, which was situated on the main road to Nidaros. Thus, the later outbreak in Toten does not indicate a slower movement of the Black Death along this main road or a later time of contamination of Oslo. The later use of the dating formula 'the summer of the great mortality' in an area 90 km south-west of Oslo fits well into this general outline of the pattern of spread in time and space.

---

[19] Source-critical problems relating to this document are discussed under Denmark and Sweden. See also Benedictow 2002: 76, and particularly n. 148.

[20] Halland is the medieval Danish (now Swedish) coastal region that stretches southwards almost from the R. Göta Älv and Lödöse almost to Scania.

[21] Benedictow 1993/1996a: 87.

Taken together, these pieces of information make it quite clear that the epicentre or feeder outbreak of the Black Death was in Oslo, and that the epidemic spread radially out of Oslo along the main roads. On the basis of the indications of the time of the Black Death's presence in the various localities given in the sources and reasonable assumptions on pace of spread, it has been possible to ascertain that the outbreak in Oslo must have taken place in the first half of April, quite likely 5–10 April. Taking into consideration the climate of the region, it is difficult to envisage an epidemic outbreak of plague significantly earlier than this date.

Theoretically, the spread out of Oslo could have started immediately after contamination, but it would be more likely to take place in the early epidemic phase when people would begin to flee and traders to hasten departure with their goods. The time horizon of these epidemiological developments is, as mentioned, normally 12 days (epizootic), + 3 days (fasting rat fleas) + 0.5–1 day (before first infective transmission), + 7 days (endemic phase), + 8 days (incubation and illness for the last endemic cases) + 8 days (incubation and illness for the early epidemic cases infected during the endemic phase), in all 39 days, or 5.5 weeks,[22] before transportation of contagion out of Oslo would become a likely occurrence. This perspective indicates that Oslo would have been contaminated by the Black Death in the second week of March. Also the assumption of quite a high average daily pace of spread of 1.5 km can now be seen to include also an assumption about improbably early ship transport from England: a sailing ship moving according to the standard assumption at an average daily speed of 40 km, would cover the distance from south-eastern England to Oslo in about 35 days, which implies that it would have set sail in early February. This most certainly, cannot have been the case; at the time commercial vessels were insufficiently developed to allow international long-distance shipping during the winter season. This line of analysis has, consequently, produced a solid line of argument in support of the scenario that the Black Death was introduced into Oslo in the late autumn of 1348, quite likely in the first half of October. About three to four weeks later, a sprinkling of endemic cases betrayed its presence and, when faced with incipient epidemic developments, the townsmen were induced to found an altar for St Sebastian, before winter cold drove plague underground into a smouldering enzootic unobtrusive presence in the rat colonies. The Black Death then re-emerged in the first half of April. This pattern of plague in Oslo is not exceptional. A plague epidemic in Oslo and the surrounding region in the autumn of 1547 was suppressed by cold winter weather and resurfaced in Oslo in time to have reached serious epidemic intensity at the end of April the following year.[23]

This means that the Black Death probably landed in Norway before it invaded southern Germany roughly 1,500 km to the south. The Black Death's early invasion of Norway shows the significance of sea transport and metastatic leaps by ship in the grand strategy of the Black Death.

*

---

[22] Cf. above the discussion (in connection with the arrival of the Black Death in Constantinople) of the normal time lag between the introduction of the contagion until it had developed epidemic form and when it was recognized by the chronicle-producing élites, and also the discussion above of the correlation between the time of contamination of English parishes and the death of parish priests.

[23] Benedictow 2002: 163–6.

While the Black Death was raging in south-eastern Norway a new and independent introduction of the Black Death by ship from England took place in Bergen, on the western coast, Norway's largest town, with quite probably about 7,000 inhabitants. Two Icelandic annals provide most of the available information on the Black Death in Bergen, namely the *Lawman's Annal*[24] and *Gottskalk's Annal.*[25] At the time, Iceland was incorporated in the Norwegian kingdom and had long constituted part of the Norwegian Church province. For natural reasons of geography, the Icelanders related mostly to western Norway, especially to Bergen. These facts are reflected also in the Icelandic annals: in so far as they take notice of events in Norway, most of their information comes from western Norway, and they usually have little to say about events in other parts of the country. It is, therefore, not really surprising that they contain scant information on the Black Death in south-eastern Norway or central Norway (i.e., the region of Trøndelag with the cathedral city of Nidaros).

On the other hand, what they can tell about concrete events in western Norway appears well-informed, especially on ecclesiastical matters. The likely informants were ecclesiastical dignitaries who lived through those terrible times in Bergen. It is generally and reasonably assumed that the former Abbot of St John's in Bergen, Gyrd Ivarsson, who was consecrated bishop of the Icelandic diocese of Skálholt[26] in 1349, and sailed to Iceland in 1351, has probably provided some of the information. The author of the *Lawman's Annal*, the Icelandic priest Einar Hafliðason,[27] can be shown to be acquainted with the Icelandic Bishop Orm of the diocese of Holar, who stayed in Norway at the time of the Black Death and also returned to Iceland in 1351. The reliability of this annal is strengthened by the description of the clinical manifestations and course of the plague illness, which, as we shall see, is consistent with a non-specialist observation, and closely related to a number of other descriptions elsewhere in Europe.

The *Lawman's Annal* renders the following account of the events:[28]

> At that time, a ship left England with many people on board. It put into the bay [of the harbour] of Bergen, and a little was unloaded. Then, all the people on the ship died. As soon as the goods from this ship were brought into the town, the townsmen began to die. Thereafter, the pestilence swept all over Norway and wrought such havoc that not one-third of the people survived. The English ship sank with its cargo and the dead men, and was not unloaded. More ships, cargo vessels and many other ships, sank or drifted widely around. And the same pestilence visited the Shetland Islands, the Orkney Islands, the Hebrides and the Faroe Islands. That was the sort of the disease that people did not live more than a day or two with sharp pangs of

---

[24] *Lögmanns–annáll*, published in *Islandske Annaler* 1888: 275–6. The name is probably a reference to the judge = lawman who owned it in the seventeenth century. The reader should here perhaps be reminded that the singular form *annal* is used in the meaning of *chronicle* in many European languages

[25] *Gottskálks Annáll*, published in *Islandske Annaler* 1888: 354. For a source-critical presentation of analysis of these annals with references to the scholarly discussion of them in English, see Benedictow 1993/1996a: 44–7; Benedictow 2002: 67–73. My translations.

[26] In Icelandic, á is pronounced as *aw* in English, for instance, in *law* or *saw*, corresponding to the pronunciation of letter å in other Nordic languages.

[27] The letter ð is pronounced as voiced *th* in *then* or the definite article *the* in English, and is also used in phonetic notation of English as the phonetic symbol for this consonant.

[28] See Benedictow 1993/1996a: 71–2. My translation from Old Norse.

pain. After that they began to vomit blood, and then the spirit left them. From this disease expired Archbishop Arne and all the canons of Nidaros [cathedral], with the exception of one who survived, named Lodin. He arranged an election, and appointed Abbot Olaf of Nidarholm archbishop. Likewise died Bishop Thorstein of Bergen. Likewise died Bishop Guttorm of Stavanger. Bishop Hallvard of Hamar also expired at the time. This pestilence did not come to Iceland.

Gottskalk's Annal contains a clue with respect to the source of some of its information. It contains a reference to an Icelandic ship with known owner and persons on board that at the time of the epidemic was ready to sail from Bergen to Iceland but was prevented from sailing because great mortality broke out on board. The implication is that this ship reached Iceland the next year, and that news about the epidemic catastrophe was learned from this source. The account implies at least one well-informed ecclesiastical source who could convey apparently trustworthy details on the number of corpses coming to a cemetery in Bergen at the peak of the epidemic (obviously the cemetery of the Cathedral's parish since there were so many clerics among them). Also the information provided on the events in the coastal parishes of the county of Agder in Sørlandet (the 'South Country') is concrete and detailed, with the different categories of personnel sent by the bishop of Stavanger in order to provide spiritual succour to the victimized population painstakingly specified. Information is also provided on prominent persons who died in the epidemic. The ecclesiastical dignitaries mentioned in connection with the presentation of the *Lawman's Annal* may also have been the source of some of this information. The account runs like this:[29]

> A large killer pestilence came to Norway and Shetland. Then died Dominus Archbishop Arne and Abbot Thorkell [Einarsson] of Helgafell [a monastery in Iceland]. Seven parishes in Agder [a county in southern Norway] were desolated in a short time. The bishop of Stavanger sent there many priests and deacons and his servants, and they all died hastily. The loss of life in Bergen was so great that eighty corpses came to one church on one day, and among them were thirteen priests and six deacons. Died Dominus Bjarne and Dominus Peter and Dominus Olaf. Died Bishop Thorstein of Bergen, Bishop Guttorm of Stavanger, Brother Hamund, Brother Thorvald, Runolf '*anima*' and many other men on Thorlak's ship so that she could not go to Iceland . . .

The reliability of both these annals on the matter under discussion is strengthened not only because good sources of information can be indicated. Their trustworthiness is also underscored by the information they furnish on the deaths of prominent Norwegian and Icelandic ecclesiastics, which in many cases can be tested and verified on the basis of independent material; in no case can they be falsified.

Yet although the two annals' accounts are probably founded, to a considerable extent, on solid information provided by known persons arriving in Iceland from Bergen in the following years, they cannot be used as scholarly accounts of high academic value. Einar Hafliðason, the anonymous author of *Gottskalk's Annal*, Bishop Gyrd Ivarsson or Bishop Orm were not modern scholars by training or ambition. In

---

29 My translation from Old Norse.

fact, the annals relate not only information that on closer examination proves to be trustworthy but also include extravagant exaggerations. Immediately before the point where the citation of Einar Hafliðason's Annal begins, he states that only fourteen persons survived the plague in London. To take a less extreme example: it must be clear that his assertion that less than one-third of Norway's population survived is not based on any sort of censuses, parish registers or any other type of systematic demographic information. It is also clear that the annal writers knew almost nothing about the epidemic events in south-eastern Norway. Accordingly, it should be considered a crude guestimate meaning unheard-of mortality and a disastrous reduction of the population.

These chronicles do not provide any specific information with respect to the time that the ship from England with plague on board put into the bay of the harbour of Bergen. Fortunately, there are a few helpful indications in the sources that point at the first half of July as the likely time of contamination, quite likely in the early part of that period, in that the change from the endemic to the epidemic phase took place in the second half of August and that the Black Death had presented itself as a fully-fledged killer epidemic around 1 September.[30]

This dating of the time of Bergen's contamination makes King Edward III's licence of 8 May for the merchants Thomas and William de Melchebourn of Lynn to export grain to Norway very interesting indeed (see above, p. 149). Only a few English ships sailed to Norway with grain on board, and this trade was generally quite small, as also illustrated by the fact that it was necessary to obtain a royal licence for quite a small amount that would take up only a small part of a ship's cargo space. It is known from the preceding years that the burghers of Lynn exported mainly grain to Bergen.[31] In the spring and summer of 1349, the Black Death raged in Norfolk and Lincolnshire, precisely in the area around the large bay known as the Wash where Lynn (now King's Lynn) is situated. It would take some time to acquire the grain from the surrounding districts, transport it to Lynn, load it and to make the ship ready to put to sea. This, then, is quite likely the very ship that brought the Black Death to Bergen.

There are no sources relating to the history of the Black Death north of Nidaros. Thus, Nidaros constitutes the northern end of the Black Death's European history. It also represents the northern end of the Black Death's known use of metastatic leaps by ship.

Gottskalk's Annal provides, as mentioned, a detailed and, it would seem, trustworthy account of the Black Death's dramatic ravages in seven parishes in Agder on the coast of Sørlandet that was in the bishop of Stavanger's obedience. The bishop of Stavanger sent priests, deacons and servants there in order to provide the local population with spiritual services, but they all died. Conspicuously, the account does not contain any hint to the effect that the plague actually was present in the small cathedral city of Stavanger at the time. Presumably, this is the reason the bishop had at his disposal extra clerical personnel and servants who could be sent there to ensure the continuity of ecclesiastical and spiritual service to the population. Thus, the

---

[30] Benedictow 2002: 73–6.
[31] Benedictow 2002: 76.

annal's account indicates that plague reached the southern coastal parishes of Agder in Sørlandet before it reached Stavanger in south-western Norway.

This pattern of events indicates that, at the time the parishes in Agder were ravaged, the epidemic had not spread the 150 km from Bergen to Stavanger that would usually be covered in about four days by ship; perhaps, the Black Death had not yet arrived in Bergen. This indicates that the Black Death did not arrive in the southern coastal parishes of Agder from Stavanger, but from the considerably earlier introduction of plague in the south-eastern part of Norway where the Black Death was in full swing in the summer months. Apparently, the plague in Agder was due to a metastatic leap by ship from south-eastern Norway, in all likelihood from Oslo. One should note that the main sea lane from Oslo along the western side of Oslofjord and Sørlandet had three important destinations along the coast of Agder.[32]

While raging in the cathedral city of Hamar and the country district of Toten, the Black Death moved further northwards along the main roads to Nidaros and to Bergen, respectively. On the holding of Hammar in the hundred of Vågå[33] at the northern end of the principal valley of Gudbrandsdalen a person died of plague on 31 October, and in Valdres, a district of south-central Norway about halfway between Oslo and the county of Sogn, the dating formula 'the autumn of the (great) mortality' is used in the aftermath of the Black Death. Reaching Vågå, the Black Death had moved roughly 300 km, almost two-thirds of the distance from Oslo to Nidaros.

In Norway, the Black Death predictably petered out in the early winter months of November and December because of increasingly cold weather. In the sources, the last reference to its active presence is the death of the bishop of Stavanger, who succumbed on 7 January 1350. This reflects the much milder and moister climate on the western coast (much like the weather in Scotland). In the mountainous inland of southern Norway, a certain Anund Helgason, we are told, died in the hundred of Tinn in the county of Numedal and Telemark before New Year's Eve and was buried in the cemetery of the parish church of Mæl. Actually, in the course of the 300 years of the history of plague in Norway comprising more than thirty waves of epidemics from 1348 to 1654 there is not a single case of a winter epidemic of plague. This constitutes decisive evidence to the effect that plague in Norway was invariably bubonic plague transmitted by rat fleas. Without exception, these epidemics of bubonic plague exhibited the characteristic features of epidemics of bubonic plague as studied in India, China, Madagascar, Indonesia and Egypt in the first half of the twentieth century. The fact that plague contagion was always imported into Norway from England and other parts of Northern Europe shows that the genetic properties of plague contagion for all practical epidemiological purposes remained unchanged throughout these 700 years.[34]

Information on Anund Helgason's death is given in the testimony of a priest who was present at his deathbed. It also provides a piece of vital evidence with regard to the Black Death's tremendous powers of spread in dispersedly settled country

---

32 See map in Steen 1934 by p. 224.
33 The letter å is pronounced as the English *aw* in, for instance, law or saw.
34 Benedictow 2002.

districts. The priest not only testifies that he was present himself when Anund Helgason died but that this also occurred

> in the presence of these persons: Ragndid Simonadottir and Alvald Sveinkason and *many other good persons* [. . .][35]

This piece of information reflects that, according to the values and norms of medieval people, it was an important social act to be present at the deathbeds of relatives and neighbours in order to show their regard and to express consolation and sympathy. After death had occurred, neighbours and relatives gathered for a commemoration. Relatives, of course, had additional motives relating to inheritance. In the case of the Black Death, this meant that quite a number of persons would normally come together in the houses of the diseased and deceased, which were swarming with dangerous rat fleas that would bite them and jump onto their clothing and ride with them back to their farmsteads. After having arrived in these new places, the rat fleas would occasion an epizootic among the rat colonies, which would subsequently translate into an epidemic at the social level of the free holding or tenement, which, in its turn, would give occasion to new gatherings of mourning and inheriting persons, and so on. Medieval people's profound social values in relation to illness and death and their thirst for inheritance were their worst enemies. Plague's tremendous powers of spread in old-time peasant society, its fearsome ability to blanket districts and even regions was owing to a unique combination of social dynamics and the special mechanisms of transmission and infection at work in plague epidemics. Only when the social element of the dynamics of spread was at least superficially understood to the effect that it was dangerous to visit houses of the diseased and deceased, and this particular set of social values began to disintegrate, was plague put on the defensive.

The process of spread by rat fleas was much slower than the spread of viral diseases by droplets as in the case of measles, mumps or chicken pox. Plague's characteristic tendency to linger in the same area for many months is reflected too in the meagre Norwegian source material on the history of the Black Death. In the same hundred of Upper Eiker, 60–80 km south-west of Oslo, where the dating formula 'the summer of the great mortality' is used, documents show that the Black Death lasted almost to New Year's Eve, as was the case in the nearby district of Sandsvær.[36]

Medieval man's religious values are also reflected in donations to religious institutions, parish churches, monasteries, cathedrals, and so on, in order to purchase chantries, intercessory prayer or obtain religiously attractive burial cites. There are 38–41 extant sources conveying such religious donations from the decade preceding the Black Death, an annual average of four, quite evenly spread out through the decade, while for the year of the Black Death alone, in 1349, there are recorded 16 such donations, four times higher than the average annual level.[37]

---

[35] Benedictow 1993/1996a: 98–9, 183; Benedictow 2002: 65–7. My translation from Old Norse.
[36] Benedictow 1993/1996a: 81, 99.
[37] *Regesta Norvegica*, Vol. 5, Nos 1113, 1120, 1129–30, 1183, 1196–7, 1200, 1201, 1206, 1207–8, 1212, 1213, 1214, 1215, 1217, 1219, 1220.

17

Denmark[1]

On the eve of the Black Death, Denmark comprised almost 70,000 sq. km and included at the time three important populous regions situated along the southern tip of the Scandinavian Peninsula that were lost to Sweden around the middle of the seventeenth century, namely Scania, Halland and Blekinge. The size of Denmark's medieval population is not known, but it was certainly much larger than Norway's or Sweden's, possibly as big as the combined populations of those two countries. That is the main reason Denmark was the great political power on the Nordic political scene in the Middle Ages. This also means that Denmark's population density was much higher than in the other Nordic countries, perhaps something of the order of magnitude of 10 persons per sq. km, which is still considerably smaller than in contemporary England or France. Around 1300, Denmark had over seventy towns and was far more urbanized than the other Nordic countries.[2]

The scholarly discussion of the Black Death's history in Denmark begins with a statement in the *Chronicle of Zealand* to the effect that 'a pestilence ravaged the country' in 1348, and that, in 1349, 'there was a great mortality in Denmark'.[3] Emeritus Professor Erik Ulsig of the University of Aarhus, who published the current standard work on the history of the Black Death in Denmark in 1991, considers that the chronicle misdates the outbreak of the Black Death, and redates it to 1349.

> It is strange that the Chronicle of Zealand, which was already written at the end of the 1350s, misdates the plague, as it is well known that there was plague in 1350, while, on the contrary, it must be excluded that it could have reached Denmark as early as 1348.[4]

It is difficult to understand why it should be impossible that the Black Death could have reached Denmark in 1348, when it had landed in southern England in May, had broken out in June, and had spread to Kent and Essex in south-eastern England in the

[1]   The standard work on the Black Death in Denmark is Ulsig 1991. I am grateful to Emeritus Professor Erik Ulsig, Department of History, University of Aarhus, and to Senior Lecturer Nils Hybel, Department of History, University of Copenhagen, who both have read the first version of the manuscript on the Black Death in Denmark and have made valuable comments.
[2]   Benedictow 1996c: 155, 178.
[3]   *Annales Danici medii ævi* 1920: 174–5.
[4]   Ulsig 1991: 22. My translation from Danish.

autumn. On the contrary, it must be considered a realistic possibility that the Black Death could have entered a ship bound for Denmark or Norway in a port in southern or south-eastern England and have gone ashore in some port in Denmark some time in the autumn of 1348. This does not, of course, constitute any sort of proof or evidence to the effect that it actually happened. On the other hand, the most conspicuous part of Ulsig's statement is that he underscores that 'it is well known that there was plague in 1350', and that he is not able to support his redating of the plague epidemic to 1349 with concrete evidence.[5] And, then, there is a source-critical point that contributes to reduce further the credibility of the chronicle: it is not extant in original but in a much later post-medieval transcript.[6]

As the chronicle states that the country was ravaged, it must be assumed that the Black Death arrived in the spring, or in the early summer at the latest, in order to have had time to become widely spread. This dating makes it as likely that the Black Death arrived in Denmark from southern Norway as from England.

In the light of this source-critical discussion, it becomes useful to revert to the 'open letter' (litteræ apertæ) King Magnus Eriksson sent to the population of the Swedish diocese of Östergötland,[7] where he relates with great alarm that the Black Death was raging 'over all Norway and Halland, and was on its way hither'. Halland is the coastal region stretching along the eastern side of the Kattegat all the way from the north-western corner of Scania along Sweden's western border almost up to Norway's south-eastern border. This reference to the Black Death in Halland is the only certain piece of evidence of plague in Denmark in 1349. The clear territorial differentiation between 'all Norway' and Halland in Denmark, makes it highly unlikely that King Magnus Eriksson knew about any outbreak of plague elsewhere in Denmark.

The dating of this 'open letter' is somewhat problematic. It is preserved in an undated transcript, so the time it was issued must be determined on textual and contextual grounds. Fortunately, it is possible to resolve this problem within quite narrow margins of uncertainty. The king informs the inhabitants of Östergötland that he has summoned the bishops of Linköping and Skara (whose dioceses were the immediately most threatened areas) and a number of lay members of the Council of the Realm, to a meeting in the town of Lödöse (the precursor to Gothenburg) in order to consider religious countermeasures to God's epidemic punishment for their sins. Royal letters issued in Lödöse on 25 and 29 September are the only evidence that the king stayed in the town that autumn,[8] and an exhaustive study of his itinerarium (travel route) makes it highly unlikely that he could have been there on any other occasion. This makes it reasonable to infer that the meeting took place around this date, which also is the conclusion of the scholar who has studied King Magnus's itinerary.[9] This indicates that the 'open letter' was written about three weeks earlier in order to allow time both for the messengers to summon the bishops and councillors

---

[5]   Cf. Ulsig 1991: 32, where he reveals obvious misgivings and a clear reservation as to the tenability of this redating.
[6]   Nielsen 1970: 326.
[7]   This document was referred to in relation to the discussion of the Black Death in Norway, and is also discussed in relation to the Black Death in Sweden. See also Benedictow 2002: 60, and n. 108.
[8]   Diplomatarium Suecanum, Vol. 6, Nos 4486 and 4488.
[9]   Grandison 1885: 99.

of the realm to the meeting, and for the time they would need to travel to the king with the utmost urgency. This suggests that the 'open letter' was written in early September in or near the town of Jönköping, about 115 km to the east of Lödöse, where the king stayed on 11 September.[10] He would obviously be on his way to Lödöse, where he had summoned the meeting.

The Black Death must be assumed to have been introduced into one of the seaports in Halland, probably, as we shall see, Halmstad in the southern part of the region, about eight weeks earlier in order to have had time to reach a degree of epidemic development that would be reported with great consternation to the king, for the time needed for the 'messenger' to ride to the king in great haste, for the king and his present councillors to discuss the matter and decide to summon an extraordinary meeting of the members of the Council of the Realm in the nearest regions, and to advise the population on the most efficient religious anti-epidemic countermeasures that should be taken in the meantime. This means that the contamination of Halmstad probably occurred around 8 July.

This time perspective indicates two possible areas of origin of the contamination. The contagion could have been transported by ship from Oslo or the Oslofjord area where the Black Death was raging in the summer after having broken out in Oslo probably in April (see above). The king could also have been frightened into writing his 'open letter' by the news that the Black Death was raging in the hundred of Idd (or nearby) in south-eastern Norway, close to the present south-eastern border with Sweden, at the end of August, indicating that the district had become contaminated around mid-July. Halland could also have been contaminated by Hanseatic ships fleeing from the ravages of the Black Death in eastern England.

One should note that the Prussian town of Elbing (Elblag) was contaminated probably in the second week of July since the outbreak there is dated to 24 August (see below), which makes it certain that the Black Death had sailed through the Sound much earlier. According to the standard assumption that the contemporary average pace of ship transport was 40 km a day, the ship that contaminated Elbing must have passed by Halmstad around 20 June in order to cover the roughly 900 remaining km in time to occasion the contamination of Elbing in the second week of July. This could have been a ship fleeing from the outbreak of the Black Death in Oslo where the Hansards had a trading station. The distance from Oslo to Halmstad is roughly 550 km, which would usually be covered by ship in a fortnight, so a ship leaving Oslo in the first week of June would usually have reached Halmstad around 20 June. A Hanseatic ship coming from England could have fled from their trading station in London around 1 May.[11]

In the Middle Ages, ecclesiastics, noblemen and gentry, burghers and other rich or affluent people considered it worthwhile to spend some of their money to shorten the time in purgatory when they thought that their days were numbered, or if the end came unexpectedly, their family would do it for them. The usual method was to endow chantries in churches or monasteries that entailed some specific religious services: the person's name would be entered in the respective ecclesiastical institution's calendar or in special registers called obituaries or anniversary books under the

---

10   *Diplomatarium Suecanum*, Vol. 6, No. 4483.
11   See below, Ch. 20 on Germany.

day of their death, so that on that day every year a priest would sing masses and perform a commemoration service that would include also intercessory prayer for the deceased person's soul. Most of the founders of chantries were burghers or ecclesiastics of the three cathedral cities.[12] Because these registers record the time of the donor's death, they will reflect the time of the outbreak, the height of intensity and the duration of the epidemic; a series of such sources will reflect also the progression of the epidemic in time and space.

In the case of the Danish history of the Black Death, three such registers are particularly valuable sources in the absence of almost all other types of evidence. The *Anniversary Book of the Chapter of the Cathedral of Ribe* in south-western Jutland records the death of 34 donors of chantries in the twenty years preceding the advent of the Black Death, corresponding to an annual average of 1.7 entries; in 1350, 17 such entries were made, ten times the annual average. Although nothing is specifically said of the cause of death, there can be no doubt that this dramatic increase reflects the brutal onslaught of the Black Death.[13]

Table 5: Deaths of donors of chantries in Ribe Cathedral in 1350, by month

J	F	M	A	M	J	J	A	S	O	N	D
1	2	0	0	2	0	3	6	1	1	0	1

The first of these 17 entries is made in January 1350 and two in February, followed by a break until two new entries are made in May, then the full brunt of the Black Death is reflected in numerous entries in July and August.[14] Epidemiologically, the most rational explanation for the time pattern of the entries is that the Black Death was introduced into the cathedral city of Ribe in the late autumn of 1349, probably first in the quarters of the poor classes. In January, it began to show its lethal might among the upper classes, killing as many donors of chantries to the cathedral in the first two months of 1350 as the usual number for two years. Then, the onset of cold weather forced the epidemic to subside and to go underground, as it were, smouldering among the rat colonies until the arrival of spring and warmer weather, when the epidemic resurged and, according to the usual seasonal pattern of the Black Death and later plague epidemics, reached the peak of its intensity towards the end of the summer and in the early autumn. The time pattern of the death of donors of chantries in Ribe Cathedral provides another piece of evidence to the effect that Denmark was invaded by the Black Death in 1349, albeit, in this case, at the end of the year, probably in October or November, and, thus, 3–4 months later than in Halland.

The cathedral city of Ribe was situated on the riverside of the R. Ribe, only a few kilometres from the western coastline. There is no indication as to where plague came from, but it could certainly have been introduced by Hanseatic or Dutch ships

---

[12] Ulsig 1991: 38.

[13] Kinch 1869: 208; Ulsig 1991: 22–4, 33, 36–8, 41.

[14] The conspicuous lack of endowments in June could reflect a temporary breakdown of clerical functions owing to the sudden violent increase in the epidemic onslaught, and have been entered later, corresponding to the pattern of events reflected in the number of wills registered in the Court of Hustings in London in 1349, cf. above, p. 136 and Table 4.

returning from Bergen in western Norway, or from the towns of Oslo or Tønsberg in the Oslofjord area of south-eastern Norway, perhaps from north-eastern England, and possibly from Scotland. It could also, perhaps, have come from the coastal area of Friesland north of the Zuider Zee in the northern Netherlands where the Black Death broke out in late 1349.[15] North-western Germany is not a possible source of origin of plague contagion. Cologne was itself contaminated at the end of the year, the recognized time of the outbreak being 20 December.[16] There is a very suspect rise in the number of wills made in Lübeck at the end of 1349, but the pronounced contemporaneity and the distance of 200 km rules out contamination from this source.[17]

So far it has been possible to identify outbreaks of the Black Death in two separate corners of Denmark in the last four months of 1349, but the question remains as to whether Denmark really was ravaged in 1349 as stated in the *Chronicle of Zealand*, according to Professor Ulsig's interpretation. In that case also the central Danish island regions of Zealand and Funen, and the south-eastern region of Scania must have been invaded, and in the summer at the latest, in order to allow time for wide-spread dissemination. A particular type of source is extant in sufficient quantity to make it possible to approach this problem. Religious institutions kept also registers in which they recorded the donations of chantries. The incidence and time pattern of such endowments would tend to reflect the time and intensity of a large epidemic crisis because people feared for their lives and prepared for the worst. Information of this type is provided by the *Book of Endowments of the Chapter of Roskilde Cathedral* in central Zealand, reflecting the often-overlooked fact that the town of Roskilde and not Copenhagen was the cathedral city of the diocese of Zealand. This book of endowments shows that 28 chantries had been founded in the preceding twenty years (1330–49), an annual average of 1.4 chantries. There is no indication of extraordinary mortality in 1349, but, in 1350, there is one entry in October and five in November, over four times as many as the annual average: the sudden surge to six entries in 1350 is clearly a statistically significant indication of the presence of the Black Death.

This material shows no reflection of a possible outbreak of the Black Death in Zealand in 1349 at all, but instead indicates that it raged in the autumn of 1350. Zealand is a relatively small island comprising an area of about 7,000 sq. km, and the cathedral city of Roskilde is situated only about 30 km from Copenhagen, by far the most populous and busiest seaport town in Zealand. The maximum length and breadth of the island are about 125 and 95 km, respectively, it was densely settled and contained a number of seaports and other urban centres. In short, even assuming that the Black Death spread at a modest average daily pace of one kilometre, the island should be expected to have been completely engulfed in three or four months, and

---

[15] Biraben 1975: 84. See also below, Ch. 21, on the Netherlands.

[16] See more about this below in Ch. 20 on the Black Death in Germany and Ch. 21 in the Netherlands.

[17] Ibs 1994: 88, 90–1. A letter from the town council of Ålborg in northern Jutland to the city council of Lübeck in 1358 contains a reference to the mortality of the year 1350 or around that year. As pointed out by Ibs, the dating is conspicuously inaccurate. However, it is compatible with an outbreak at the end of 1349 in Ribe that was suppressed by the winter, followed by a resurgence in spring, which made 1350 the real plague year. This is the only additional piece of evidence relating to the Black Death in Jutland. Ibs 1994: 90–1. *Urkundenbuch der Stadt Lübeck*, Vol. 3, doc. no. 300, 20 May 1358. Therefore, nothing more can be said on the origin of the Black Death and the spread of the epidemic in time and space in Jutland.

this assumption of pace in this densely settled and (for its time) highly urbanized island is rather on the low side. More realistically, the Black Death would have spread at an average daily pace of 1.5 km and have engulfed the island in 2.5 months. In epidemiological terms, it is inexplicable that the Black Death should have broken out in Zealand in mid-1349 and not have reached or threatened Roskilde until the next autumn. In fact, even the evidence presented so far makes it clear that the Black Death could not have been introduced into Zealand in 1349 at all, but was introduced in the summer or early autumn of 1350.

Professor Ulsig is certain that the *Chronicle of Zealand* provides an incorrect dating that must be changed. This fact invites, of course, further suspicion. This suspicion is strengthened by the fact that the original manuscript is lost and it is now known only in post-medieval transcripts, making the spectre of scribal error diminish its reliability and credibility and, therefore, its usability as a historical source.[18] However, the original manuscript of the *Book of Endowments of the Chapter of Roskilde Cathedral* is also lost and its contents are also known only in later transcripts, a fact that introduces some uncertainty of its own for the same reason.

Professor Ulsig points out that the *Anniversary Book of Our Lady's of Copenhagen* contains too few entries on the deaths of donors of chantries to constitute valid statistical material on its own. However, conspicuously and interestingly, the anniversary book contains three entries under 1350, two of them in late August and late September. Although this material cannot be allotted validity on its own, it fits remarkably well into the indicated time pattern, that the Black Death was introduced into Copenhagen in the second half of June and ravaged Zealand I. in the late summer and autumn of 1350. It is also reassuring that these two clerical sources taken together and seen in contextual perspective provide a coherent epidemiological pattern of introduction and spread: in Zealand I., the Black Death was, as would be expected, introduced into Denmark's by far largest town, namely Copenhagen, and, taking into account the quite developed epidemic form that would scare members of the upper classes into making donations to religious institutions or endowments of chantries, this occurred probably in the second half of June. From Copenhagen it spread to Roskilde, a distance of 30 km, with a delay comprising the ordinary time for development into epidemic form in Copenhagen, about three weeks to cover the distance, and about six weeks to develop into an epidemic form in Roskilde, around fifteen weeks in all. This fits nicely indeed with the dates of the entries in the respective sources, late August and September in Copenhagen, late October and November in Roskilde. This means that the Black Death in Zealand I. probably originated in northern Germany where the Black Death by now was in full swing, for instance, in Lübeck where the Black Death had flared up in May after a first outbreak in the late autumn of 1349 that was suppressed by the arrival of cold winter weather (see below).

The Danish archbishop resided in the cathedral city of Lund in Scania on the eastern side of the Sound. Scania is the southernmost region of the Scandinavian Peninsula and is one of the regions that were conquered by Sweden from Denmark in the mid-seventeenth century, together with the adjacent regions of Halland (on the

---

[18] Nielsen 1970: 326.

Sound) and Blekinge (on the Baltic Sea). For the period 1300–90, the *Obituary of the Cathedral of Lund* contains 79 entries giving the date of death of individuals, an annual average of 1.2 entries, the entries being quite evenly distributed among the first five decennials (1300–49). However, in the year 1350, six entries are recorded.[19] It appears incontrovertible that this sudden surge in entries reflects the ravages of the Black Death. The entries are spread throughout all the year, a feature that suggests that Scania was invaded by the Black Death around the turn of the year, quite possibly at the end of 1349, and that it had spread southwards from Halland to Lund. An earliest introduction in the southern town of Halmstad (as suggested above and enlarged upon in the next chapter on Sweden) may contribute to explain the quite early invasion of north-western Scania at the end of 1349.

These conclusions can be tested on documentary material consisting of all known donations by deed or will to religious institutions in Denmark, to parish churches, cathedrals, monasteries, and so on, in the years under discussion as compared to the previous years. The distribution of these donations in time and space in the plague year(s) could also reflect the disease's pattern of spread under the assumption that members of the donation-making social élites were inspired to do so when they suddenly realized that their own lives were at risk. This approach has not been attempted before, but it yields, as will be seen, valuable results.

Because donations to religious institutions are an ordinary feature of pre-epidemic and post-epidemic social and religious life, it is a fallacy of methodology to assume that any specific donation was caused by fear of imminent death by the Black Death – it is all a question of statistics. The paucity of direct evidence on the Black Death in Denmark makes the indirect manifestations of people's despair in the face of massive mortality, and the obvious fact that their own lives were very much at risk, useful for historians. It persuaded members of the social élites to make donations to religious institutions in a last-ditch effort to avoid perdition and to shorten the time of horrors and tortures in the purgatory. The material on donations by deed and will is presented in Tables 6 and 7, and the information that it can provide is discussed below.

The documentary material presented in Table 6 shows an annual average of 5.6 donations to religious institutions in the nine years 1340–8. In 1349, there is a sudden surge to 13 donations, 2.3 times the average. Unfortunately, the material breaks down into three almost equally large parts, distributed between the two halves of the year and donations with unknown dates within the year. This makes it technically impossible to identify the time when the surge started that caused the doubling in the number of donations in that year compared with the annual average of previous years.

In 1350, the number of donations increases tremendously, by a factor of 5.5 times in relation to the average of 1340–8. There cannot be any doubt that this great rise in the incidence of religious donations reflects people's despair at the ravages of the Black Death, although there is not the slightest reference to the epidemic. The reason is that such documents were couched in a very traditional formal language.

This documentary material on donations to religious institutions confirms the

---

[19] Ulsig 1991: 22–4, 33, 36–8, 41. Cf. Kinch 1869: 208–9, n. 3.

Table 6. Donations to Danish religious institutions 1341–50[a]

Year	No. of sources	No. of donations	1st Half- year	2nd Half-year	Without date
1340	103	6	3	0	3
1341	82	5	4	1	0
1342	82	4	2	1	1
1343	118	3	0	2	1
1344	114	5	5	0	0
1345	100	5	2	2	1
1346	94	7	1	4	2
1347	103	9	3	6	0
1348	110	7	1	3	3
1349	123	13	4	5	4
1350	134	31	10	15	6

[a]   Danish medieval sources are published in a special series called *Diplomatarium Danicum*, abbr. *DD*. There is also a parallel series with translations called *Danmarks Riges Breve* published with the same succession of volumes and the same numbering of the sources as in *DD*. Tables 6 and 7 are based on the following sources: *DD* 3rd Series, Vol. 1: 7, 32, 33, 86, 89, 92, 149, 163, 168, 177, 196, 216, 222, 269, 284, 338, 340, 404; Vol. 2: 10, 13, 28, 46, 56; 120, 148, 191, 198, 206, 244, 266, 271, 276, 280, 307, 317, 341, 346, 360, 372–3, 375, 395, 397, 407; Vol. 3: 5, 58, 59, 61, 93, 97–8, 103; 134, 139, 159, 180–1, 192, 196, 198, 201, 207–8, 222, 225, 227, 229, 240, 255, 260, 263–6, 285, 292, 301, 304, 306, 308, 310, 316, 317, 320–1, 323–4, 326, 332, 340, 341, 348, 352–6, 367, 370, 376. King Magnus's and Queen Blanca's wills, from 1346, 1347 and 1348, have been omitted from the material because of their very special, and highly unrepresentative character, but the material includes ordinary donations of religious institutions by the king. In some cases, especially when sources are known only from brief abstracts in religious institutions' cadasters or registers of holdings, it is not stated whether the property in question has been acquired by donation or purchase. There could, consequently, be a few additional donations, but the uncertain cases are too few to affect the statistical significance of the material. There is no discernible difference in the use of deeds or wills; their relative distribution is, therefore, not presented in the table.

conclusion of the previous analysis. The doubling of the number of donations in 1349 confirms that the epidemic invaded Denmark in 1349, and, compared to the number of donations in 1350, it supports an inference to the effect that the invasion occurred in the second half-year, otherwise the numerical distribution of donations between 1349 and 1350 would have been more balanced. It also shows that 1350 was the great year of the Black Death in Denmark. The place names in the material from 1349 contain no indication of an outbreak of the Black Death in Zealand I.

Almost 150 years ago, C. Lange was intrigued by the fact that Denmark's political life seemed unaffected by any disastrous event throughout the year 1349. In that year, there were large political assemblies of royal councillors and lay and ecclesiastical dignitaries both in the town of Ringsted in the heart of Zealand I. and in the town of Nyborg on the coast of eastern Funen. Also in 1349, King Valdemar led a military expedition into northern Germany to support his brother-in-law King Ludvig of Brandenburg against his enemy.[20]

[20]   Lange 1862: 121.

Table 7. Donations to Danish religious institutions 1349–50, according to time, number in consecutive order, locality and region

Date	No.	Locality/institution	Hundred/town	Region
22.10.49	1	Sale parish church	Ginding	Jutland (north-central)
31.10.49	2	Lund Cathedral	town	Scania (west)
13.11.49	3	Söndrum parish	Halmstad	Halland (south)
5.1.50	4	Roskilde Cathedral	town	Zealand (central)
26.2.50	5	Ribe Cathedral	town	Jutland (south-west)
26.2.50	6	Ribe St Peter's[a]	town	Jutland (south-west)
1.3.50	7	Ribe Cathedral	town	Jutland (south-west)
8.3.50	8	Bavelse	Tybjerg	Zealand (south)
17.3.50	9	Lund Cathedral	town	Scania (west)
31.5.50	10	Ribe Cathedral	town	Jutland (south-west)
31.5.50	11	Roskilde Cathedral	town	Zealand (central)
31.5.50	12	Ribe Cathedral	town	Jutland (south-west)
27.6.50	13	Our Lady's, Copenhagen	town	Zealand (east)
14.7.50	14	Bosjö Monastery	Frosta	Scania (central)
22.7.50	15	Ribe Cathedral	town	Jutland (south-west)
23.7.50	16	Haglösa	Skytts	Scania (south-western tip)
10.8.50	17	Sæby	Volborg	Zealand (central)
29.8.50	18	Lund Cathedral	town	Scania (south-west)
1.9.50	19	Halmstad, monastery	seaport town	Halland (south)
23.9.50	20	Lund Cathedral	town	Scania (south-west)
23.9.50	21	Västra Skrävlinge par. ch.	Oxie	Scania (south-west)
28.9.50	22	Ribe Cathedral[b]	town	Jutland (south-west)
28.9.50	23	St Clara Convent, Roskilde	town	Zealand (central)
29.9.50	24	Gammelby, to a parish ch.	Svansø	Schleswig[c]
13.10.50	25	Ribe Cathedral	town	Jutland (south-west)
28.10.50	26	Lund Cathedral	town	Scania (south-west)
31.10.50	27	tenement in Lillöd[d]	Gärd	Scania (central)
6.12.50	28	tenement in Årsjö[e]	Herrestad	Scania (central)

[a] Both these donations were made by the bishop of Ribe on 26 February, but are known from documents issued on 24 March.

[b] Donation of land in the hundred of Hvidinge in south-western Jutland, quite near Ribe.

[c] Schleswig belonged to Denmark until 1864 when most of it was conquered by Prussia; Svansø (in German, Schwansen) is a peninsula east of the cathedral city of Schleswig.

[d] Donation to Bosjö Monastery in the nearby hundred of Frosta.

[e] The Archbishop of Lund testifies that the priest Niels Frendesen, clerk in his chamber, for the benefit of his soul has endowed the altar that he possesses in Lund Cathedral with his tenancy in Årsjö.

The time pattern of the donations to religious institutions presented in Table 7 indicates that the first two outbreaks of the Black Death in Denmark are reflected in the three donations made in the three weeks from 22 October to 13 November 1349 for two main reasons: this number of donations corresponds to the average for six months in the preceding years, and their territorial distribution is co-ordinated with the known areas of invasion. The donation to Lund Cathedral on 31 October and the donation on 13 November of tenancies to the parish church of Söndrum outside the seaport town of Halmstad in southern Halland should be considered with keen interest, because they can easily be coupled with King Magnus's reference to the presence of the Black Death in Halland in his 'open letter' from September. Halmstad has above been indicated as the likely place of entry of the Black Death in Halland on independent grounds, and this is supported also by the analysis of the Black Death's spread in western Sweden after having been introduced from Halland (see below). The donation to the parish church of Söndrum fits nicely into the picture and supports the inferences made above on the basis of other source materials as to the time and areas of invasion.

Other interesting indications of the pattern of spread can be discerned in the material from 1350 when these donations are presented according to time and locality. These donations used as indirect evidence of people's fear of being struck by the Black Death produce a somewhat distorted picture for several reasons. Some people will contract plague and die before having had time to make a donation or will, but would have extracted a promise from relatives in attendance at their deathbed that they would attend to it as soon as possible. Plague is a disease that tends to linger for months in the same district, a characteristic epidemiological feature that will tend to blur the pattern and pace of spread as reflected in the sources. Many of the deeds are produced in religious institutions and do not indicate where the donor is resident. In these cases, the whereabouts of the Black Death can be indicated with varying accuracy according to a couple of alternative considerations: in a number of cases, the donor is a parson, in which case his parish will be entered as the locality; if the donor's place of residence cannot be identified, the locality of the recipient institution will be entered on the assumption that people would most likely make donations to institutions to which they had some sort of personal devotional relationship, and that would very probably be within the confines of the diocese to which they belonged, be it to the local church, the cathedral or a religious house. The governing principle must be to attempt to come as close as possible to the donors' place of residence.[21]

The place names in this specific documentary material of endowments contains, as mentioned, no indication of an outbreak of the Black Death in Zealand I. in 1349 (Table 7). Instead, it shows clearly that the Black Death ravaged the island in 1350. It indicates, as mentioned, the start and the locality of the first incursions of the epidemic by donations to religious institutions in Lund and Halmstad, which coincide in time and location with King Magnus's account. At the start of 1350, there is a conspicuous flurry of donations to Ribe Cathedral (nos 5–7) that accords with our knowledge of the Black Death's outbreak there, probably at the end of 1349. Later, several other

---

21 Table 6 contains four donations with unknown date within the year that have been left out of Table 7.

donations to the cathedral are made (nos 10, 12, 15) when the epidemic broke out again or increased greatly in intensity after having been dampened or forced underground to an enzootic existence in the rat colonies by cold winter weather.

The second clear feature is the spread of the epidemic in Scania, which accords well also with other findings. Donations to Ribe Cathedral and to religious institutions in Scania throughout the year reflects plague's tendency to linger in areas owing to the special mechanisms of dissemination, and could also reflect the realization of promises of donations given at deathbeds.

Summing up, for a number of reasons it may appear difficult to retain the orthodox opinion that the Black Death's conquest of Denmark began with an invasion of Zealand I. in the summer or the early autumn of 1349, and next broke out in Jutland and Scania in 1350. The earliest outbreak of the Black Death in the Kingdom of Denmark was in the region of Halland on the eastern side of the Kattegat, more specifically probably in the seaport town of Halmstad, and this outbreak was probably known by King Magnus at the beginning of September and no later than at the end of the month. It is likely that the Black Death broke out in Ribe at the end of 1349, and, as it seems, at about the same time also in the opposite corner of the Denmark, on the eastern side of the Sound, in the region of Scania. The outbreak in Scania is indicated by an increasing incidence of donations to religious institutions, a development obviously connected with the spread into Scania of the forces of the Black Death that had moved out of the epicentre in Halmstad in southern Halland. Excepting the source-critically problematic dating in the *Chronicle of Zealand*, all evidence supports inferences to the effect that 1350 was the year when the Black Death ravaged Jutland, Zealand I. and Scania.

18

Sweden

On the eve of the Black Death, Sweden's territory did not include the present-day regions of Scania, Halland and Blekinge, which were conquered from Denmark in the middle of the seventeenth century, nor the counties Bohuslän, Jämtland and Härjedalen, which were conquered from Norway at the same time, in all 74,000 sq. km. The vast northern parts of Sweden, which also had some quite obscure territorial delimitations, were extremely thinly populated, the overwhelming majority of the population living south of the region of Medelpad (south of the present-day county of Västernorrland), i.e., within a territory of about 185,000 sq. km.

The size of Sweden's population on the eve of the Black Death is not known. In order to throw a glimmer of light into the reign of demographic darkness, it could, perhaps, be useful to make an estimate based on a quite reasonable assumption of comprehensive social and economic similarity between Norway and Sweden. Around 1330, Norwegian parishes contained on average c. 62.5 households, at the time population growth had tapered off and an overall stationary population size had developed, called the high medieval population maximum, which still prevailed on the eve of the Black Death.[1] If this correlation of average number of households within parishes is tentatively applied to contemporary Sweden, which at the time contained about 1.750 parishes, the following estimate can be made: 1,750 parishes multiplied by 62.5 households gives a total national number of 105,000 households, which, assuming a stationary population with an average household size of 4.5 persons, suggests a population of around 492,000 persons. In addition, there were some small social categories of people living outside the parish system, fleeting underclasses in the towns, indigents and vagabonds, hunter-gatherers, and so on. Thus, a population size of roughly 500,000 persons may possibly be discerned. The tentative nature of

[1] Medieval Norway contained about 73,250 tenancies in the period 1300–30 (cf. above under Norway), distributed in 1,200 parishes. Norwegian agrarian historians agree that these tenancies and free holdings were normally inhabitated by one household. There was undoubtedly a small or tiny incidence of joint families, which means that the number of households was slightly higher than the number of tenancies and free holdings, and a small addition is therefore warranted. According to Sandnes 1971: 63, 202, central Norway (Trøndelag) contained 6,925 households distributed in 119 churches, which gives an average of 58 households. Subsequent research has increased somewhat the number of tenancies and free holdings in Norway, although quite little in central Norway. Taking into account both this increase and a small incidence of joint families, this figure could usefully be rounded upwards to 62.5.

this estimate, its character of guestimate, must be strongly underscored, and it should be related to with great circumspection and caution. It may, however, be of some interest that the estimate fits nicely into the picture of the relative political and military strength between the Nordic countries at the time.

The territorial estimate and the population estimate (minus the minuscule population of the northernmost counties) suggest an average population density south of Medelpad of 2.7 persons per sq. km. This figure should be handled with similar circumspection and caution but is useful for epidemiological studies within great margins of uncertainty. However, it is also true that much of the countryside south of Medelpad consisted of woods, lakes, moors, hills and mountains, and the population was therefore in reality living in considerably greater density, concentrated in areas that were well suited for arable and animal husbandry. The agricultural population was partly settled in village communities and partly on scattered detached or semi-detached holdings.

One sobering point has been made several times already: as we move northwards and north-eastwards in Europe, the historical evidence that can be used in the study of the Black Death becomes increasingly poor. The Black Death's history in Sweden reflects the continuation of this unfortunate development, which means that attainable insights into this momentous event in its history are severely limited. The sources also tend to take on the character of pieces of epidemic structures that have been atomized by history in the sense that the outcome of dedicated endeavours to collect sources for the history of the Black Death in Sweden consists of a number of dispersed pieces of information that can only with great difficulty be correlated in a meaningful way to produce a rough outline of the temporal and spatial dimensions of the event.

Sweden's history of the Black Death begins with a so-called 'open letter' (*litteræ apertæ*) from King Magnus Eriksson of Sweden and Norway to the inhabitants of the Swedish diocese of Linköping (province of Östergötland). Similar letters were undoubtedly sent to the populations of the other Swedish dioceses, but only this specimen is known. This letter has been mentioned above under Norway, and has been discussed more thoroughly in connection with the history of the Black Death in Denmark. The present discussion in relation to Sweden will therefore contain some reiteration, a fact that also reflects the paucity of sources on the history of the Black Death in the Nordic countries. In the 'open letter', the king informs the inhabitants of the diocese about the gruesome 'sudden death' and 'plague' that wrought havoc on people in the countries to the west of their country, and was raging 'over all Norway and Halland, and was on its way hither'. He also informs the inhabitants that he had summoned the bishops of Linköping and Skara, whose dioceses comprised the immediately most threatened areas, and a number of named lay members of the Council of the Realm, to a meeting in the town of Lödöse (the precursor to Gothenburg) in order to consider religious countermeasures to God's epidemic punishment for their sins. In this 'open letter' Magnus conveys the decisions of the meeting, and similar letters must be assumed to have been sent to the populations of the other dioceses, although only this specimen is extant today.

This 'open letter' is preserved in an undated transcript, but was produced in the autumn of 1349. Royal letters issued in Lödöse on 25 and 29 September are the only evidence that the king stayed in the town that autumn.[2] Because these are the only sources on the king's whereabouts this autumn that link him to this town, it is reasonable to give priority to an inference to the effect that the meeting took place around this date and that the 'open letter' was written about three weeks earlier, which also is the conclusion of the scholar who has studied the king's itinerary.[3] King Magnus stayed near the town of Jönköping, about 115 km east of Lödöse, on 11 September, and the 'open letter' may have been written in or near this town whence he journeyed to Lödöse.[4] Also on more general grounds, one could have presumed that the meeting could be held about three weeks later, which would allow time both for the messengers to summon the bishops and councillors of the realm to the meeting and for the time these dignitaries would require to travel to the king with the utmost urgency.

In the cited phrase, it is not clear whether or not the word 'all' relates only to Norway or also to Halland. It appears, however, almost inconceivable that King Magnus Eriksson would have dared to summon a meeting of bishops and councillors in Lödöse a few miles upstream on the R. Göta Älv a few weeks later if the Black Death had already crossed the narrow corridor of Swedish land on both sides of the river's last kilometres that divided Norway and Denmark, and had moved into the Danish region of Halland from this direction.

Instead, the Black Death must be assumed to have been introduced into one of the seaports in Halland. As pointed out in Chapter 17, on the Black Death's history in Denmark, the contagion was probably introduced in the seaport of Halmstad in the southern part of the region. Additional evidence relating to the spread of the Black Death in the adjacent Swedish areas will be adduced below in support of this view. In order to allow time for the epidemic to reach a stage of development that would be reported with great consternation to the king, and for the time needed for the 'messenger' to ride to the king and present his awesome news, for the king and his present councillors to deliberate on the matter and decide how to handle this extremely grave situation, it becomes likely that the plague was introduced 8–9 weeks earlier, in the first week of July. This could have been brought about by Hanseatic ships fleeing the onslaughts of the Black Death in Oslo or in the Oslofjord area, or in English ports, calling desperately at some harbour on the Sound when the Black Death revealed its murderous presence on board, or the mortality among the crew made it difficult or impossible to sail on homewards.

A recognized outbreak of the Black Death in Halland at the end of August would understandably make the king jumpy. In addition, the 'open letter' should be seen in the light of a likely reference to the Black Death in the hundred of Idd in south-eastern Norway, about 170 km north of the border, and of Lödöse at the end of August. The terrible presence of the Black Death in the long and narrow south-eastern Norwegian border counties with Sweden and in the similarly long and narrow Danish border region make it very easily understandable that the king and his councillors got the jitters and considered how this unparelleled epidemic manifestation of

---

[2]   *Diplomatarium Suecanum*, Vol. 6, Nos 4486 and 4488.
[3]   Grandison 1885: 99.
[4]   *Diplomatarium Suecanum*, Vol. 6, No. 4483.

the Lord's mighty anger could be prevented from being unleashed on Sweden or at least be moderated.

Unfortunately, this exhausts the source material that relates explicitly to the spread of the Black Death in western Sweden and in the neighbouring Norwegian and Danish areas. Sadly, there is not the slightest direct piece of information on when and where the Black Death actually entered western Sweden, and it can only be inferred that Sweden was first invaded from the west and that this event occurred at some time in the autumn, probably in October or November. This makes it also clear that the Black Death would not have made much headway before its advances were stopped by the onset of cold winter weather.

The second piece of direct information on the Black Death in Sweden relates to the outbreak of the Black Death in the town of Visby in Gotland I., off Sweden's Baltic coast south of Stockholm, at Easter 1350, i.e., in the week starting on Easter Sunday, 28 March. According to the standard assumption on the developmental processes of plague epidemiology, with some addition for the social attitudes and behavioural characteristics of the chroniclers, the time of the outbreak in Visby implies technically that the Black Death was introduced into local society around 7 February and no later than around mid-February. At that time, winter still reigned. One should note that this is an area characterized by a very cold winter climate, and shipping under medieval conditions would be prevented not only by fear of winter storms, but also because the Baltic Sea is normally covered by ice in the period January–early March.[5] The Hanseatic cities and towns therefore prohibited merchant ships from putting to sea in the months November–February.[6] Importantly, the Black Death had only just invaded the south-western part of Sweden so that the contagion could not have been passed on from the mainland. Thus, the Black Death must have been introduced into Visby in the late autumn, had been prevented from developing into a full-blown epidemic by the onset of the usual severe winter cold, and finally made its presence observable by an increasing number of cases some time during Easter week when spring was in the air.

In our context, the outbreak in Visby is important not only because it reflects a process of dissemination of plague contagion in the Baltic Sea area in the autumn of 1349, but also because Visby was to a considerable extent a town dominated by Hanseatic Germans and therefore played a vital part in the commercial network in the Baltic area. In short, it shows that the Black Death was spread by Hanseatic ships in the autumn of 1349. The Black Death could thus have been introduced into Visby by ships from Prussia or Pomerania, or by Hanseatic ships coming from England or Norway (cf. below p.199). Nothing more appears to be known about this outbreak in Visby, and for some intriguing reason it does not seem to have been a source for the contamination of Sweden's south-eastern coast.

The evidence indicates unambiguously that the Black Death invaded Sweden from the west, from Norway and from Halland, and moved eastwards across Sweden all the way to the Baltic Sea (see below). This pattern can be discerned in a special type

---

[5]   In winter, a thick and durable layer of ice is normally formed on the Baltic Sea, caused not only by the quite severe winter climate but also by the very low salinity of the water. The Baltic area does not draw climatic benefit from the Gulf Stream as north-western Europe and particularly Norway do.

[6]   Hansen 1912: 127.

Table 8. Donations to Swedish religious institutions 1341–50[a]

Year	No. of sources	No. of donations	1st Half-year	2nd Half-year
1341	80	7	3–4[b]	3–4
1342	60	8	3–4[c]	4–5
1343	80	5	3	2
1344	117	8	6	2
1345	143	11	5–6[d]	5–6
1346	107	9	7	2
1347	148	4	3	1
1348	114	5	2	3
1349	125	7	4	3
1350	147	28	10	18

[a] Swedish medieval sources are published in a special series called *Diplomatarium Suecanum*, abbr. *DS*. Tables 8 and 9 are based on the following sources: *DS*, Vol. 5, Nos 3534, 3544–5, 3560, 3569, 3584, 3599, 3604, 3614, 3619, 3629, 3632, 3649, 3651, 3661, 3672, 3678, 3691, 3705, 3708, 3730, 3758, 3765, 3774, 3786, 3790, 3791, 3827, 3860, 3886, 3911, 3921, 3951, 3957, 3970, 3983, 3996–7, 4013, 4016, 4023, 4039, 4045, 4055, 4064, 4073, 4082, 4090, 4095, 4154, 4164, 4190, 4269; *DS*, Vol. 6, Nos 4335, 4339, 4369, 4373–4, 4402–3, 4419, 4441, 4495, 4498, 4512, 4523, 4526, 4537, 4539, 4546, 4550, 4576, 4579, 4590, 4606, 4608–9, 4613–15, 4618, 4620, 4631–3, 4635–36, 4639, 4641–3, 4651, 4654.
  King Magnus's and Queen Blanca's wills, the second from 1347 and the third from 1348, have been omitted from the material because of their very special, and highly unrepresentative character. The material includes ordinary donations to religious institutions by the king: there are three of them in the whole material, two in 1346, and one in 1350. There is no discernible difference in the use of deeds or wills, which is why their distribution is not presented in the table.
[b] Source No. 3534 contains no dating within the year 1341.
[c] Source No. 3613 contains no dating within the year 1342.
[d] Source No. 3875 contains no dating within the year 1345.

of source material, namely donations to religious institutions, parish churches, cathedrals, monasteries, and so on. Donations used as indirect evidence of fear of being struck by the Black Death present methodological and source-critical problems that have been discussed in relation to the use of this type of sources in the study of the Black Death's Danish history. It will therefore suffice in this context to reiterate a few central points. This material can be used to confirm the presence of the Black Death if it reveals an abrupt surge in the number of religious donations, even though the epidemic is not mentioned, because such documents are couched in a heavily traditional, formal language. Donations to religious institutions are an ordinary feature of pre-epidemic (and post-epidemic) social and religious life, and it is a fallacy of methodology to assume that any specific document was caused by fear of imminent death by the Black Death – it is all a question of statistics. The distribution in time and space of a large increase in such acts can indicate the pattern of territorial spread and local duration. This material is presented in Tables 8 and 9.

The material gathered and processed in Table 8 reveals a large increase in the number of donations to religious institutions in 1350 compared to normal pre-plague years. As reflected in the extant source material, the annual average number of donations to religious institutions in the pre-plague years is seven, while in 1350 alone 28 such documents are known, a fourfold increase. Despite the fact that the Black Death is not mentioned even once in the sources relating to the Swedish mainland, this huge and abrupt surge in the number of donations must be a reflection of people's overwhelming fear of imminent death. People who had not considered themselves likely victims of death in the near future suddenly acquired overwhelming motives for avoiding dying intestate, to ensure a more promising passage from life to death, and to demonstrate their contrite hearts and fervent religious devotion by making a donation to a religious institution. The almost hibernating phase of plague in the winter months is the main reason that there are nearly twice as many donations in the second half of 1350 as in the first half of the year, a feature that contrasts sharply with the preceding years in which donations are quite evenly distributed between the first and second six-month periods of the year.

A rough outline of the Black Death's pattern of spread in time and space across Sweden can be discerned in Table 9, which organizes all documents containing donations to religious institutions in 1350 according to time and locality.

There is one possible, or rather likely, reflection of the presence of the Black Death in 1349, a donation by the vicar in the parish of Hvalstad in the region of Västergötland to Skara Cathedral issued on 20 December. Presumably, the reason for this is, as mentioned, that the Black Death had only had time to make short incursions into Swedish territory before the onset of winter weather forced it underground, so to speak. However, after having smouldered in local rat colonies during the winter, this prepared the ground for a violent resurgence of the Black Death in the spring. This outline of the epidemic process may appear quite similar to what probably happened in Norway one year earlier.

It is a significant feature of Table 9 that the donations to religious institutions start in Västergötland and in western Småland, and end up on the eastern coast, in Uppland, Södermanland and eastern Småland. The usual assumption that Stockholm was ravaged in the autumn of 1350 is, therefore, in all likelihood correct.[7] Donations to institutions in the large region of Småland begin at the end of February in the south-western part of the region, in Finnveden, close to Halland's south-eastern border and reflect quite possibly contamination at the very end of 1349. This means that they probably were associated with the Black Death's progression from the outbreak in Halland that King Magnus Eriksson refers to in his 'open letter', which again indicates the seaport town of Halmstad as the place of introduction, as was also suggested above in the discussion of the king's letter.

Significantly, the religious donations in Småland end in a parish church in the easternmost part of the region, close to the Baltic Sea. Thus, the pattern of spread is clear: the Black Death entered Sweden in Västergötland and south-western Småland from south-eastern Norway and southern Halland, respectively, and moved relentlessly eastwards until it reached the Baltic Sea and completed the conquest of Sweden. The number of donations in 1351 is about the same as before the Black Death, namely eight, which in view of the population decline indicates that a few made early in the year may still reflect some belated action on behalf of persons who died under circumstances that did not permit the issue of a personal deed or will.

---

[7] Ahnlund 1953: 173; Dahlbäck 1988: 25.

Table 9. Donations to Swedish religious institutions, December 1349–50, according to date, number in consecutive order, locality and region. Hundred = 'härad',[a] ch. = church, insts. = religious institutions

Time	No.	Locality/institution	Hundr./town	Region
20.12.49	1	Hvalstad parish ch.	Vartofta	Västergötland (east)
1.2.50	2	Gökhem parish ch.	Vilske	Västergötland (central)
12.2.50	3	Vreta Convent	Gullbergs	Östergötland (north-central)
21.2.50	4	Rakkeby Convent	Kullings	Västergötland (south-west)
28.2.50	5	Burseryd parish ch.	Västbo	Småland (Finnveden)[b]
		Båraryd parish ch.	Västbo	Småland (Finnveden)
		Biälbo parish ch.	Göstring	Östergötland (near Alvastra)
16.3.50	6	Skara Cathedral	town	Västergötland (north-central)
20.3.50	7	Nydala Monastery	Västra	Småland (Njudung)
3.5.50	8	Svenarum parish ch.[c]	Västra	Småland (Njudung)
22.5.50	9	Alvastra Monastery	Lysings	Östergötland (south-west)
25.5.50	10	Vista parish ch.	Tveta	Småland, north-central
23.6.50	11	Klokkarike parish	Boberg	Östergötland (north-west)
		Linköping Cathedral	town	Östergötland (central)
14.8.50	12	Linköping Cathedral	town	Östergötland (central)
15.8.50	13	Risberga Convent	Edsberg	Närke (central)
18.8.50	14	Nydala Monastery[d]	Västra	Småland (Njudung)
28.8.50	15	Nydala Monastery	Västra	Småland (Njudung)
1.9.50	16	insts. in Jönköping	town	Småland (north of Njudung)
7.9.50	17	Sko Convent	Hagunda	Uppland (central)
12.9.50	18	several parish chs.	Västbo	Småland (Njudung)
		Byarum parish ch.	Östbo	Småland (Finnveden)
21.9.50	19	Nydala Monastery	Västra	Småland (Njudung)
		Åker parish ch.[e]	Östbo	Småland (Finnveden)
26.10.50	20	St Nicholas ch.	Stockholm	Uppland (south-east)
27.10.50	21	Vreta Convent	Gullberg	Östergötland (north-central)
29.10.50	22	Våla parish	Våla	Uppland (north-east)
3.11.50	23	Knifsta parish	Ärlinghundrad	Uppland (south-central)
10.11.50	24	Linköping Cathedral	town	Östergötland (north-central)
23.11.50	25	Botnaryd parish ch.	Mo	Västergötland (east)
24.11.50	26	Alvastra Monastery	Lysing	Östergötland (south-west)
30.11.50	27	Nydala Monastery	Västra	Småland (Njudung)
26.12.50	28	Vimmerby parish ch.	Sevede	Småland (east)
31.12.50	29	Strengnäs Cathedral	town	Södermanland (north-central)

[a] See presentation of important administrative structures in the Nordic countries under Norway, Ch. 16 above.
[b] Småland is such a large region, reaching from Halland's south-eastern border to the Baltic Sea, that it will be useful to indicate the main territorial divisions within the region. Finnveden is a south-western area bordering on the Danish province of Halland, Njudung is a north-central area, and Värend a south-central area.
[c] Donation from the vicar of Svenarum parish to Nydala monastery close by.
[d] In No. 14 and No. 15, two different men donate tenements in the parish of Svenarum to Nydala monastery nearby, which suggests that they are local men reacting to the presence of the Black Death in the locality or in the vicinity.
[e] The donor is the parson of Åker parish.

Interestingly, there is no indication of any independent introduction of the Black Death on Sweden's eastern, Baltic coast. The donation to Vreta Convent in Östergötland on 12 February 1350 is too early and far inland in Östergötland; Alvastra Monastery, which was endowed at the end of May, is situated on Östergötland's western border. It could be that the inhabitants of Östergötland really got the jitters already in the autumn of 1349 when King Magnus's 'open letter' to them was recited in churches and market places, relating the gruesome events that took place in the countries to the west: people had died in such mind-boggling numbers that there was not enough space for them in the consecrated cemeteries in which their bodies had to be buried if they were to have any hope of salvation; and, death came so fast that there was no time for the priests to administer the last rites, which also meant that good Christian people would be doomed to eternal perdition and punishment. For these extremely frightening reasons, the king ordered them to walk barefoot to their parish churches and to process around the cemeteries carrying holy relics, and to fast completely on Fridays except for bread and water.

The strong position of the cloistered people in the religious outlook of the time is also reflected, with 13 of the 28 donations being made to religious houses, and these donations are quite evenly spread throughout the year. Interestingly, in the face of the horrors of the Black Death, donors appear to have had a clear preference for nuns over monks.

The late donation to Nydala Monastery in central Småland could be a reflection of plague's tendency to linger in the same area for many months owing to its special mechanisms of spread. This pattern has also been observed in Norway, where the Black Death can be seen to linger in the districts of Eiker and Sandsvær south-west of Oslo from the summer until the end of the year.[8] The great mortality caused by the Black Death is reflected in the sudden appearance of numerous deserted holdings: in the cadaster of Vadstena Convent, it is stated about a number of vacant tenements that they had been 'deserted since the great plague'.[9]

There remains a central epidemiological question that must be considered, the conspicuous fact that Sweden was not also invaded across the waters of the Baltic Sea by Hanseatic merchant ships or German refugees from the ravages of the Black Death. Instead, the Black Death had to move slowly all the way from the western coast to the Swedish shores of the Baltic Sea. Why did the Black Death not succeed in engulfing the country rapidly by two separate plague fronts that were established in opposite regions of the country, as happened for instance in Norway, Germany, England and the Low Countries? Even more remarkably, the Black Death raged in Visby from the early spring of 1350 and spread out over Gotland I., but did not manage to invade Swedish coastal districts on the Baltic Sea from this seemingly splendid operational base. There can be only one explanation for this shape of the epidemic events, namely that trade and travel broke down in 1350 under the ferocious onslaught of the Black Death. In the ensuing 150 years of the Late Middle Ages, Sweden was frequently invaded by plague, and apparently more often from the east across the Baltic Sea than from the west.

---

[8] Benedictow 1993/1996: 81, 99.
[9] Sandnes 1981: 85.

Except for Gotland I., which at the time of the Black Death and for a few more years belonged to Sweden (until it was reconquered in 1645), there is not a single extant contemporary source that refers to the Black Death in Sweden, and if we change our frame of reference slightly to mainland Sweden, this statement can be unequivocally asserted. This presentation of the Black Death's history in Sweden shows that it is, nonetheless, possible to glean proof of its widespread presence, and evidence of its pattern of spread in time and space from indirect reflections in a category of sources in which there is no reference either to the Black Death or of any other epidemic. However, it is often stated in the wills that it is made in illness ('licet corpore debilis'), and in one case it is also specified that the donor was in his final death throes ('corpore debilis et in extremis vite laborans'). It is also specified that the donation was made to secure especially attractive burial sites, in the parish church, in a monastery or to fund a chantry. When Kristina Siggesdotter, Olof Kase's widow, on 23 November 1350 made a donation of a tenancy to the church of Botnaryd parish to obtain a 'privileged' burial site for her husband and their children, it is reasonable to assume that it was the Black Death that had swept away this little family, and that she was the only survivor. She may here serve to symbolize the great tragedy of thousands upon thousands of people who fell victim to the Black Death this year, but will remain anonymous to posterity.

Another very specific sort of tragedy occurred that can serve to reflect people's despair in the face of the unprecedented epidemic carnage as it unfolded on Gotland I. and in eastern Sweden. A document that is preserved in an undated version in the Hanseatic city of Rostock contains a warning from the mayors and town council of Visby: In Gotland, they had apprehended several 'traitors', and had forced them to admit their diabolic plot against Christendom. Among them was an executed peripatetic player of a regal (a 'medieval portable organ') who had confessed in his last hours that he had poisoned the wells in Stockholm, Västerås and Arboga, and indeed, all over Sweden where he had been travelling. Incidentally, here, we also learn that the Black Death hit the town of Västerås, 90 km north-west of Stockholm, and the small town of Arboga, 130 km west of Stockholm.

The letter shows that suspicions were also directed against the Jews, an attitude that obviously was imported to Visby from abroad, because there is no indication in the sources of the medieval Nordic countries of a Jewish presence at any time. In all likelihood, this anti-Jewish attitude was kindled by rumours of the comprehensive persecution of Jews that was taking place in Germany on the basis of similar accusations. However, the ground may have been prepared for the internalization of prejudiced attitudes from paintings on church walls, from the iconography of triptychs, and from religious legends.[10]

The Black Death's conquest of Sweden constituted the final phase of the conquest of Western and north-western Europe.

---

[10] Ahnlund 1958: 173. On the absence of Jews and on anti-Jewish attitudes in the medieval Nordic countries, see Gad, Berulfsen and Kilström 1963: 73–8.

19

Austria

Introduction to the final phase

At the same time as one of the armies of the Black Death emerged victorious in the western parts of Europe, all the way from Spain to Norway, another formed a broad, although sharply zigzagged plague front that moved northwards in Europe's central regions. This plague front was made up by the massed forces from the original epicentres in Marseilles, northern Italy and on the Dalmatian (Croatian) coast. Austria was invaded about the same time as Switzerland, in August 1348. This heralded the beginning of the conquest of Central Europe. Austria and Hungary, together with eastern Germany, Prussia, Pomerania and the Baltic states, formed the deployment areas and staging areas for the campaigns against Eastern Europe and against Russia, where the Black Death finally petered out after having conquered the continent of Europe.

Austria[1]

The present-day Austrian state was only in the making at the time its territory was invaded by the Black Death. Politically, it was part of the so-called Holy Roman Empire of the German Nation, a fiction dating back to Charlemagne's great conquests, his coronation by the pope in A.D. 800 as emperor and the establishment of the propaganda myth that he had resurrected the Christian Roman Empire of the Late Antiquity. More realistically, Charlemagne had united Frankland (the Kingdom of the Franks) and most of the continental lands and countries that developed a Germanic language, and a number of other regions, areas and countries as well, including a large part of present-day northern Italy.

Austria is the latinized form of the Austro-German name *Österreich*, composed of two words that mean east(ern) ('Ost') and Realm ('reich'), respectively. This was the name of a margravate[2] that Charlemagne established on the eastern border of his empire after he had defeated the mounted Mongol people called Avars in A.D. 788. Later, the margravate was expanded to include the land to the west of the R. Enns,

---

[1] The central work on the Black Death in Austria is Klein 1960, although he relates mainly to the events in the regions of the Eastern Alps.
[2] A margravate is a border province ruled by a margrave.

called Upper Austria in contrast to the original area that was now called Lower Austria where also Vienna is situated, and together these two areas were to constitute the Duchy of Austria.

In the 1280s, Rudolf of Habsburg, who in 1273 had become the monarch of the Holy Roman Empire of the German Nation, transferred to his son Albrecht and his son's father-in-law Count Meinhard of the Tyrol the duchies of Austria, Styria, Carinthia and Carniola on feudal terms. From now on, these duchies formed the core of the emerging Austrian state and, excepting Carniola, they are today 'Lands', i.e., provinces in Austria. Today the larger part of Carniola constitutes the Republic of Slovenia.

The present-day Austrian province of the Tyrol largely corresponds to the former region of Northern Tyrol. Southern Tyrol and a small part of the area of the former Duchy of Carniola belongs today to Italy (the provinces Trentino-Alto Adige and Friuli-Venezia Giulia, respectively), because their populations are predominantly Italian. Northern Tyrol and Southern Tyrol and the present-day province of Salzburg were at the time of the Black Death episcopal fiefs: they were at the same time administrative divisions of the Catholic Church and fiefs of the Holy Roman Empire, meaning that their archbishops were simultaneously in the obedience of the pope and tenants-in-chief holding their respective coextensive areas as fiefs directly from the Holy Roman Emperor of the German Nation with appurtenant lay administrative and military functions. Only much later did they become integrated parts of the Austrian state. The small westernmost province of Vorarlberg, which borders on Bavaria in the north and on Switzerland in the west and south, belonged at the time to the house of Habsburg, but economically and ethnically/nationally the local population had quite strong affinities to the Swiss, so strong that even in the twentieth century there was a political movement in favour of joining Switzerland as a new canton. The small easternmost province of Burgenland, a narrow band of land stretching all along the border on Hungary, belonged to the Kingdom of Hungary until after the First World War.

Finally, one should keep in mind that the territory of the present Austrian state emerged in the aftermath of the First World War as a consequence of the dissolution of the Habsburg Empire.

Arguably, it is anachronistic to discuss the arrival and spread of the Black Death in this region in terms of the territory of the present-day Republic of Austria. However, the modern state of Austria comprises its present territory exactly because it constitutes a natural ethnic and economic entity. In epidemiological terms, this means that Austria is a territory integrated by the rational and advantageous movement and exchange of people and goods, and such movements also have a concomitant territorially integrative function with respect to the dissemination of epidemic disease, whatever its feudal or political status. Furthermore, as in the case of Switzerland, Austria is a modern national entity, and the inhabitants of this country and its historians all relate to the history of the Black Death within this national geographical framework.

The Austrian national territory comprises 84,000 sq. km; the size of its medieval population is not known, and population density at the time of the Black Death cannot be estimated.

As the history of the Black Death moves into the German-speaking regions of Europe, chronicles (annals) become the prevailing type of source available. In these chronicles, datings are conspicuously associated with central religious feasts that chroniclers could easily relate to, and the authors probably also wished to be pedagogically nice to prospective readers who quite likely would not have calendars. Consequently, one should suspect that these datings are only approximate indications of time. A more serious drawback is the fact that even severe epidemics were peripheral in the classical humanistic education that moulded the chroniclers' mind and horizon of interest. Many chroniclers do not mention the Black Death or refer to it only in brief and often insouciant statements.

The time and place of the Black Death's arrival in Austria were closely associated with the Italian territorial connections. Venetian ships played an important part in the transportation of the Black Death from Kaffa or Constantinople to Mediterranean ports in Southern Europe, and especially along the coasts of the Adriatic Sea. As should be expected, the city of Venice was one of the original bridgeheads or epicentres that the Black Death established in this part of the world. The outbreak in Venice was recognized on 25 January 1348, which means that it was introduced probably at the end of November 1347 (see above).

The very early outbreak of the Black Death in the great commercial and industrial city of Venice, and this city's close territorial proximity to the (Italian-speaking) episcopal fief of Southern Tyrol and the Duchies of Carinthia and Carniola, made for an early invasion also of modern Austria proper. This Venetian connection is also mentioned in the contemporary *Annal of Neuberg*.[3] However, the early invasion of Austria does not only reflect the close commercial and national ties between the Venetian city state and northern Italian regions under foreign domination, but also the vital commercial integration of these territories that made the eyes of their lords glitter. People and goods moved in substantial numbers and amounts along the main roads across these areas, over the mountain passes into Austria proper and also, to a considerable extent, further on across Austria and into southern Germany. For these reasons, the Black Death moved with ease along these roads, riding silently and imperceptibly in goods or luggage or in the clothing of people who had not the slightest inkling about the service they perforce performed for this gruesome enemy of humankind.

On its way from the original epicentre in Venice towards various parts of Austria, the forces of the Black Death marched north-westwards in the direction of Southern and Northern Tyrol, northwards in the direction of Carinthia and north-eastwards in the direction of Styria. On its way north-westwards, its outbreak in the episcopal city of Trent (Trento) in Southern Tyrol was recognized on 2 June 1348, corresponding to a probable time of invasion in mid-May. This is the first indication that the Black Death would invade Austria in the early autumn, and first in the Duchy of Northern Tyrol, i.e., the modern Austrian province of the Tyrol. From Trent, the Black Death marched northwards via Bolzano across the northern parts of Southern Tyrol, over the Brenner pass and into Inntal in the Duchy of Northern Tyrol. Already in September, it demonstrated its lethal epidemic might in these southern mountain areas of the (Northern) Tyrol, and had ravaged Vintschgau thoroughly, which indi-

---

3   Klein 1960: 94.

cates that the invasion probably had occurred already in July. In the Benedictine monastery of Marienberg, all the inmates died except two priests, a lay brother and a novice, the dying day of one of the priests being specified to 13 September 1348.[4]

From this area, the Black Death moved further northwards, breaking out in Upper Inntal (Oberinntal) west of Innsbruck in the late autumn. This development was roughly as would be expected, since the distance from the Brenner pass to Innsbruck is only 30 km. In early October, the Black Death broke out somewhat further to the east, in Pusteria/Pustertal, which today is the northernmost part of Southern Tyrol/ Trentino-Alte Adige, but at the time was part of Carinthia, which means that it probably invaded the area at the end of August.

The Black Death also moved out of the city of Venice along roads leading northwards across the area of the Venetian city state that today comprises the provinces of Veneto and Friuli-Venetia Giulia towards Carinthia, and north-eastwards through the Duchy of Carniola (present-day Slovenia) in the direction of Styria. In August, the Black Death is reported both in Istria and in Friuli[5] in the north-eastern corner of Italy, which borders on Carinthia. In January, the Black Death is reported to be raging in Villach, about 20 km into Carinthia from the north-easternmost corner of Friuli.[6] At the time the epidemic had probably been rife for some months. According to the chronicle of the monastery of Neuberg situated in Mürztal in Styria,[7] the Black Death originated in Venice, then moved into 'Upper Italy' whence it slipped into Carinthia and next into Styria, raging in these 'Lands' from Michaelmas to Easter, i.e., from 29 September 1348 to 12 April 1349. In the monastery's local area, in Inner Mürztal, the Black Death broke out on Martinmas, i.e., 11 November 1348. Suddenly, the Black Death had appeared in the very territorial centre of Austria.

The Black Death's movement along this route appears to have been performed at a somewhat quicker pace than along the roads leading into Austria over the Tyrolese mountains, which suggests a somewhat higher traffic density.

At the same time, the Black Death also appeared in the Salzburg mountains after having moved along the main roads across Carinthia and over the Tauern mountain passes.[8] According to the account books of the Benedictine monastery of St Peter in the cathedral city of Salzburg, the Black Death broke out in Pongau, a mountain area situated immediately south of Bischofshofen in central Salzburg, on 11 November 1348.[9]

At the end of 1348, the Black Death had conquered important bridgeheads and deployment areas in Austria, especially in the mountain areas, but it had also advanced deeply into Austrian territory in some areas. It was now poised to complete its conquest. 1349 was the year of the 'great mortality' for most of Austria, and now also the plains stretching from the foot of the mountain areas were overrun.

According to the *Annal of Klosterneuburg*, in the city of Vienna in the eastern corner of Austria, the Black Death lasted from Easter to Michaelmas, i.e., the outbreak was

---

4   Klein 1960: 95.
5   Sticker 1908: 50.
6   Biraben 1975: 77.
7   About 35 km north-west of the town of Graz.
8   Klein 1960: 100.
9   Klein 1960: 114.

recognized on 12 April and ended on 29 September.[10] Taken at face value, this implies that the Black Death should have arrived in Vienna about seven weeks earlier (around 23 February), or rather some days earlier if we also take into account the climate of the season. However, the *Annal of Neuberg* states that the Black Death broke out in Vienna at Whitsuntide, i.e., 31 May, and lasted until Michaelmas.[11] On the other hand, sporadic cases were reported also in 1350[12] – this feature, a long-drawn-out final phase with sporadic cases, is quite typical for plague epidemics in large cities.

It is quite usual to assume that the invasion of Vienna and Lower Austria was implemented by the army of the Black Death that moved up the R. Danube and had begun to ravage the Kingdom of Hungary in January and February.[13] The paucity of sources for the Black Death's history in south-eastern Europe precludes any certainty about the origin of the army of the Black Death that at the time moved up the R. Danube in Hungary proper. However, it cannot conceivably have moved all the meandering way from the estuary of this mighty river, because present-day Romania's coast on the Black Sea was not contaminated until 1348, and because a 130 km-long unnavigable stretch south-east of Belgrade, where the R. Morava joins the R. Danube, prevented the continuity of all transport of goods on the river for a considerable distance. This great river would, therefore, probably not take on a significant disseminative role until the contagion reached Belgrade or invaded the county of Vojvodina that borders on present-day Hungary in Yugoslavia's north-eastern corner.

This highlights two other alternatives. The Black Death in Vienna could have originated in its early bridgeheads on the Dalmatian (Croatian) coast created by Venetian ships on their way home from Kaffa or Constantinople. Outbreaks are registered in Spalato (Split) on 25 December 1347 and in Ragusa (Dubrovnik) a fortnight later (see above). At the time, these important seaports were under the Venetian city state, while the coastline and inland belonged to the Kingdom of Hungary. This means that the Black Death would have had 15–17 months, or roughly 450–500 days, to spread north-eastwards across these politically integrated territories of the Kingdom of Hungary up to the Danube. The distance from Spalato to the Danube on the border of present-day Hungary and the distance from Ragusa to the R. Danube in Belgrade is roughly 330 km as the crow flies. This corresponds to an average daily pace as the crow flies of about 0.7 km, or on the ground roughly 1 km per day. Having reached the mighty river with its lively commercial shipping activities, it would be easy to find opportunities for river transport.

However, the distance from Mürztal in the heart of Styria, where the Black Death broke out 11 November 1348, to Vienna is only about 120 km. The Black Death reached Vienna either at the end of February or in the second week of April (outbreak either on 12 April or 31 May) 1349. This means that the Black Death would have had 100/150 days to travel the 120 km, a distance that would be covered with an average daily pace of spread of 1.2 or 0.8 km, respectively. This alternative is, therefore, a

---

[10] Neumayr, Mazakarini and Potuzhek 1964: 260–1; Klein 1960: 96; Velimirovich and Velimirovich 1989: 811, 816.

[11] Hoeniger 1881: 15.

[12] Velimirovich and Velimirovich 1989: 811.

[13] Sticker 1908: 51; Biraben 1975: 81, 83. See above, p. 76.

serious competitor for the doubtful honour of being the source of contamination of Vienna and much of the Duchy of Austria.

Eggenburg, situated about 80 km north-west of Vienna and close to the border of the Kingdom of Bohemia, may, as has been suggested, have been attacked some time in the summer of 1349, which implies that the territorial spread in Austria was nearing completion at the time.[14]

Probably, the armies of the Black Death that marched out of the original epicentres on the Dalmatian (Croatian) coast and the army that exited the original epicentre in Venice towards the Duchy of Carniola and reached Mürztal in November 1348 met somewhere in eastern Austria.

[14] Biraben 1975: 83.

20

Germany

In 1349, the armies of the Black Death closed in on the territories of the present-day Federal Republic of Germany from several quarters – from the south across Austria and Switzerland; from the west by forces that in the summer and the autumn were moving up along the R. Rhine in Alsace in north-eastern France; and from the north by armies of the Black Death engaged in the murderous conquest of England and Norway from where ship transport was easily available. Metastatic leaps by Hanseatic ships coming from their trading stations ('Kontors') in London, Oslo or Bergen could easily have brought the Black Death to German towns and cities on the North Sea and Baltic Sea in the summer or the autumn of 1349.

At the time of the Black Death, the territories of Germany constituted the core areas of the Holy Roman Empire of the German Nation. The Empire comprised a great number of principalities and lay and ecclesiastical fiefs held directly in homage to the emperor (above, p. 179). It comprised also a considerable number of so-called free cities and towns that were not in the possession of some feudal lord or magnate but were formally subordinated directly to the emperor himself. However, this subordination was of little concrete significance; in reality, they functioned largely as independent republican city states governed by their own city councils. A considerable number of these principalities, fiefs and free cities have since joined other states or have become sovereign states. The notion that this area was united under the auspices of the German emperor was largely fictitious. According to the notions of modern social science with regard to the constituting structures of statehood, the Holy Roman Empire of those times appears as a relatively artificial construction. This means that the territory was politically fragmented, not only according to feudal principles of organization, but also, in reality, in the case of some principalities, according to semi-developed structures of statehood. However, at the time, this political fragmentation did not much affect the commercial integration of the Empire or the movement of pilgrims that are so important to the spread of epidemic disease.[1]

In the context of the subject of this book it is important to note some changes in borders and German settlement. Most of the Netherlands and the Kingdom of

---

[1] Denecke 1986: 207–23.

Bohemia belonged to the Holy Roman Empire, and, at the time, the Kingdom of Bohemia comprised not only the present-day territory of the Czech Republic, but also the Duchy of Silesia, a region that is today incorporated in south-western Poland, and, in addition, a couple of small areas to the west, so that the Kingdom reached almost to Nuremberg. Almost all the southern coastline of the Baltic Sea, from its beginning near Lübeck to the Gulf of Finland, belonged either to the Empire or to the Order of the Teutonic Knights, comprising the German provinces of Mecklenburg, Pomerania, Prussia and the present-day Baltic states.

Along the Baltic coasts lay a string of commercial cities and towns, of which several of the most important had the status of free cities, among them Lübeck, Rostock and Stralsund. A few years after the Black Death, they organized formally the Hanseatic League together with German free cities and towns on the North Sea, such as Hamburg and Bremen. This reflected increasing political co-operation and the development of well-organized trading stations in important commercial centres abroad, among them London, Bergen, Oslo and Novgorod. Lively exchange of goods by sea all the way from Novgorod in Russia to Lübeck, Bergen, London and Bruges in Flanders, and in the opposite direction, meant that epidemic disease would be easily disseminated between urban centres facing the North Sea and the Baltic Sea, and that disease would spread from them into their hinterlands along the commercial road and river systems.

The urban developments along the coasts of northern Germany in the High Middle Ages were related to sustained general population growth that gave momentum to brisk urban growth in the Empire as a whole. It meant that increasing amounts of goods were transported along the inland routes of communication, either along the large waterways or on the main roads. This increasing traffic density that reflects a more general trend towards the modernization of Europe intensified the dissemination of contagion and the incidence of epidemics.

The source material on the history of the Black Death in the German territories must be considered quite poor, and consists almost entirely of short statements and assertions in chronicles.

A glance at the map would spontaneously suggest that the Black Death first penetrated into Germany in south-western Bavaria from the Austrian province of the Tyrol as early as the late autumn of 1348. The Black Death invaded Austria over the Brenner pass probably in July 1348. The distance from the Brenner pass across the Tyrol to the German border is only about 50 km, which could presumably be covered in 2–2.5 months, corresponding to an average daily pace of spread of 0.8–0.6 km. Actually, the Black Death can be seen to have moved further northwards roughly at this pace, because it broke out in Upper Inntal (Oberinntal) west of Innsbruck in the late autumn, and must be assumed to have reached Innsbruck sometime in October. The distance from the Brenner pass to Innsbruck is only 30 km, about halfway to the German border and about 45 km from Garmisch Partenkirchen in Bavaria. Thus, one could reasonably assume that the Black Death would continue its northwards march, and have reached Garmisch Partenkirchen at the end of 1348. However, this appears not to have happened. In all likelihood, the reason is that the winter weather in the mountain areas was too cold to allow epidemic spread of a disease dependent on transmission by fleas and high degrees of bacteraemia in rats. In the lowlands, the epidemic process of spread could proceed at a normal pace: as shown above, forces sent westwards by this army of the Black Death invaded Pfäfers in eastern Switzerland in April 1349, after having marched roughly 200 km from the Brenner pass and the Austrian Tyrolese mountains via Innsbruck and Upper Inntal at an average daily pace of c. 0.8 km. The onset of cold winter weather may also be the reason the Black Death did not proceed directly from its outbreak in November in Constance on the Swiss–German border into Germany's south-western province of Baden-Württemberg. The Black Death was forced to postpone its invasion of southern Germany until the arrival of spring brought warmer weather.

These developments meant that when the spring of 1349 arrived, the Black Death was poised to strike into southern Germany on a broad front stretching from Basle in the west to Upper Austria in the east. Strategically, this massive deployment of epidemic forces along the borders of southern Germany meant that, when the invasion got under way, Germany would be attacked both in a vast pincer-like movement formed by armies marching from opposite southern corners into the south-western province of Baden-Württemberg and into the south-eastern province of Bavaria, and, in addition, on a broad central front over the Tyrol's northern mountain range.

Also in this case, developments on the ground did not conform to well-founded assumptions. One would normally assume that the western arm of the pincer would consist of several armies that had marched together northwards out of Lyons in April 1348. One of these armies took off into Switzerland and invaded Basle, where the Black Death broke out in early May the following year, which also means that it had reached that great river Rhine on the German border. The other western armies had marched on to Chalon before, at the important crossroads there, in the summer of 1348, they split into three armies that were sent in three main directions: one headed north-westwards towards Paris, another marched on northwards in the direction of Rheims and Nancy, and a third army took off north-eastwards from Chalon. The north-eastbound army entered Besançon probably at the end of September 1348, and marched relentlessly on; after having reached Mulhouse it marched along the R. Rhine, outbreaks being recognized in Colmar in June and in Strasbourg on 8 July, respectively. From Mulhouse, the distance to the Rhine is only 10–15 km, and this distance to the river is steadily decreasing so that Strasbourg is situated on the western river bank. Despite this fact, there is no indication that the Black Death on this march northwards close to the Rhine actually crossed it into Germany.

Instead, it was forces from Basle that opened the German front and carried out the conquest of the western regions of Germany all the way from the Black Forest to the city of Cologne, about 500 km farther north. Again, metastatic leaps by ship transport, this time on the R. Rhine, were the pivotal part of the strategy that allowed it to move northwards at much greater pace than forces moving by land. While the epidemic presence of the army of the Black Death that marched north-eastwards from Chalon was recognized in Strasbourg on 8 July, the epidemic presence of the water-borne army from Basle had already been recognized in May (unspecified day) in the town of Lichtenau, almost 20 km further north, but on the German side of the river. In Frankfurt on the R. Main, 200 km north of Strasbourg, the outbreak of the Black Death was recognized on 22 July, implying a time of invasion in the first week of June. The Black Death would then first have had to invade the city of Mainz, at the conjunction of the R. Rhine and the R. Main, where it broke out 'in the summer', and next move 35 km eastwards up the Main to Frankfurt.[2] This demonstrates again the great significance of metastatic leaps by ship transport in the strategy of the Black Death: in three months, the Black Death had leapt 300 km northwards, almost halfway across Germany.

The eastern arm(y) of the pincer movement employed the same strategy of metastatic leaps along a great river, in this case the R. Danube, which, in Germany, runs from its original sources in the Black Forest in the province of Baden-Württemberg north-eastwards to the city of Regensburg in central Bavaria, where it turns south-eastwards and leaves Bavaria and Germany for Upper Austria near the border town of Passau. The Black Death moved upstream: the contemporary author Konrad von Megenburg states in his *Book of Nature* that it moved on from Vienna 'towards Bavaria and to Passau'.[3]

Konrad von Megenburg is clearly of the opinion that the town of Passau was the first place in Bavaria to be invaded by the Black Death. It is therefore unfortunate for our endeavours to uncover the pattern and pace of spread that the time of the outbreak in Passau is not given. The usual dating of the Black Death's outbreak in the city of Regensburg to 25 July 1350[4] has made the epidemic process incomprehensible and left scholars pretty much confused. At the time, Regensburg was the only city situated on the Danube in Bavaria, actually on its northernmost bend. Being by far the most important hub of trade and travel in the region, it must be considered of special importance also in an epidemiological perspective. This importance is increased by the frequently held opinion that the region of Franconia that stretches northwards from the other bank of the R. Danube should have escaped the Black Death. It has been something of a breakthrough in the study of the Black Death in Bavaria that Amalie Fößel has succeeded in showing that the dating of the outbreak of the Black Death in Regensburg to 25 July 1350 is owing to a misinterpretation of a notice in the *Lawbook of the City of Regensburg*, which, seen within a wider textual context, makes it clear that the year referred to is 1349.[5]

The distance from Passau to Regensburg is about 115 km. It is, however, difficult to combine our new knowledge of the time of the outbreak in Regensburg with our knowledge on the plague's usual pace of spread for estimating the time of the outbreak in Passau, because of the possibility of metastatic leap(s) by ship transport. Whatever the case, ship transport upstream this distance would take some time; furthermore, according to the standard assumption, depending on the size of the urban centre, six–seven weeks would normally elapse from the introduction of contamination until a disquieting number of conspicuously rapid deaths would attract the attention of the chronicle-producing social elites and lead to recognition of the presence of the Black Death. Quite likely, then, the Black Death had invaded Regensburg around 8 June, which may suggest that Passau was contaminated probably at the end of April. Cross-infection of ships or boats in Passau's harbour could easily have happened; for this reason transport of the contagion from Passau to Regensburg could possibly have started before the outbreak of the epidemic proper.

---

[2] Fößel 1987: 10; Hoeniger 1881: 20.
[3] Fößel 1987: 7.
[4] See, e.g., Hoeniger 1881: 17; Biraben 1975: 76–7.
[5] Fößel 1987: 8.

This means that, by a solid margin, this is the earliest identifiable outbreak of the Black Death in Bavaria, which could have been as early as the outbreak in Lichtenau north of Strasbourg in May (see above).

The lack of accuracy that characterizes so much of medieval chronicle-writing, and the problems historians face in their endeavours to turn their accounts and opinions into historiography will be illustrated by the following discussion of the Black Death's history in Bavaria. The bare essentials of the epidemic events are related in an elementary way in the *Annals of Matsee*, where it is stated that, in 1349, the plague ravaged Vienna cruelly and, then,

> comes to Bavaria, namely in Mühldorf where at Michaelmas [= 29 September] the preceding year there died 1,400 of the inhabitants [. . .] likewise in Braunau, and in Munich, and in Landshut [. . .] it raged as much.[6]

This statement is clearly problematic for several reasons. First, the dating of the outbreak in the town of Mühldorf to the autumn of 1348 must be erroneous on two grounds: (1) at the time, the plague was only on its way down from the Brenner pass towards Innsbruck; (2) the datings are irreconcilable because it is first said that the plague ravaged Vienna in 1349 and then came to Bavaria and to Mühldorf; consequently, an outbreak in Mühldorf in the autumn of 1348, long before the outbreak in Vienna, is illogical and untenable.

The author could be understood to the effect that the outbreak had started some unspecified time earlier and had killed 1,400 persons by Michaelmas, but the year must still be incorrect.

This does not end the historian's woes, because in the *Annals of Mühldorf* it is actually asserted that the epidemic broke out on 29 June 1348. In this case too, the year given must be wrong, because at the time the Black Death was in the process of marching out of Trent in northern Italy in the direction of the Brenner pass. However, the day given for the recognized outbreak can be accepted. The conclusion must be that the outbreak is misdated by one year. Summing up the evidence, it appears likely that the outbreak of the Black Death in Mühldorf was recognized on 29 June 1349, and that the town was probably contaminated six weeks earlier, i.e., c. 18 May; furthermore, that the epidemic was considered finished at Michaelmas after having killed a great portion of the population.

A similar problem is associated with a notice in the *Chronicle of Augsburg* to the effect that the Black Death broke out in this city in the summer of 1348. The same objections that have been marshalled against other datings of the Black Death's arrival in Bavaria to 1348 hold good in this case too, which means that it must be redated to the summer of 1349.

The datings of the epidemic events given in various chronicles are few and without exception so problematic that they must be redated, either from 1350 to 1349 as in the case of Regensburg, or from 1348 to 1349 as in the cases of Mühldorf and Augsburg. This fact inevitably diminishes the validity of any account of the Black Death in Bavaria. However, it can to some extent be strengthened again if the data

---

6   Hoeniger 1881: 15–16. My translation from Latin.

that have emerged on the basis of this heavy input of source criticism provide a consistent and realistic pattern of epidemic spread in local time and space.

Realistically, the Black Death could have used two main strategies of spread into Bavaria. First, it is an established fact that the Black Death moved north-westwards upstream the R. Danube and crossed into Bavaria at the town of Passau, and then moved on to the city of Regensburg, where its outbreak was recognized at the end of July. This means that on its way north-westwards up the Danube the Black Death could have branched off south-westwards and upstream the large tributaries that flow into the Danube, up the R. Inn from Passau in the direction of Braunau and Mühldorf, and up the R. Isar in the direction of the town of Landshut and the city of Munich. Alternatively, the forces of the Black Death that conquered the Austrian province of the Tyrol in the autumn of 1348 and on a broad front were frustrated in their endeavours to cross over the mountain passes into Bavaria by the the advent of winter, could have succeeded with the arrival of spring and warmer weather. This means that the Black Death could have sailed downstream on the same rivers.

Is it possible on the basis of the sparse source material to distinguish between these two strategies and indicate which of them was actually realized on the ground? One usable approach is to assume that the successive order in which the various towns and cities are mentioned in the *Annals of Matsee* is not fortuitous but reflects the chronicler's opinion with respect to the succession of the epidemic outbreaks. In that case, Mühldorf would have been infected before Braunau, and Munich before Landshut. Using this criterion, a clear and consistent pattern of spread in time and space emerges: in addition to the established invasion along the Danube from Passau to Regensburg, Bavaria was invaded from the Austrian province of Tyrol over several mountain passes, whence the epidemic forces moved downstream along the large local tributaries.

The criterion of order of urban centres mentioned in the main source cannot be allotted decisive weight on its own for determining the territorial progression of the Black Death in southern Bavaria, but its indications are strengthened by two facts. The epidemic presence of the Black Death in Augsburg was recognized in the summer of 1349 and it was, therefore, almost certainly invaded no later than Regensburg. Obviously, the Black Death could not have moved farther upstream on the R. Danube from Regensburg and have branched off along the tributary R. Paar that flows south-westwards in the direction of Augsburg more than 130 km away, and have broken out there before or, possibly, at about the same time as it emerged in Regensburg itself. Instead, the origin of infection must be forces of the Black Death that had crossed the mountains near the town of Füßen and had moved on to the R. Wertachs or the R. Lechs, which join in the city of Augsburg. Secondly, it is strengthened by the consistency of the findings that the case of Augsburg independently implies the same pattern as suggested by the succession of urban centres mentioned in the *Annal of Matsee*, and that the Black Death in all three cases moved downstream and not upstream on the local rivers.

What happened further becomes increasingly unclear. The Black Death continued to move upstream on the R. Danube until, later in the year, it had crossed Bavaria's territory and broken out in the town of Ulm in Baden-Württemberg, immediately across Bavaria's western border. Presumably, it moved further on in the direction of the Black Forest in the south-western corner of this province. On general epidemiological grounds, one would like to assume that forces of the Black Death also marched on slowly by land into the south-western corner of Baden-Württemberg from Basle, that other forces moved out of Constance on the Swiss side of L. Bodensee and entered the province at the middle of its southern border, and that yet other forces moved into the south-eastern corner of the province from the westernmost Austrian province of Vorarlberg and from the Swiss canton of St Gallen. One would also like to assume that, at the same time, other forces marched into the heartland of the province from bridgeheads established on the Rhine's eastern bank, from Lichtenau, for instance. From the spring of 1349, the province of Baden-Württemberg can be seen to have been increasingly surrounded by hostile epidemic forces. However, regrettably, no additional information on the epidemic events has reached posterity.

According to Hoeniger, Zaddach, Fößel and some other scholars, a large area around the axis Nuremberg–Würzburg should have escaped the ravages of the Black Death altogether.[7] This view is based on a selection of what they consider to be the best available chronicles. Some alternative evidence to the contrary is provided in other chronicles, but is dismissed on grounds of low quality. As this area was severely ravaged by a great plague epidemic a few years later, and repeatedly throughout the Late Middle Ages, an escape from the Black Death cannot have been owing to any structural obstacles to the dissemination of the disease.

In this case, a contributory or partial explanatory factor relating to season and climate can be established: it has already been pointed out that, as the Black Death moved on northwards in inland Europe, winter weather tended to slow down its pace of spread, as it did between Besançon and Montbéliard, or to stop its spread temporarily for the cold season, to be resumed with the advent of spring and warmer weather, as in the case of the invasion of Bavaria from the Tyrol. Another quite general feature that has emerged is a strong slowdown in the average daily pace of spread by land, from around 2 km from Marseilles to Lyons to between 0.5–1 km. Assuming an average daily pace of 0.66 km by land, the Black Death would not succeed in reaching Nuremberg from Regensburg or Würzburg from Frankfurt on the R. Main before the onset of the winter. In this area in the north-western half of Bavaria (mainly central Franconia), the Black Death could have found itself epidemically extinguished by cold inland winter weather, although it would most likely preserve some enzootic activity (see Glossary), smouldering on in local rat populations.

In addition, the Black Death could easily have moved in from several quarters. There was a southern plague front of joint forces that had moved over the Tyrol and along the Danube and, after having reached Regensburg in the early summer of 1349, was about 100 km from Nuremberg by land; Würzburg, at the other end of the axis, was situated on the R. Main about a hundred km by land south-east of the city of Frankfurt that likewise was invaded in the early summer of 1349. The distance along the river is somewhat longer, but could be covered at a much higher pace. Hoeniger clearly envisages that the forces of the Black Death that moved inland along the R. Main formed a plague front somewhat farther to the north, roughly along the borders between Hesse and Bavaria in the north-west and between Thuringia

---

[7] Hoeniger 1881: 31–2; Zaddach 1971: 11; Fößel 1987: 12–18.

(Thüringen) and Bavaria[8] in the north, which, in 1350, moved into north-western Germany.

Although a temporary stop in the epidemic activity and progression can be explained on seasonal grounds, epidemiologically, it appears inexplicable that the Black Death should not have either recrudesced from the microbiological embers smouldering in local rat populations or have moved into the area from the surrounding regions in the spring and finished the job in north-western Bavaria.

None of the scholars who argue in favour of the view that this area in north-western Bavaria escaped the Black Death attempts to present an epidemiological explanation, and indeed, in this case it does not appear possible to construct one. While chance can be accepted as an explanation for the narrow escape of some town or village that the Black Death passed by, chance cannot explain why a large area or region should be spared. A scholarly position that takes on the character of a conundrum is clearly unsatisfactory. As long as this epidemiological enigma stands undefeated, the validity of this position remains seriously undermined.

This impasse highlights the fact that this position is weaker than its proponents admit. First, it is based on what, in the methodology of historical science, is called an inference *ex silentio*, i.e., an inference from silence in the sources. But inference from the fact that some social phenomenon is not mentioned in some sources to an assertion to the effect that this phenomenon did not occur or exist is a fallacy of methodology, unless the sources in question are of such a kind that it would be exceptional or unusual if such a phenomenon was passed over in silence. However, what medieval chroniclers do not find occasion to mention is a perennial source of amazement for historians. However strange this may seem to modern man, there are a large number of contemporary chroniclers who did not bother to mention that their community, or any other community, had been ravaged by the Black Death, or by later plague epidemics, notwithstanding that they must have observed unspeakable tragedy and misery. Blockmans makes the same point in relation to the chronicles of the Low Countries, although he fails to relate it more specifically to the humanistic culture, tradition and mentality that formed the content of chronicles:

> One could remark, that, although we have a series of firm evidence about an abnormal high mortality at our disposal, the data are nevertheless scarce. Most of the narrative sources simply are silent about death or plague in 1348–52, although they mention the ones of 1360–61 and of 1368–70. Is the unknown phenomenon here being ignored from fear or from ignorance?[9]

One should also take note of the fact that the selected chroniclers do not comment on the Black Death at all generally, not even in Frankfurt or Regensburg, although news of the catastrophic events in the surrounding cities, towns and rural districts would undoubtedly have made a great impression on modern people.

---

[8]   Hoeniger refers to a line that could roughly be drawn along the mountain range called Spessart, via Rhön and the Thuringian Forest (Thüringerwald). 1881: 25.

[9]   Blockmans 1980: 845. This subject has not been discussed systematically, but is often referred to in connection with concrete analyses of certain non-political subjects, and particularly often in relation to the Black Death and later plague epidemics. See also, however, Halsberghe 1983; Despy 1977: 195; and comments above, Ch. 13, on Belgium.

Comments by Fößel about one of the two chronicles she has selected as the evidential basis for her discussion are clarifying. *The Annal of Ulman Stromer* is divided into
two parts, one that contains memorable events and one genealogical part containing
information relating to his biological family and relatives. Fößel states that the first
part 'does not contain general news on catastrophes', but that in the second part of
the *Annal* the word 'pestilence' is mentioned three times as the cause of death, first for
the author's brother in 1362, and, next, in relation to two persons in 1395.[10] These
cases show that this chronicler did not mention serious epidemics in the general part
of his *Annal* that is said to relate to 'memorable events', although he was perfectly
aware that serious epidemics hit his city. This is exactly the same intellectual attitude
to the notion of memorable events that Blockmans identifies in the chronicles of the
Low Countries. Thus, Fößel has actually selected to constitute her evidential basis a
chronicle (annal) that as a general rule does not mention epidemic events or other
calamities that might befall Nuremberg. Fößel's approach is methodologically flawed,
since silence about the Black Death is exactly what should be expected.

Stromer is not an eccentric, atypical chronicler; on the contrary, his approach to
the writing of a chronicle belongs to a broad humanistic tradition that provides a
quite simple general explanation: epidemics are peripheral to the humanistic education and culture that have shaped the chronicle-producing men's minds and social
outlook. This is the main reason that there are so few chronicles containing information about the Black Death; that when information is given it is usually in the
form of brief, careless notices containing frequent slips of the pen, often without indication of time; and that when time is indicated, it is often in some way flawed, as
shown above. Unfortunately, there is reason to assume that the most highly educated
and socially ambitious chroniclers will conform more to the humanistic ideals of classical learnedness, and precisely for this reason omit information on events that was
not entirely in line with their high standards and social ambition. Men of less education and learning or with more modest social ambition would not be so reluctant to
include more 'vulgar' news, so to speak. Arguably, therefore, the criteria used to
single out the best chronicles are flawed in their social and cultural analysis of the
chronicle-producing classes, and, for this reason, poorly suited in relation to a subject
that is peripheral to the humanistic ideals of learned writing. Correspondingly,
Roman classical chroniclers provide almost no information on the great epidemics
that ravaged the Empire from the time of Emperor Marcus Aurelius at the end of the
second century A.D., and in the following centuries. This is also the reason that when
medieval chroniclers occasionally give accounts of the Black Death, they are often not
based on personal observation but legitimized by rendering Thucydides' literally classical account of the so-called 'Plague at Athens' during the Peloponnesian War about
1,800 years earlier.[11] Of course, these arguments and comments do not at all prove
anything with respect to the actual events; they serve only to undermine the usability
of the selected chronicles as sources for negating the presence of the Black Death in
the region centred on the axis Nuremberg–Würzburg.

---

[10] Fößel 1987: 12.
[11] Thucydides, *The Peloponnesian War*, Book Two, sections 47–55. The disease described by Thucydides is
certainly not plague, and the Greek word used has the meaning of epidemic without reference to any specific
disease. See also Bulst 1977: 57–8.

In this scholarly state of affairs, priority will be given to evidence that contributes to an outline of the epidemic process that is reconcilable with the basic premises of epidemiology and the historical sociology of the area at the time. Both Sticker and Biraben assume that both Nuremberg and Würzburg were attacked by the Black Death in 1350, and, thus, have accepted the validity of the information provided in the alternative sources, albeit without displaying any source-critical interest in the obvious problems relating to the usability of these sources.[12] Although the sources on which this view are based are deemed to be of modest or poor quality, the fact that, in this case, they provide information that conforms with the basic epidemiological requirements for valid explanation strengthens their case for level of tenability over and above non-explanatory interpretations based on silence in the selected sources. In conclusion, at this stage of research, the view that Würzburg and Nuremberg and the region centred on this axis were invaded by the Black Death in 1350 should have priority over the view that this did not happen.

How did the epidemic events develop in the northern half of Germany? The Black Death's rapid advance downstream the Rhine from Basle where its outbreak was recognized in early May, all the way to the city of Cologne, about 500 km down the river, where it arrived around 1 November (epidemic presence recognized c. 20 December), was a significant event in its German history. Along this mighty river, the Black Death disseminated contagion in towns and cities, contaminations that formed new small or large epicentres of spread by land, e.g., from Lichtenau a little north of Strasbourg (see above), but on the German side of the river, into central Baden-Württemberg, or by water along the many small and large rivers that intersect German territory, e.g., invading the town of Limburg, about 50 km upstream on the R. Lahn from the Rhine, and so on.[13] Of particular importance is the Black Death's spread out of the city of Mainz upstream the R. Main, both because this is the Rhine's largest tributary flowing westwards, almost all the way from the Bohemian (Czech) border across the German territory to the Rhine, and because it occurred so early. We are told somewhat imprecisely that the epidemic in Mainz took place in the 'summer'; it started probably around mid-May, since the outbreak in Frankfurt, 75 km upstream, was recognized on 22 July, which indicates a time of contamination in early June. However, contagion could have been disseminated with goods from Mainz's harbour to Frankfurt's harbour in an early stage of the epidemiological developments, which implies that the disseminative transport could have taken place some time in the second half of May. Dissemination of plague contagion along the R. Main must be the origin of the plague front that was formed in this central part of Germany and that moved slowly (and southwards). *The Chronicle of Limburg* states tersely that, in the summer of 1349, the Black Death spread across the province of Hesse from Mainz to Limburg, a statement that can inspire scepticism about the local chronicler's horizon of knowledge and interest.[14]

According to Sticker and Biraben, the Black Death broke out in the town of Erfurt

[12]   Sticker 1908: 67; Biraben 1975: 76–7, 84, 408. Biraben does not indicate his source, and is, probably, in this case dependent on Sticker's information.
[13]   Biraben 1975: 76–7.
[14]   Sticker 1908: 67.

in the early months of 1350, but no source is indicated. Hoeniger cites *Chronica Sampetrinum*, which with great accuracy dates the time of the epidemic to 25 July 1350–2 February 1351.[15] Hanni Spiegler, who has written a dissertation on 'The History of Plague in Erfurt', argues in favour of a dating of the outbreak to the summer of 1350.[16] At first glance, this may appear confusing, because the plague front that moved northwards from southern Germany could not have reached so far; on the other hand, by the summer of 1350, the Black Death had spread over large parts of northern Germany. This pattern is explicable only if the plague front in this north-central part of Germany actually moved southwards. There are also other epidemic events in northern Germany that imply landings of the Black Death on the coasts of the North Sea and the Baltic Sea.

The few and dispersed pieces of information that have been handed down to posterity with regard to the Black Death's pattern of spread in Germany are difficult to interpret and to shape into a clear and consistent picture of the process(es) of spread. The only realistic scholarly objective is to construct an explanatory hypothesis that will be able to reconcile the bits of information on the Black Death's spread in time and space with the epidemiology of plague and the movement in time and space of people and goods along the existing systems of communication.

Seemingly, a north-western plague front was formed by a similar process east of the R. Rhine to that which arose along the R. Main. It is possible to glean information from the sources to the effect that, in the early months of 1350, the Black Death broke out in the north-western towns of Paderborn and Osnabrück and in Minden, which is situated halfway between Osnabrück and Hannover. Next, we are informed that, in May, the Black Death broke out in a string of cities comprising Bremen, Hamburg and Lübeck on the coasts of the North Sea and the Baltic Sea, and, at the same time, in Hannover, Halberstadt and Magdeburg in inland northern Germany.

In an epidemiological perspective, the contemporaneity of these quite widely dispersed outbreaks is puzzling, as is the relationship between these outbreaks and the earlier outbreaks, and the origin or origins of contagion appear puzzling as well. The distance from Cologne, where the Black Death is said to have broken out c. 20 December, to Osnabrück and Paderborn, is roughly 150 km by land as the crow flies, and 200 km to Minden. Thus, the Black Death would have had to move at a daily pace of *at least* 1.7–2.25 km using this definition, and considerably faster on the ground, to achieve this feat. On the background of the accumulated knowledge of the Black Death's pace of spread by land, and taking into consideration basic demographic and economic circumstances, it is difficult to accept that the epidemic should attain its highest pace of spread in this part of Europe under these circumstances (perhaps with exception of the pace of spread from Marseilles to Avignon).

On top of this problem comes the fact that this rapid advance would have occurred from the end of December to the end of March, i.e., in mid-winter. Winter weather slowed down the Black Death's pace of spread in Burgundy, it stopped the Black Death from crossing the mountain passes into Bavaria, and it ended the spread of the Black Death in Norway. Cold weather in exactly the same period of time has been

---

[15] Hoeniger 1881: 26.
[16] I have not had access to this dissertation, but it is cited by Zaddach 1971: 12, 166.

used above to explain the fact that the Black Death's advance in Bavaria stopped somewhere between Regensburg and Nuremberg and between Frankfurt on the R. Main and Würzburg. This seasonal argument is even more relevant for northern Germany, although it will allow for endemic cases and occasional small outbreaks in the winter months, especially in spells of mild winter weather.

Another conspicuous complicating feature of the pattern of spread in northern Germany, especially from a seasonal perspective, is the fact that outbreaks of the Black Death were recognized also in the Hanseatic coastal cities of Bremen, Hamburg and Lübeck in May, in Lübeck on Whitsunday, 16 May. Epidemiologically, this pattern raises some urgent questions relating to the structure of spread in time and space, to pace of spread, means of spread and the origin(s) of contagion. The fact that the outbreaks in Halberstadt and Magdeburg far inland were recognized in the same month of May as in the coastal cities remains inexplicable in epidemiological terms on assumptions of interrelated processes of contamination. Erfurt is too far away, and even an assumption to the effect that the Black Death, nonetheless, broke out in Erfurt at some time in the winter months will not provide a realistic origin for the outbreaks in Halberstadt and Magdeburg. Consequently, the early infection of these northern commercial cities as the result of spread from the north-western plague front appears impossible.

This conclusion highlights the fact that there are realistic alternatives. Importantly, outbreaks of the Black Death were first recognized in the south-eastern Baltic area, in Prussia and Pomerania, before the outbreaks in Lübeck, Hamburg and Bremen in May. At the time, Prussia was the south-western part of the Baltic territories ruled by the Order of the Teutonic Knights. It faced the Gulf of Danzig (Gdansk) and stretched farther northwards so that it included the Memel area (Klaipeda) north of Königsberg (Kaliningrad).[17] Hoeniger cites a notice in the *Book of Citizenship*[18] of the town of Braunsberg to the effect that, in 1349, the Black Death broke out in Elbing, where it raged from the feast of St Bartholomew to Christmas Day, i.e., from 24 August to 25 December, and that, in the same year, a multitude of people succumbed in Königsberg, and in Frauenberg, in 'Molhusin' and in Samland, northwest of Königsberg.[19] Elbing, Frauenberg, Braunsberg and Königsberg[20] are all situated along the Frisches Haff, a sort of vast lagoon[21] on the eastern side of the Gulf of Danzig. The dating of the outbreak in Elbing shows that the Black Death had been introduced into the town probably in the second week of July 1349.

This information is corroborated in a notice written in the autumn of 1349 in the *Chronicle of Oliva* to the effect that the Black Death raged 'all over Prussia and Pomerania'. The corroboration with respect to Prussia is important. Important too is

---

[17] After the Second World War, Prussia was divided between Poland, Russia (the enclave around Kaliningrad/Köningsberg) and Lithuania.

[18] In this book, the names of persons were entered who paid a certain sum of money to attain the rights of citizenship, primarily the rights to perform craftmanship or commerce and to hold office.

[19] Hoeniger 1881: 24.

[20] Modern names are Elblag, Frombork, Braniewo and Kaliningrad, and the new name of Frisches Haff is Zalev Wislany (the estuary of the R. Wisla/Vistula).

[21] Frisches Haff is about 80 km long, 2–18 km wide and 3–5 metres deep, and is separated from the Baltic Sea by a 52 km-long, 2–3 km-broad peninsula stretching north-eastwards, and a smaller peninsula stretching southwards from Samland, allowing only a small opening through which ships can enter the lagoon.

the addition of the Duchy of Pomerania, which, at the time, stretched westwards from the Prussian border along the Baltic Sea's southern shores to a point halfway between Rostock and Stralsund. Also the reference to Pomerania is corroborated by an independent source, for its major western commercial city of Stralsund was in all likelihood contaminated at the end of 1349, since the Black Death's presence is recognized in a bill of exchange issued by the city councillor, Arnold Voed, on 20 March 1350.[22] This means that, as should be expected, the Black Death spread also westwards from the outbreak in Elbing that seems to be indicated as the original epicentre in this region.

At this early date, the infection could have been brought to Prussia by ships coming from England or from the Oslofjord area. The average distance travelled by ships sailing along the coasts at the time is assumed to be about 40 km per day (see above), so the ship that contaminated Elbing must have passed through the Sound around 20 June in order to cover the remaining roughly 900 km in time to occasion contamination in the second week of July. One could suspect that this was a ship fleeing from the outbreak of the Black Death in Oslo where the Hansards had a trading station. The Black Death appears to have broken out in Oslo in April and was raging in the Oslofjord region in the summer (see above). The distance from Oslo to the Sound is roughly 550 km, which would usually be covered by ship in a fortnight; a ship leaving Oslo in the first week of June would be passing through the Sound two weeks later on schedule to reach a town in Prussia on the Frisches Haff in the second week of July. Correspondingly, a Hanseatic ship coming from England must be assumed to have fled from the trading station in London around 1 May in order to contaminate Elbing in the second week of July. In London, the Black Death had flared up in a gruesome epidemic disaster with the arrival of warmer spring weather.[23] One should, however, keep in mind that the longer the voyage, the less likely that a ship with plague on board would reach its destination.[24]

This means that the larger part of the northern German coastline all the way from Samland in present-day Lithuania to far into western Pomerania was ravaged by the Black Death in the autumn of 1349. Importantly, this information makes it clear that southern Germany and northern Germany were invaded almost at the same time, with a northern time lag of only three months, and that also a north-eastern plague front had been formed that was on the march westwards and southwards deeper into German territory. These developments can be enlarged upon and become better understood.

Such a wide spread of the Black Death along the coasts of north-eastern Germany, Pomerania and Prussia with their comprehensive commercial network must have constituted a grave danger for further spread. This seems to be corroborated by a study of wills in Lübeck. The annual average of extant wills in the pre-plague period was slightly below six, whereas in 1350 the number sky-rocketed to 127 (or 129).[25]

---

[22] Lalla 1999: 34, referring to Techen 1926. Pomerania's other important city, Stettin (Szczecin), seems not to have been ravaged until later in 1350. Biraben 1975: 76–7.

[23] Cf. the figures on the number of wills proved in the Court of Hustings, above, Table 4.

[24] In the sixteenth and seventeenth centuries, no European ship with plague on board ever reached America. Iceland was contaminated twice, at the beginning and end of the fifteenth century, which indicates that this island was at the extreme range for transfer of plague contagion by ship (from Norway or England).

However, this figure does not include the start of the increase, an abrupt surge that took place at the end of 1349, bringing the total for that year up to 25.[26] This development must surely reflect at least an incipient outbreak of the Black Death that was suppressed by cold winter weather but, conspicuously, surfaced again in March, probably caused by a spell of mild weather, when 12 wills were made, double the yearly average of the preceding period. This figure is similar to the 11 wills that were produced in May, when the presence of the Black Death was explicitly acknowledged in the extant source material, and which was a prelude to the big epidemic bang in the following months. Interestingly, this also means that the time and progression of the epidemic in Lübeck, according to wills, is quite similar to the time and progression of the epidemic in Ribe in south-western Jutland according to the entries in the *Anniversary Book of the Chapter of the Cathedral of Ribe*. In both cases, ostensibly after having started at the end of 1349, the epidemics reached the height of their impact on the chantry-producing and will-producing social classes in July and August. The majority of city councillors in Lübeck died in these months.[27] This time pattern reflects that the upper classes and social elites were victimized with a significant delay compared to the lower social classes.

This analysis of wills in Lübeck highlights the real epidemiological significance of the fact that Bremen and Hamburg, like Lübeck, had recognized outbreaks in May, although the exact date is not known. These outbreaks can now be seen in the same perspective: the contagion was introduced quite late in the autumn, the outbreaks were, therefore, suppressed in an early phase by cold winter weather, but re-emerged in the spring. The wills in other large cities have not been thoroughly studied, but it is known that there was an abrupt surge in the number of wills in Hamburg in June 1350.[28] It appears, therefore, that the coasts of north-western Germany were widely contaminated with a delay of a couple of months in relation to north-eastern Germany, namely at the end of the shipping season in 1349, probably sometime in October.

On 24 June, the archbishop of Bremen permitted the clergy in the small town of Kiel, 70 km north-west of Lübeck, to establish a new cemetery and a chapel outside the town gates.[29] This must reflect dramatic epidemic mortality that had required several weeks to reveal its real character and to fill up the cemeteries. This event comprises elements of time that come in addition to the time consumed by the ordinary epidemiological developments of plague, namely the time required for the epidemic to cause such huge mortality that the local authorities had to consider what to do in order to ensure all inhabitants burial in a consecrated cemetery, time to send a letter to the archbishop, and the time needed for the archbishop to handle the request administratively. The Black Death in Kiel must have broken out no later than in Lübeck, but would probably have been recognized earlier because of the smaller size of the urban structures. In all likelihood, Kiel had also been contaminated at the end of the shipping season in 1349.

[25] Von Brandt 1973: 127.
[26] Von Brandt 1964: 5–6.
[27] Peters 1940: 92.
[28] Ibs 1994: 94.
[29] Ibs 1994: 91.

On the other side of the Baltic Sea, almost halfway to Stockholm, the epidemic presence of the Black Death was recognized in the town of Visby in Gotland I. in the Easter week of 1350, starting on Easter Day, 28 March.[30] This means that the outbreak in Gotland I. was recognized six to seven weeks earlier than the outbreak in Lübeck, which was recognized on 16 May. According to the standard assumption relating to the time pattern of plague epidemics in towns, a recognized outbreak on 28 March will usually reflect contamination about six weeks earlier, but with some further delay in winters, indicating in this case contamination around 7 February. However, in this case, it must be ruled out that contagion could have been introduced at that time because it precedes the shipping season by many weeks: the cold winters and the very low salinity of the Baltic Sea regularly produce a thick, ice-covered surface that breaks up slowly and disappears with the arrival of spring weather, so generally the months January–March did not allow sailing to Gotland. Actually, the league of Hanseatic cities and towns prohibited merchant ships from putting to sea in the months November–February on safety grounds.[31] There can hardly be any doubt that the Black Death was introduced in the late autumn and had been prevented from developing into a full-blown epidemic by the onset of the usual cold winter weather in the Baltic area. A sudden surge in epidemic deaths in Easter week disclosed its presence. In our context, the outbreak in Visby is important for two reasons: (1) because it provides another instance of a process of wide dissemination of plague contagion in the Baltic Sea area in the autumn of 1349; (2) because this town was dominated by Hansards and, therefore, played a vital part in the commercial network in the Baltic area. When Lübeck and Visby were contaminated in the late autumn of 1349, it appears unlikely that the contagion was not spread even further around by ship within the prevailing system of regional and international trade.[32]

The Hanseatic cities of Bremen and Hamburg on the North Sea, and Lübeck in the south-western corner of the Baltic Sea, were more likely to have been contaminated by ships returning from England, Oslo or Bergen in the autumn of 1349 than from Prussia. The large number of ships involved would make it likely that some contaminated ships for more or less fortuitous reasons would manage to reach their return destinations. The likelihood that contaminated ships would succeed in making it to the cities of Bremen, Hamburg or Lübeck must be considered much greater than that they would make it all the way to Prussia for three main reasons: they were situated at appreciably shorter distances from plague-infected areas in England or Norway; much larger numbers of ships were calling at their harbours and unloading vast amounts of goods, because their burghers owned far more ships and were much more numerous and ran larger and more active businesses; and they had particular emphasis on trade with England and Norway.

These ships would often arrive at their return destinations so late that imported plague contagion would not develop from the endemic phase into an incipient epidemic phase before November. Generally, plague (like other contagious diseases) would usually first break out among poor working-class people in the harbour areas.

---

[30] Peters 1940: 34. At the time, Gotland I. still belonged to the Kingdom of Sweden. Shortly afterwards, the island came under the Danish Crown and did not revert to Sweden until 1645.
[31] Hansen 1912: 127.
[32] See also above p. 173.

The first phase of the epidemic developments would for this reason often be unnoticed or ignored by the chronicle-producing upper classes who were resident at a distance. In these great commercial cities, it would quite likely take additional time for the epidemic to assume proportions that would make contemporary observers among the social elites cognizant of the Black Death's presence and its inherently disastrous character. In short, incipient plague epidemics based on contagion unleashed by ships returning at the end of the shipping season would quite likely be suppressed by the advent of cold winter weather, and their presence would quite likely remain unnoticed or ignored by the chronicle-producing classes. The epidemics would revert to an enzootic phase and smoulder on in the rat colonies until the arrival of spring and warmer weather allowed them to develop into a full-blown plague epidemic. (This type of development could be called the *Visby-pattern.*)

In these endeavours to construct an explanatory hypothesis for the Black Death's pattern of spread in time and space in northern Germany one crucial question remains to be explained: How did the Black Death reach Magdeburg and Halberstadt in time to produce recognized outbreaks in May? Any valid answer to that question will also be applicable to the outbreaks in Hannover, Minden, Osnabrück and Paderborn. Northern Germany's large river system and the vital role it played in the commercial exchange between the great cities along the northern coasts and inland towns and cities will stand at the centre of epidemiological explanation: Magdeburg is situated on the R. Elbe upstream from Hamburg; Halberstadt is situated on Holzemme, which belongs to the R. Elbe's system of tributaries; Hannover is situated at the end of the navigable part of the R. Leine, which is a tributary to the R. Aller, a large navigable tributary that flows into the R. Weser about 35 km north-west of Bremen; Osnabrück is situated on the R. Hunte, the Weser's largest western tributary, which is navigable up to a distance of c. 30 km from Osnabrück. The town of Münster, about 40 km south-west of Osnabrück, where the Black Death broke out in May, is situated near the R. Ems, which flows into the North Sea in eastern Friesland (hypothetically, it could have been contaminated by refugees from Friesland late in 1349). The close economic interaction between these towns and cities and the great Hanseatic cities Bremen, Hamburg and Lübeck is shown also by the fact that they all joined the Hanseatic League. Northern Germany was also criss-crossed by a system of roads that saw the movement of substantial amounts of goods and numbers of people.

Thus, for reasons of plague's special epidemiological properties, the arrival and spread of the Black Death along the northern coasts of Germany in the autumn of 1349, and its wide dissemination in northern Germany during the winter and early spring of 1350 took on a concealed or veiled character so that the process of contamination and spread came only episodically to light and even more episodically became reflected in the extant chronicles.

Finally, the types of goods Bremen, Hamburg and Lübeck sent up along the rivers and along the roads merit interest. Grain, cloth, stockfish (dried cod) and salted fish, hides and furs were important commercial goods. All these products were either very attractive foods for rats or provided fine echological niches for fleas under transport. One point of particular interest that has so far been overlooked is a finding by Dutch physicians combating plague in Java in the first decades of the twentieth century: they discovered that black rats liked to travel with shipments of stockfish.[33] Stockfish was the valuable product Hanseatic merchants endeavoured to acquire in large amounts in Bergen (because they were prohibited from sailing farther north).[34] The Catholic Church's prohibition of the consumption of meat on Fridays, and the numerous religious feasts comprising fasting, not to forget the forty days of Lent, meant that stockfish was in great demand all over Northern and Western Europe.

Summing up, the gist of the explanatory hypothesis that has been formed above is that the commercial cities on the coasts of northern Germany were invaded by the Black Death in the late autumn of 1349 but that this occurred so late in the year that the Black Death did not succeed in producing major outbreaks before they were suppressed by cold winter weather, and, after having reverted to an enzootic phase in the rat colonies, resurged and developed into full-blown epidemics in May. In the meantime, in the winter months, contaminated goods were distributed along the commercial networks, especially along the rivers but also along the commercial roads that criss-crossed northern Germany, so that the contagion became quite widely distributed in this period. An instance illustrating this process is that Hannover appears to have been contaminated along the waterways from Bremen, and Minden may have been contaminated by goods forwarded there by land from Hannover. The reported outbreaks in some towns in the winter months of 1350 must be assumed to reflect both the ongoing process of contamination of northern German towns and spells of mild weather that allowed plague to shift from the enzootic phase to an observable early epidemic phase. This shift revealed the presence of the Black Death before it again was forced underground by the return of cold weather (or continued as a sprinkling of endemic cases) until the arrival of spring and warmer weather when the Black Death ravaged the populations in its typical fashion. Now, it also formed a broad plague front that moved southwards towards central Germany where it met the plague armies that moved northwards from the invasions across the borders of Austria and Switzerland.

The Black Death invaded the March of Brandenburg, a region situated mainly south of Pomerania, at the end of 1350, which shows that the Black Death was also on the march southwards from its landings on the south-eastern coasts of the Baltic Sea. However, also in this region transport by boat on large navigable rivers was considerably faster. The town of Thorn (Torun) situated on Prussia's southern border with Poland, about 150 km upstream on the R. Vistula (Weichsel/Wisla), was ravaged earlier that year.[35] Frankfurt on the R. Oder (the present-day border river between Germany and Poland) was not attacked until the following year.[36]

The territory of Germany is quite large, the distance from the border in the south to the northern coasts being 750 km as the crow flies. Nonetheless, taking into consideration that plague is a disease spread by rats and rat fleas, and that the progress of the epidemic therefore stopped or at least slowed down very strongly in the cold season,

---

[33] Van Loghem and Swellengrebel 1914: 468.
[34] Bruns 1900.
[35] Biraben 1975: 80.
[36] Hoeniger 1881: 27.

the Black Death's conquest of Germany was achieved quite rapidly: the observable campaign as manifested in outbreaks started in June 1349 and tapered off at the end of 1350. There were two main reasons for this. Firstly, Germany was invaded by two plague fronts, from the south and a northern plague front that was formed with a delay of only a few months. Secondly, the systems of navigable rivers are very extensive and allow comprehensive movements of barges, boats and ships. These could easily be infested with rats or with rat fleas, in the clothing of members of the crew, or unwittingly loaded with goods. The infection was thus transported over considerable distances. The two plague fronts can schematically be said to have covered roughly 375 km each in the about the same length of time, corresponding to a daily average pace in the crow-flying perspective of roughly 0.75 km. The much higher pace of movement along the main German rivers than by land played a major role in the Black Death's dynamics of spread. The vitality of the large Hanseatic commercial cities must also be counted among the substantial contributory factors. However, the spread eastwards was at a considerably slower pace, with the Black Death not reaching Frankfurt on the R. Oder until 1351, obviously for the reason that the intensity of transport of goods and people was much smaller in this direction than along the north–south axis.

21

The Netherlands[1]

In the chapter on the Black Death's history in Belgium, it was explained why the history of the Black Death in the Low Countries has not only been divided between the two constituent countries, but has also been separated in time and space: the territory of the southern part of the Low Countries, here inaccurately called Belgium, was invaded in the main from France, while the territory of the northern part of the Low Countries, here inaccurately called the Netherlands, was invaded by forces coming from other directions (see below).

Formally, the historical territory of the modern state of the Netherlands consisted, like Belgium's, of a number of dukedoms and countships, in this case all held in the German emperor's hand, mainly the duchies of Utrecht, Geldern, Overijssel, Zeland, Friesland and Groningen, and the countships of Holland and Drenthe.[2] These territorial divisions correspond largely to the present-day division into provinces. The territory of the present-day Kingdom of the Netherlands comprises 32,600 sq. km but, historically, the northern half of the Low Countries did not include the province of Northern Brabant or some small areas on the southern shores of Western Schelde that at the time constituted the northernmost parts of the 'Belgian' County of Flanders. Thus, on the eve of the arrival of the Black Death, the northern part of the Low Countries, here inaccurately called the Netherlands, comprised about 27,000 sq. km.

With a population of roughly 1 million inhabitants in 1469, and, presumably, at least double that figure on the eve of the Black Death, the population density must have been at least 80 persons per sq. km before the great epidemic catastrophe, more than double the figure for England, France or Italy. In the Low Countries as a whole, the degree of urbanization in 1469 was a remarkable 34 per cent, in Southern Holland even 54 per cent. On the eve of the Black Death, when at least twice as many people were living within the same territory, the degree of urbanization must have been significantly higher.[3] In the century preceding the Black Death, many former

---

[1] As in the case of Belgium, the most important work on the history of the Black Death in the Netherlands is Blockmans 1980. Holland was a countship in the Netherlands, and today roughly the same the area constitutes the two provinces of Northern and Southern Holland.

[2] The continental title of count is said to correspond more to the English title of earl; a continental county would thus correspond to an English earldom.

[3] See Ch. 13 on Belgium for this demographic information. The cautious phrasing of the point on the degree of pre-plague degree of urbanization reflects the fact that the dynamic economic developments in the Low Countries in the Late Middle Ages must have stimulated urban growth.

villages would have grown to contain more than one thousand inhabitants, perhaps several thousand inhabitants, and would have made the sociological transition from village community to (small) town. In many cases, this urban status would be lost as a consequence of the dramatic diminution of the population in the ensuing century, although the dynamic development of proto-industrialization in the Late Middle Ages would have stimulated urban development. Modern research on plague epidemics in Italy and France in 1630–2 and 1720–2, respectively, and also in India in the early twentieth century, indicates that morbidity rates (and consequently mortality rates) in plague epidemics are particularly low in towns, and are still, on average, much lower in cities than in typical rural environments.[4] It should, consequently, be expected that the mortality caused by the Black Death was not so dramatic in the Netherlands as in less urbanized countries and regions.

In 1950, Van Werveke maintained, as mentioned, that the Low Countries were only marginally affected by the Black Death. Under the presentation of the Black Death's history in Belgium it was shown that subsequent research had rendered this view untenable. In the case of the Netherlands, Van Werveke had to accept research showing the presence of the Black Death in the northern duchies of Friesland and Groningen: a very sharp and sudden increase in mortality in seven monasteries occurred in 1350–1. In Friesland, the Black Death appears to have begun its onslaught at the end of 1349.[5]

The city of Deventer on the border between Overijssel and Geldern was infected already in the early spring of 1350, and the epidemic continued into 1351. It is *The Necrologium of the Chapter of St Lebuinus' Church in Deventer* that provides evidence on the sudden onset of extreme mortality. A necrologium is a register of much the same kind as an obituary, namely a register in which a religious institution entered notices on the death of spiritual members and of donors who had endowed chantries with specification of date of death, because at that day a priest should sing masses and perform a commemoration service and intercessory prayer for the dead person's soul (see Ch. 17 on Denmark). In the preceding twenty years, the names of 2.25 persons had, on average, been entered each year. In 1350, 52 names were entered, all in the short period May–September.[6]

The neighbouring Duchy of Overijssel was also ravaged in 1350 and into 1351. This fact emerges clearly in a document issued by the bishop of Utrecht on 12 January 1351 concerning a dispute between the parish church and the monastery at the town of Zwolle in the north-western part of the duchy about the rights of inhumation (because it produced income). The dispute had become acute because of 'the epi-

---

[4]   See Benedictow 1987; above pp. 31–34.
[5]   Meinsma 1924: 401, 404–9, 433–5. For Friesland, see also Biraben 1975: 84; Hoeniger 1881: 23–4.
[6]   Blockmans 1980: 843–4. In view of the fact that we are relating to upper-class persons, who would become victims later in the epidemic process than the poor classes, it must be certain that the contagion could not have been introduced later than in March. This could suggest the alternative scenario that Deventer was contaminated at the end of 1349, but that the epidemic process was arrested by cold winter weather so that it regressed into a enzootic phase, re-emerging in epidemic form in the spring. However, contamination of Deventer at the end of 1349 presupposes a metastatic leap that cannot be plausibly coupled with a place of origin and a means of transportation.

demic or mortality that has already for quite some time been raging in the said town of Zwolle and in surrounding places'.[7]

Next, studies in the count of Holland's account books from 1350 uncovered clear reflections of the ravages of the Black Death, although in the form of rather peripheral indications. Greatly increased mortality was reflected in greatly increased income from the inheritances of serfs, illegitimately born children and foreigners who had died without heirs in western Friesland, which is the northernmost part of the present-day province of Northern Holland, and in Kennemerland, a district in the south-western part of the same province. Thus, all sides of the Zuider Zee (IJsselmeer) were ravaged by the Black Death. The count's account books reveal also a great general contraction in economic activites in 1351 accompanied by a sharp diminution of income. Furthermore, in the districts of Dordrecht in the south-eastern part of the modern province of Southern Holland, the number of deaths doubled in 1352–3.[8]

A charter from 1352 refers to an 'enormous mortality' in the cathedral city and diocese of Utrecht.

The pattern of spread has some conspicuous features, and appears to be moving from the north and southwards: the earliest known outbreak is in Friesland at the end of 1349; next, it broke out in Groningen and in the northernmost districts of Northern Holland. In the following months, plague fronts appear to have been moving southwards on both sides of the Zuider Zee: both Kennemerland in the south of Northern Holland and the city of Deventer on the border between Overijssel and Gelderland were invaded in 1350. The last-known phase of the Black Death is the epidemics in the districts around Dordrecht and in the diocese of Utrecht that reportedly took place as late as in 1352–3. There is no concrete indication of movement northwards by the broad plague front in Belgium, not even in the cases of the outbreaks in Dordrecht or Utrecht, a feature that is, actually, rather intriguing.

This raises the question of the origin of the Black Death in the Netherlands. The usual assumption that the contagion had been introduced from Germany is by no means clear; in fact, it stands up badly to closer scrutiny. The point of departure of this discussion must be the fact that it was Friesland and not Groningen that was attacked first, as should be expected if the contamination had moved in from Germany. The fact that Friesland was infected in late 1349 appears crucial, because it cannot be co-ordinated with the earliest and nearest German outbreak of the Black Death, the outbreak in Cologne that was recognized on 20 December. Thus, it appears reasonable to assume that Groningen was infected from Friesland and not from north-western Germany.

If the Black Death had moved down the R. Rhine from Cologne, the central Netherlandish provinces would have been attacked first, but there is no indication of spread downstream from Cologne into the Netherlands at all, not even in 1350. Contamination of the central and southern parts of the Netherlands appears to have occurred in 1352–3 as a result of the spread southwards of infection from the original

---

[7] Cited by Blockmans 1980: 844, n. 16. My translation from Latin.
[8] De Boer 1978: 34–6, 65–6.

introductions in Friesland and in Groningen that took on the character of original plague fronts. The usual assumption that the Netherlands was infected by offshoots from the German plague fronts appears untenable. This activates once more the question of origin.

It has been argued above in the chapter on the Black Death's history in Germany that there was widespread infection of northern Germany all the way from Bremen and Hamburg to Lübeck and to the Hanseatic town of Visby on Gotland I. in the late autumn of 1349,[9] and also the town of Ribe in south-western Jutland was infected at the end of 1349 (see Ch. 17 on Denmark). It appears to be the most fruitful and likely scenario to assume that the contamination of Friesland, i.e., the original introduction of the Black Death in the Netherlands, should be put within this broader picture as being connected with the return of Hanseatic and Netherlandish ships from places where the Black Death is known to have been raging in the autumn. In late 1349, the Black Death could have been introduced in Friesland from several places, perhaps from northern England, possibly from Scotland, and certainly from Norway where the Black Death was rife in the whole of southern Norway through the summer and autumn of 1349, and it raged in Bergen in western Norway from about mid-August. Ships returning from the important Hanseatic trading station ('Kontor') in Bergen on Norway's western North Sea coast and from the smaller but bustling trading station in Oslo must be put in focus as the most likely sources of the contagion. From these towns appreciable numbers of Hanseatic and Dutch ships returned bound for Hamburg or Bremen, or the cities and towns in the Zuider Zee area and on the coast of the Countship of Holland. The substantial number of ships involved would ensure that at a significant number of contaminated ships would reach their destinations, and increase the risk of multiple infections.

Like Germany, the Low Countries were also conquered by two plague fronts that started in the southern and northern ends of this territorial entity, respectively, starting in the north with a time lag of a few months relative to the southern plague front.

Although more evidence on the Black Death's history in the Netherlands has been gleaned from the extant contemporary source material, it is still quite deficient in many respects. Nonetheless, glimpses of its presence and mortal effects cover most of the country. It is, therefore, clear today that also the Netherlands was broadly ravaged by the Black Death. Van Werveke's assertion to the effect that the Low Countries were only marginally affected has again been shown to be untenable, this time for the northern half.

Blockmans points out that such comprehensive account books and tax registers as were produced by the domain administrations of the counts of Holland and Hainault containing crucial evidence on the presence of the Black Death, were not created in the Countship of Flanders or the Duchy of Brabant because of the prevailing lease-holding system in these principalities. It is a sad fact for historians that in many principalities all over Europe, including the Low Countries, account books and tax

---

[9] See also Ch. 18 on Sweden.

registers were often not produced in the years of the Black Death precisely because the administrations broke down under the impact of the gruesome epidemic onslaught.

This demonstrates again the inherent fallacy of methodology implied in inference from silence in the sources to assumptions to the effect that a phenomenon did not occur or exist, when it cannot be argued that the sources used should be expected to include such information. In the case of the Low Countries, the total lack of notices on the Black Death in chronicles and other narrative sources is conspicuous. Despite the fact that these areas were characterized by high standards of education and literacy for their time, the sources that contain information on the Black Death are all incidental in nature; no source is produced with the objective of handing down information on this exceptionally grisly event to posterity. As I have had occasion to point out several times, and have discussed particularly in relation to the German source material, the classical and humanistic ideals and education that moulded the mind and mentality of the chronicle-producing elites did not include epidemic events. Consequently, it is not really surprising that no narrative source containing such information is preserved in the Low Countries. Because silence in the sources on epidemic events is what should be expected, the sort of inference made by Van Werveke is a fallacy of methodology. Interestingly, it seems that the Black Death was such a mind-stretching event that the recurrence of plague epidemics persuaded chroniclers to realize their noteworthiness. From the next plague epidemic, which broke out about ten years later, notices on them become quite frequent.

In this situation, when the application of source criticism produces arguments to the effect that information on the subject under study will surface only incidentally in the sources, more generalized types of arguments will carry more weight. In this case, the central tenets of plague epidemiology make it impossible to explain why the Black Death should not have spread all over the Low Countries. These countries were characterized by high population density and intensive economic and social interaction both locally and regionally, and by importation of large amounts of grain from various directions in order to satisfy the needs of this large, densely settled and highly urbanized population.

This line of argument does not contradict Blockmans' view that the Low Countries, as also the Netherlands, did not suffer such great losses of population in the Black Death as Italy or England did. This is, on the contrary, in accordance with the established epidemiology of plague, which predicts substantially lower morbidity and mortality rates in urban environments than in rural environments.

However, the Low Countries' intensive engagement in international trade and shipping implies that plague contagion would be imported particularly often. This appears to be reflected also in the *Necrologium of the Chapter of St Lebuinus' Church in Deventer*, which indicates recurrent epidemics of plague in 1359–60, 1364, 1367–8, 1375 and 1384–5. And, then, there was a new great wave of plague in 1400–1, and so on.[10] Thus, the diminution of the population of Belgium and the Netherlands in the following hundred years was quite likely of the same order of magnitude as in other

---

[10] Sivéry 1966.

countries, despite the likelihood that each epidemic caused a somewhat lower level of mortality.

While the Black Death's pattern of spread across Europe separates the two main parts of the Low Countries, the patterns of internal spread and long-time demographic effects unite them.

22

The Baltic Countries

The present-day Baltic states, Estonia, Lithuania and Latvia, are situated along the south-eastern shores of the Baltic Sea. In addition, after the dissolution of the Soviet Union, a small Russian enclave came into being around the present-day city of Kaliningrad, the Hanseatic city of Köningsberg from the Middle Ages until after the Second World War. On the eve of the Black Death, there was still a significant Baltic-speaking population element in Prussia, an area that after the Second World War was ceded to Poland. Historically, the whole of the area should be included in the concept of the Baltic countries.

At the time of the Black Death, the area covered by the present-day Baltic states was mainly dominated by the Order of the Teutonic Knights. A number of commercial towns and cities containing German populations with close ties to the Hanseatic towns and cities further to the west had also grown up.

Very little is known about the Black Death in the Baltic areas, except, perhaps, in Prussia, where the main events have been commented on in connection with the presentation of the events in north-eastern Germany and Prussia. The reason for this is a notice in the town of Braunsberg's *Book of Citizenship* to the effect that the Black Death broke out in the town of Elbing (Elblag) on the Bay of Danzig (Gdansk) as early as 24 August 1349, a date that implies that the contagion was introduced in the second week of July. It is further stated that the Black Death broke out also in several commercial towns along the vast lagoon called Frisches Haff (Zalev Wislany), an area that today partly belongs to Poland, partly to the Russian enclave of Kaliningrad: Frauenberg (Frombork), Braunsberg (Braniewo) and Königsberg (Kaliningrad). There appear to have been new outbreaks in this area in the following year, for instance in the town of Marienburg (Malbork), 30 km south-west of Elbing. The Black Death had also travelled 150 km upstream on the large R. Vistula (Weichsel/ Wisla) and ravaged the town of Thorn (Torun),[1] situated on Prussia's southern border with the Kingdom of Poland.

Not much is known about the further spread of the Black Death in the area of the

---

[1] Biraben 1975: 80.

present-day Baltic countries, at the time, the lands of the Teutonic Order. However, the pace of spread was quite slow, for it did not invade the area of modern Latvia until 1351.[2] It is, therefore, not certain, that the Black Death completed the conquest of the Baltic countries that year.[3]

---

[2]   Hoeniger 1881: 27.
[3]   Biraben 1975: 85.

23

Russia[1]

Today, the concept of Eastern Slavs comprises three nationalities speaking three versions of eastern Slavonic language, namely Russians, Belorussians and Ukrainians, of which the Belorussians and Ukrainians achieved statehood and sovereign states only after the dissolution of the Soviet Union in the early 1990s. In the Middle Ages, peoples of all branches of the Eastern Slavs were known as Russians.

There was no unified Russian state at the time of the Black Death. The terms Russian and Russia refer, therefore, to the territories that came to be dominated by the emerging Russian state, later Imperial Russia, and were settled by peoples speaking the contemporary versions of the eastern Slavonic languages. The use of the terms Russia and Russian in this book refers to distant history, not to modern politics and recent state formation.

Russian territories were divided into a number of principalities and the city state of Novgorod, which possessed a large territory and was called Great Novgorod in the fourteenth century. These Russian territories were conquered by the Mongol armies in the years 1237–40 that established the Golden Horde and devastated the principality of Kiev. The remaining Russian principalities and Great Novgorod became subjugated dependencies of the Golden Horde, paying high tributes in the form of taxes and young recruits for the Mongol-led army. The most important of the Russian dependencies at the time of the Black Death were the principalities of Tver', Ryazan', Nizhniy Novgorod,[2] Moscowy, Vladimir, Suzdal' and Great Novgorod. Some of the areas settled by Russians in the west had at the time of the Black Death chosen to

---

[1] The scholarly history of the Black Death in Russia, as in other former Communist countries, is in a sad state. Because the idea that large diminutions of populations could have had a considerable impact on societal processes and have moulded an historical period, i.e., the Late Middle Ages, was assumed by Communist ideologues and party watchdogs to represent a challenge to Marxist-Leninist orthodoxy, this field of historical study was laid waste. Consequently, the best presentation of the history of the Black Death in Russia was written before the Russian Revolution, namely Dörbeck's account from 1906, which contains a general history of plague in Russia, and this book is available in a contemporary German translation. However, in their book on the history of epidemics in Russia (1960) Vasil'yev and Segal have made valuable contributions both with respect to the collection of sources and their interpretation. This book is, unfortunately, only available in its original Russian version. Scandinavians can benefit from Akiander's translations of Russian chronicles.

[2] Novgorod simply means 'Newtown' and Nizhniy means 'Lower'. The addition of this adjective reflects an obvious need to differentiate the reference to this town from the city of Novgorod.

recognize the authority of the grand dukes of Lithuania, a strong new state that had developed from the thirteenth century, and that was independent of the Mongol khanate, in order to avoid the hardships of Mongol domination.

For the purpose of conscripting recruits and collecting taxes the Mongols took three censuses of the male population of Russia in the years 1245–74, and these censuses also formed the basis of the administrative divisions and subdivisions of the Russian lands. On the basis of these censuses and administrative divisions a population guestimate of 10 million inhabitants has been made, a figure that should be treated with the utmost caution, although there is nothing inherently unreasonable about it. Considering the vast territories in question, it is clear that the population density was very low indeed.

Russia was blessed with a great number of large, navigable rivers that facilitated trade and travel over the vast distances.

A very important religious development within the vast Russian area of Mongol political dominance fortuitously came to affect the history of the Black Death in a decisive way. Khan Uzbeg (1313–41) converted to Islam and made it the official state religion. With the zeal of new converts and the political objectives embedded in a new state religion his successor Khan Janibeg (1342–57) launched military campaigns to drive the Christian merchants out of the area of the Golden Horde. This severed the lines of trade along the caravan routes between China and the Italian trading stations on the Sea of Azov and the Black Sea. In 1346, Janibeg's ambition led to the fateful siege of Kaffa where the Black Death first was introduced into the Mongol camp, then slunk into the town. The Italians fled in panic from the epidemic onslaught, and thus allowed it to sail triumphantly with them to Asia Minor, the Middle East and Europe.

Religious zealotry and violent anti-Christian sentiments appear to have led to an intermission or a temporary radical reduction in trade between the Golden Horde and Christian merchants in the Russian principalities. There can hardly be any other explanation for the fact that the Black Death did not move north-westwards into the Russian areas from its original outbreak in the south-eastern lands of the Golden Horde on the Caspian Sea (see above). Instead, the Black Death had to move by the long route from Europe's Mediterranean coasts to the Hanseatic towns and cities on the Baltic Sea, and to the areas of the present-day Baltic states, before it could launch its attack on Russian territories. This must be the reason that Russia was conquered from the north-west and not from the south-east, and was the last region of Europe to be attacked by the Black Death rather than the first.

In the case of the Black Death's history in Russia, we are entirely dependent on chroniclers for information. In Russia, it broke out in the town of Pskov in Great Novgorod.[3] Unfortunately, the year of the outbreak cannot be pinned down with certainty because the chroniclers disagree to such an extent that it cannot be identified. Several of the chroniclers are anonymous, their respective chronicles are named

---

3   *The Chronicle of Nikon* contains a short notice to the effect that there was a 'great mortality' in Polotsk in 1349. Polotsk is situated on R. Dvina near Belorussia's north-eastern border to Russia, 600 km to the north-east of Elbing in Prussia, where the Black Death was probably introduced in the second week of July 1349. It is not possible that the Black Death could have spread that far in 1349. The brief notice contains nothing that allows identification of the disease, and it could refer to a local outbreak of some other epidemic disease with high mortality. For these reasons, this notice is disregarded by most scholars.

after the town of origin, and numbered consecutively by Roman numerals. The depressing scholarly situation has the following shape: in *The Chronicle of Pskov II* and *The Chronicle of Nikon* the outbreak of the epidemic is mentioned under the year 1351, while in *The Chronicle of Pskov I* and *The Chronicles of Novgorod I and IV* it is mentioned under the year 1352.

Because the year in question cannot be decided on the basis of the written sources, the only remaining approach to resolve this question is to consider possible territorial sources of infection and routes of spread. If the Black Death was introduced into the area of Great Novgorod through trade relations with the Hansards, it would presumably first be brought to the city of Novgorod, which had much larger and intensive commercial interaction with them, rather than to the much smaller town of Pskov. Thus, the fact that Pskov was contaminated first becomes decisive: Pskov is situated roughly 250 km closer to the Baltic countries than Novgorod, and is almost a Russian border town to the areas of Baltic settlement. In 1351, the Black Death invaded Latvia from the south, moved after some time into Livonia, i.e., the northern half of Latvia, and invaded the territory of Great Novgorod in the north-east late in 1351 (see above). The territorial analysis of the possible sources of infection and routes of spread makes it likely that Russia was infected by spread by land to Pskov from the area of the present-day Latvia.

The structure of epidemic-related events shows that the outbreak in Pskov began in early spring, probably in the second half of April 1352. This indicates that the contagion had been introduced at the end of the previous year, and had been prevented by cold weather from developing into full epidemic form until the arrival of spring weather.

Although the chroniclers disagree on the year of the outbreak, they provide quite similar accounts of the epidemic events. In *The Chronicle of Novgorod IV*, the account of the outbreak in Pskov runs as follows in a mixture of citations and paraphrasing:

> 'In the same year, there was such a disease in the town of Pskov and in the villages that death brought down many. All sorts of people died, men and women, old and young, children and priests, monks and nuns.' Panic-stricken and not knowing and not seeing any measures for their defence from this misery, the Pskovians turned to Novgorod, and entreated Archbishop Vasiliy to visit Pskov, hold a divine service and give the town his benediction, because they 'were without any means of averting this punishment from God'. The archbishop arrived in Pskov at the end of May, led a splendid and solemn procession around the town, and after a few days he began the journey back to Novgorod. However, on the road he fell sick and died from the plague. The Novgorodians gave him a solemn funeral that attracted large crowds of people, and after a short time, the plague was very much in evidence with no less force than in Pskov. 'That autumn, the disease struck forcefully in Novgorod and in the towns on the L. Ladoga.'[4]

This account can be supplemented by the other chronicles, indicating that the epidemic lasted in Pskov through the summer, began to subside in the autumn and

---

[4]   My translation and paraphrasing of the Russian text.

ended with the arrival of the winter. Archbishop Vasiliy died on 3 July; the outbreak in Novgorod commenced on 15 August and continued to Easter. Several of the chronicles stress too that the disease spread as easily in the countryside as in the towns, and all over the Russian territories:

> This did not only take place in Novgorod, but in all lands [. . .] In the same year, there were severe epidemics in Smolensk, and in Kiev, and in Chernigov, and in Suzdal', and in all Russian lands. And there was great fear and trepidation in all human beings. In Glukhov, at that time not a single human being was left, all were dead; this was also the case in Belozersk.[5]

Nothing is said about Moscow in the chronicles. We are told that in that year the Metropolitan Feognost, the leader of the Russian Orthodox Church, died in Moscow, and that, in 1353, Grand Duke Simeon Gordiy of Moscowy died there with seven children and his brother Andrew (Andrei). This is usually taken as a confirmation that the Black Death also ravaged Moscow. It is also pointed out that the chronicles repeatedly stress that the Black Death spread over all Russia.

Unfortunately, the chronicles do not contain any indications as to the pattern of spread, means of spread by contact or transport, and in which order the various regions and towns were invaded. Because such great distances are involved, it appears unrealistic that the Black Death should have spread across these vast Russian areas in one year. Possibly, the Russian Orthodox metropolitan may have died as an old man, while the great mortality in the ruling family reflects that the Black Death broke out in Moscow in 1353. This scenario could reflect a larger pattern, that the Black Death continued to spread across the Russian territories throughout 1353, reaching Kiev, Chernigov and Glukhov in the present-day Ukraine in the south, Suzdal' east of Moscow and Belozersk in the north in that year. As in the case of the Black Death's pattern of spread in Germany, one would like to assume that transport along the many great rivers also played an important part in the process of dissemination in Russia.

Contrary to what is often asserted, there is no significant evidence to the effect that the Black Death in Russia took on the character of primary pneumonic plague. The usual duration of the disease is, for instance, said to be three days, which corresponds to the lower end of the average of 3–5 days characteristic of bubonic plague, reflecting that the rapidity of the course of illness from onset to death impressed the high-strung minds of people who lived through inconceivable carnage. The average duration of primary pneumonic plague cases is much shorter, 1.8 days, the characteristic phase with bloody expectoration lasting only 0.8 day (see also below). The high proportion of fulminating cases that die within 24 hours would most likely have impressed themselves greatly on people and would have been noted in the chronicles. Thus, the pattern of spread of this epidemic in Russia must be assumed to be quite similar to the broad European pattern. which reflects the characteristic disseminative mechanisms and properties of bubonic plague.

The chronicles contain also dramatic expressions of the unbelievable mortality.

---

5   *The Chronicle of Nikon.* My translation from the Russian text.

The unrealistic assertions to the effect that there were no survivors in Glukhov and Belozersk must be seen in the light of extreme mortality that made rumours about towns where all inhabitants were swept away not seem far-fetched to the contemporaries who lived through this terrible ordeal.

24

Did Some Countries or Regions Escape?
What Happened in Iceland, Finland, Poland
and the Kingdom of Bohemia?

In a famous slight among scholars studying the Black Death, Hoeniger states that 'It is, actually, later historiography that has let in the plague [i.e., the Black Death] in Bohemia, Silesia and Poland.'[1] Later, a further two countries have been added to the list that are supposed to have escaped from the Black Death, namely Finland and Iceland. At the end of this long march in the historical wake of the Black Death through the Caucasus, Asia Minor, the Middle East, North Africa and across Europe the validity of these assertions must be discussed. Did some countries and regions escape from the horrors of the Black Death completely or mainly? If so, how should it be explained?

Iceland
In Icelandic annals it is flatly stated that the Black Death did not reach the island. This has been confirmed by modern scholarship. The reason was that no ship came to Iceland from Norway in 1349, with an Icelandic homebound ship ravaged by the Black Death shortly before it should have put to sea from Bergen. Did the Black Death miss out also on other countries or regions?

Finland
Modern Finland comprises a large territory, but in the High Middle Ages only a small part of this territory was settled at all. People of Finnish stock speaking a Finno-Ugrian language lived inland or in the south-western coastal region called Finland Proper (Egentliga Finland), while Swedish peasants had trickled in across the Baltic Sea over a number of centuries and had settled mostly in the western and southern coastal districts and in the numerous islands outside the shoreline. Professor Eljas Orrman, the leading Finnish agrarian historian, has made a tentative estimate of 13,100 holdings in Finland on the eve of the Black Death, which means that popula-

---

1   Hoeniger 1881: 31. My translation from German.

tion size may have been in the order of magnitude of 65,000 persons.[2] There was only one small town (or perhaps two).[3] Population density must have been minute.

Already by 1846 Ilmoni had published a study of the history of epidemics in the Nordic countries in which he noted that he had not been able to adduce evidence to the effect that the Black Death had invaded Finland.[4] This negative finding has been confirmed by later research. There are indications of deserted farms in some districts in the fifteenth century, especially in south-western districts,[5] but this phenomenon could, of course, have been caused by a later plague epidemic or, conceivably, by some other serious epidemic.

How can this special feature of Finland's history in the time of the Black Death be explained? And, in particular, why did the Black Death not manage to invade Finland? It is certainly not for lack of black rats, as pointed out above. One useful approach to this question is to focus on the conspicuous fact that not even Sweden was invaded across the waters of the Baltic Sea; the Black Death had to move slowly all the way from the Norwegian and Danish border areas in the west to the Swedish shores of the Baltic Sea. Since it did not succeed in establishing a second plague front at the eastern coasts of Sweden, it could not rapidly engulf the country by the action of two separate plague fronts, as happened in Spain, Germany, the Low Countries, and in Norway, for instance. The Black Death did not even manage to cross the quite narrow waters between Gotland I., where it had raged in Visby from the early spring of 1350, and the Swedish coastal districts on the Baltic Sea. There can only be one explanation for this shape of the epidemic events, namely that trade and travel broke down under the ferocious onslaught of the Black Death in this horrible year.

There are two other important points that should be made: firstly, the quite isolated geographical position of Finland, and secondly, its tiny population at the time of the Black Death, with a correspondingly insignificant urban sector, the almost trifling extent of trade, and, therefore, a very low level of contact with the outside world.

There is certain evidence of plague in Finland at the end of the fifteenth century. However, it is also certain that Finland has not been frequently visited by plague,

---

[2]   Orrman 1996: 140. Average household size is assumed to be 5 persons, since there was fairly strong population growth, while most European populations in the first half of the fourteenth century were stationary or receding slowly. In the Early Modern period, there was a significant proportion of joint households on Finnish farmsteads in some areas, especially in areas where slash-and-burn agriculture or animal husbandry were the dominant forms of production, and it was most common among well-to-do peasants. Carelia (in the south-eastern corner of Finland) is the only part of Finland where the joint family has been common as an alternative system of family organization that can be shown to go back into the end of the late-medieval period. Around 1500, the proportion of joint families and multiple families was 23 per cent in all. For a summary on the research on joint families in Finland, see Benedictow 1996b: 104–6; Benedictow 1996c: 174–6. Otherwise, nothing is really known about the family structure in Finland in the Middle Ages. In the case of a typical European and Nordic family structure based on the nuclear family, a household multiplier of five persons presupposes significant population growth, which must be assumed generally to have been the case in medieval Finland. If there has been a significant component of joint families and multiple families, the average size of households as the basis for making population estimates must be increased significantly, probably in the range of 5.5–6 persons per household, indicating a population of 72,000–80,000.
[3]   Törnblom 1993: 376–9.
[4]   Ilmoni 1846: 130–1.
[5]   Sandnes 1981: 89–90.

which must be the reason that Finland's population, in sharp contrast to the populations of other European countries, grew strongly through the Late Middle Ages. The number of agricultural holdings in Finland increased from the guestimated 13,000 on the eve of the Black Death to 34,000 in the 1540s, which, assuming the same average household size, indicates that the population increased by 2.5 times; also urban growth was quite brisk although the urban sector still remained quite tiny at the end of this period.[6]

The strong population increase and the corresponding settlement expansion must have caused fundamental change in Finland's social and economic structures that also brought about considerably increased commercial interaction with Sweden and the Hanseatic towns and cities along the Baltic Sea. The essence of this line of reasoning is that Finland's exposure to importation of plague contagion and other diseases must have increased considerably throughout the Late Middle Ages.

Poland

According to Hoeniger, 'Poland [remained] almost untouched by the Black Death.' The borders of the medieval Kingdom of Poland were, of course, very different from those of our days. After some tumultuous and tragic centuries, modern Poland emerged after the First World War. However, the end of the Second World War caused comprehensive redrawing of borders and large-scale movements and resettlements of nationalities. At the time of the Black Death, Poland comprised a smallish landlocked territory stretching south-eastwards from the border on Prussia in the north in the direction of Moldova, and from the borders with the Eastern German regions of Brandenburg and Silesia in the west to the borders of present-day Ukraine. Because there have been comprehensive border changes in this part of Eastern Europe, some aspects of the Black Death's spread within the present-day territory of Poland have been commented on in connection with the discussion of its history in Prussia and the Baltic countries. Nonetheless, the only practical approach is to discuss the question of the Black Death's history in this part of Europe within the present-day borders of Poland, because this will provide a better picture of the strategic situation and the disseminative process.

Actually, the area of present-day Poland was hit early by the Black Death, namely the parts of Prussia and Pomerania on the Gulf of Gdansk (Danzig) that had already been invaded at the end of July 1349. Later in the autumn it reached Elblag, Frombork, and Braniewo. In the following year, Malbork and Gdansk were also attacked in this part of present-day Poland. The R. Vistula (Wisla/Weichsel), which flows for more than a thousand kilometres through almost the whole of the country until it reaches the Gulf of Gdansk, is navigable for many hundreds of kilometres, and large amounts of goods were transported in both directions on this mighty river. When Prussia and commercial centres situated near the river, like Elblag and Malbork, were invaded by the Black Death, it would be surprising if the contagion was not passed on upstream by trade relations with inland Poland. It comes as no

6   Orrman 1996: 140; Törnblom 1993.

surprise that the Black Death broke out in Torun (Thorn) about 150 km upstream in 1351.[7] And Torun was almost halfway to Warsaw.

Sticker cites two chroniclers who assert that the Black Death had invaded Poland from Hungary, i.e., from the south across the territory of present-day Slovakia, at the end of January 1350, and caused incredible mortality in Poland: more than half of the population is said to have died, and whole villages and towns were said to have been emptied of people.[8]

In 1351, the Black Death reached the German city of Frankfurt on the R. Oder. This city is situated on the large border river between present-day Germany and Poland, about 40 km north of the point where it turns eastwards and flows into Silesia. Frankfurt on the Oder may at this time have been infected from the west but it may even more likely have been infected by Hanseatic goods moving upstream from the Baltic Sea. This city prospered as a commercial centre for exportation of German goods eastwards into Polish territory, and further away to Russia, and for importation of goods from Russia and Poland for sale in its large hinterland or for sale in regions to the west. From this city on the R. Oder's western bank, the Black Death would easily cross into Poland with goods and tradesmen; it could also sail further upstream deep into Polish territory. As should be expected, this year the Black Death invaded also Silesia in the south-west of Poland and the main city there that used to be called with its German name Breslau but today is called Wroclaw.[9]

As can be seen, the Black Death was well established within the borders of the present Polish state, or, as in the case of Frankfurt, on the border, and could penetrate into Poland from the north, the west and the south. As the Black Death spread in Russia, it would, of course, also spread westwards, and it is difficult to see how invasions of Polish territory from the east could be avoided, if it had not already been ravaged.

Communist authorities and ideological watchdogs prevented serious research on the Black Death and the following plague epidemics, suspecting (correctly) that this study could establish disturbing alternative demographic views to Marxist orthodoxy on important historical developments in the Late Middle Ages. The Late Medieval Crisis was for all practical purposes unknown when Marx, Engels, Lenin and Stalin phrased Communist orthodoxy, and historical demography in general was only in an emergent phase of development. Historical demographic perspectives and Malthusian theory have been disregarded and discarded by almost all Marxists, not only by politicians but also by scholars working on the basis of Marxist theory with various later dogmatic additions and adjustments. For this reason, the study of the Black Death, later plague epidemics and historical demography more generally has been thoroughly neglected in the Communist period, and that was also the case in Poland.

However, shortly before the outbreak of the Second World War J. Pelc, the Polish economic historian, published a book on the price developments in Krakow in southern Poland in the Late Middle Ages and the Early Modern period.[10] The

---

[7] Biraben 1975: 80.
[8] Sticker 1908: 67–8. Actually, the text states that the invasion occurred in January 1349, but this is at variance with Sticker's account of the spread of the Black Death in Central and Eastern Europe and must be a misprint.
[9] Biraben 1975: 78–9.
[10] Pelc 1938.

comprehensive price material collected and organized by Pelc has since been reworked by Wilhelm Abel, the German economic historian, and organized in transparent figures. He has succeeded in showing that developments of prices and wages were the same in Krakow as in England, France or Germany. These price developments are characterized by, among other things, a great fall in the real price of grain and a great increase in real wages (the price of labour).[11] These developments are explained by the great diminution of population in Europe caused by the Black Death and recurrent plague epidemics. The great increase in real wages reflects a sudden dramatic deficit of labour. The concomitant fall in grain prices reflects that, as populations now were much smaller, poor agricultural lands were abandoned (or used for grazing), and productivity in grain production consequently increased, which put pressure downwards on prices. However, as people now had much better earnings than before, they would eat less grain-based foodstuffs and use their extra money to purchase meat, butter, wine, beer, and so on, which would put additional pressure downwards on grain prices.

The price movements in Krakow reveal that at least in large regions of southern Poland the demand for labour was much stronger than the supply, and that this was a continuous feature throughout the Late Medieval period – indeed, one that contributes to giving this period its special character. If this had not been the case at least for large regions, people would, of course, have streamed down to Krakow and the surrounding regions in order to work for much better wages and acquire a much higher standard of living than they would be able to find in local society. In fact, people were much more mobile in those days than is usually assumed. If the Black Death had not decimated populations in vast areas of Eastern Europe, population pressures there would have remained unaffected and have found outlet in comprehensive work migration to the ravaged regions. Probably sooner than later, these demographic developments would have re-pressurized the demographically decompressed areas, for instance in the regions around Krakow, and the favourable developments of real wages would have been turned around into a gradually deteriorating trend that would eventually re-establish the pre-plague economic realities and hardships. Pelc's price material must be taken to reveal a more general and lasting demographic crisis in Eastern Europe caused by the Black Death and recurrent plague epidemics.

Pelc's material also reveals that fundamental change in these socio-economic parameters begins around 1500, or rather at the beginning of the sixteenth century. The price curves of labour and grain were inverted in Poland, as in England, Germany and France. This was a clear reflection of the beginning of sustained demographic growth, which gradually changed the situation in the labour marked from a deficit of labour to a surplus, and drove wages downwards. Population growth increased demand for foodstuffs like grain (or beans) that consistently provide more calories

---

11 Abel 1935: 32–5; Abel 1955: 100–1. Actually, because there was an immediate sharp fall in population size while the amount of silver money was the same, there was a sharp inflationary movement in the first two decades following the Black Death. Then, the surplus of silver money had been depleted and a long-term fall in prices commenced. What is of real significance in this pattern is that, from the very beginning, real wages show strongly increasing purchasing power, especially in relation to grain/flour. The demographic basis for this development is a consistent feature of these developments in the real economy.

per money unit than meat or other alternatives, more marginal agricultural land was reactivated for corn production and productivity declined, factors that combined to produce a long-term trend of rising grain prices. Sustained decrease or increase in population respectively will in old-time societies produce consistently diverging development patterns of the prices of labour and basic foodstuffs like grain. In the Late Middle Ages and the Early Modern period, these socio-economic patterns in Poland were consistently similar to those that obtained in Western Europe, and this similarity was caused by similar dynamic forces, primarily by demographic developments in interaction with the available agricultural resources and the prevailing agricultural technology.

In the light of these pieces of information, I find it hard to accept Hoeniger's assertion that the Black Death only made itself felt on the fringes of Poland. An important additional consideration is that Hoeniger's view appears inexplicable in epidemiological terms. Now that times have changed and serious research into these questions is possible once more, we must hope that other sources can be found that can enlarge and deepen our knowledge of Poland's economic and demographic history in the Late Middle Ages.

The Kingdom of Bohemia

The Kingdom of Bohemia was part of the Holy Roman Empire of the German Nation in the east. On the eve of the Black Death, it comprised the regions Bohemia and Moravia, representing roughly the territory of the present-day Czech Republic, Upper and Lower Silesia (which today belong to Poland), and, in addition, two small areas in the west that gave it a sort of long territorial nose protruding almost all the way to Nuremberg.

At the time, it was a quite prosperous country, with the city of Prague at its administrative and political centre. The relative prosperity was not least derived from a large mining industry, especially silver mines. In the High Middle Ages and still into the fourteenth century, there was a steady stream of German settlers that contributed to a rapid growth in agricultural and urban production. This stimulated the growth of towns and the integration of the country in an elementary market economy that was among the most advanced in Central and Eastern Europe at the time of the Black Death. In the words of Hoensch: 'there was a rapid development of a dense network of new towns. Older settlements situated, e.g., at crossroads, fords and other strategically important places and secured by fortifications grew briskly as places of trade and craft production'. By the time of the Black Death, the Kingdom had been successfully integrated in the European networks of long-distance trade.[12] This view is confirmed by Pounds who, in his standard work on European economic history in the Middle Ages, underscores the economically developed character of these countries: 'Bohemia, Moravia and Austria [. . .] were relatively developed. They tended to approximate the Western European model.'[13] In the countryside, the peasantry would have to acquire necessities they could not produce themselves, like salt for preservation of meat and

---

[12] Hoensch 1987: 100–1. My translation from German.
[13] Pounds 1974: 113.

butter for later consumption, and iron for tools. This need could only be met by a relatively fine-meshed commercial network in which small traders would play a major part.

The population of the Kingdom of Bohemia has been estimated at 1.5 million around 1300, of which about one-sixth were Germans. In the following decades, Lower Silesia and the two small areas in the west were added to the Kingdom. It is also reasonable to assume that the population continued to grow up to the time of the Black Death both by natural increase and by continuing immigration by German settlers.[14] This indicates that the Kingdom of Bohemia, which at the time of the Black Death covered roughly 120,000 sq. km, was quite densely settled according to the medieval standards of Central Europe, roughly in the order of magnitude of 15 persons per sq. km. If the Kingdom of Bohemia was left mainly untouched by the Black Death, as asserted by Hoeniger, that would be very difficult to explain on epidemiological grounds. One should keep in mind that Hoeniger, who wrote his much-used standard work about 1880, related to epidemiology in miasmatic and not in microbiological terms.

Hoeniger found no trace of the Black Death in the archives or in the chronicles. He concluded, therefore, that 'with respect to [the Kingdom of] Bohemia we should assume that there occurred at the most a few dispersed cases of the disease in the border areas'.[15] However, in 1908, Gasquet cited an account rendered in the *Chronicle of Prague* (*Chronicon Pragense*) of some students from Bohemia who at the time of the Black Death journeyed back to their country from Bologna (where they in all likelihood had been studying at this city's famous school of law[16]):

> At this time, some students coming from Bologna into Bohemia saw that in most of the cities and castles they passed through few remained alive, and in some all were dead. In many houses also those who had escaped with their lives were so weakened by the sickness that one could not give another a draught of water, nor help him in any way, and so passed their time in great affliction and distress. Priests, too, ministering the sacraments, and doctors' medicines, to the sick were infected by them and died. So many passed out of this life without confession or the sacraments of the Church, as the priests were dead. There were generally made great, broad and deep pits in which the bodies of the dead were buried. In many places, too, the air was more infected and more deadly than poisoned food, from the corruption of the corpses, since there was no one left to bury them. Of the foresaid students, moreover, only one returned to Bohemia, and his companions all died on the journey.[17]

This chronicle asserts that the Black Death wrought as much havoc in Bohemia as in the rest of Europe. Because the account begins by referring to what the students saw after they had crossed into Bohemia, the last sentence must be taken to mean that

---

[14] Hoensch 1987: 95, 98–101.
[15] Hoeniger 1881: 31–5. My translation from German.
[16] Prague's university was founded in 1348, and achieved its high reputation later.
[17] Gasquet 1908: 37–8.

only one of the students survived the journey in Bohemia, and succeeded in returning home.

Also in 1908, Sticker published his pioneering work on the history of plague. In this work, he refers, albeit in a quite general fashion, to sources that allow him to assert that the Black Death invaded the Kingdom of Bohemia in 1350.[18] Biraben also refers to general statements in the sources to the effect that Bohemia, Moravia and Silesia were invaded by the Black Death in that year.[19]

In addition to these more general statements, there is also some specific evidence. In 1351, the margrave of Moravia promised tax exemption for four years to all those who would settle in the city of Brno and the town of Znojmo, which had been emptied of people by the plague.[20] Brno was the largest town in Moravia and situated in the heart of the province, while Znojmo is situated 55 km south-west of Brno, quite close to the border with Austria. Moravia was invaded from Austria where the town of Eggenburg, 30 km south of Znojmo, was attacked in the summer of 1349 (see above). Bohemia was probably invaded from Bavaria in south-eastern Germany.

In a paper published in 1987, Eduard Maur, the Czech demographic historian, refers briefly to the history of the Black Death in his homeland: 'The Black Death 1349–1350, occurred mainly in southern Moravia. Owing to the area's position on the European watershed and distance from the most important trade roads, Bohemia was almost completely spared.'[21] Maur does not relate to the sources, and, even more importantly, his view on the isolation of the Kingdom of Bohemia from the European networks of trade and travel, and his neglect of the bustling networks of towns and cities, trade and travel within the Kingdom, are clearly untenable. On economic and epidemiological grounds, his view appears inexplicable. He points out himself that, in the period 1348–1415, the Kingdom of Bohemia was ravaged by plague in 1357–60, 1362–3, 1369–71, 1380, 1390, 1403–6 and 1413–15. Considering that the Kingdom's position in relation to the European watershed can hardly have changed in the meantime, and considering that a flourishing internal and external market economy can hardly have sprung up suddenly between 1350 and 1357 or 1362 or 1367, Maur's arguments appear contradictory and arbitrary.

Although the source material relating to the history of the Black Death in the Kingdom of Bohemia is unsatisfactory and does not constitute the base for arguing a strong case, it indicates that this country also was actually ravaged by the Black Death.

Summing up, this discussion of assertions to the effect that some countries were spared the ravages of the Black Death has confirmed that this was the case in relation to Iceland and Finland but probably was not the cases with respect to the kingdoms of Poland and Bohemia. It has been shown in the chapter on the Black Death in Germany that similar assertions in the case of the region of Franconia are also untenable. Quite likely, the real problem in relation to Poland and Bohemia in this context,

---

[18] Sticker 1908: 67.
[19] Biraben 1975: 76–9.
[20] Hoeniger 1881: 16–17. It appears that Hoeniger has forgotten this piece of important evidence when, twenty pages later, he asserts that the Kingdom of Bohemia was not invaded by the Black Death and that there at most were a few cases of plague on the border.
[21] Maur 1987: 163–4. My translation from German.

as have been pointed out repeatedly above, is the continuously deteriorating quality and quantity of the extant sources to the history of the Black Death as we move northwards and eastwards in Europe, and the impossibility of performing serious research on the subject in the Communist period.

Part Three
Patterns and Dynamics of the Black Death

25

Patterns of Conquest, Dynamics of Spread

Introduction

For obvious reasons, epidemics, like ideologies and religions, are disseminated by people and spread first and most rapidly along main routes of trade and travel to large urban centres, whether by land or sea. In medieval times, ship transport was by far the most efficient and rapid way of transporting goods and disseminating disease at a distance. Epidemic disease, consequently, first invaded seaports, cities and commercial hubs along the coasts of the Mediterranean and the western coasts of Europe or situated on large navigable rivers.

Next, epidemics would radiate from them to local towns in the region, and from them further into the countryside by horse and carriage or by pack horses along secondary and tertiary lines of local communication. In this way a highly contagious disease would in the end tend to blanket entire areas and regions.

Seaports would also serve as points of departure for other ships, which would take disease as well as cargo on board and carry it to other destinations and commercial centres that would serve as new epicentres for the spread of disease in their regions, and so on. This principal pattern of epidemic spread in the Middle Ages holds good for the Black Death.

Metastatic leaps

In the Black Death's strategic approach to the conquest of Asia Minor, the Middle East, North Africa and Europe the combination of ship transport and metastatic leaps is most conspicuous. It starts with the ships that transported the Black Death from Kaffa to Constantinople. From Constantinople, the Black Death sailed triumphantly all the way to Alexandria whence it launched its attacks on the Middle East and North Africa, although Tunis was also attacked by a metastatic leap by sea from Messina in Sicily that established a second plague front in North Africa.

Other metastatic leaps from Kaffa or from Constantinople by ships carried the Black Death to Greece and to a substantial number of cities and towns on the Mediterranean Sea (including the Adriatic). These urban centres were contaminated at this early point exactly because they were important nexuses in regional and international trade. They functioned as epidemic epicentres, passing on contagion in many directions to other towns and cities by ship along the coasts, or up navigable rivers, and over land by horse and carriage and by pack horses in a process that eventually resulted in the blanketing of the countrysides where the vast majority of medieval populations lived.

The epicentre that was recognized in Marseilles on 1 November 1347 appears to have been of particular significance both for spread along the coasts and for spread inland. Another important epicentre was established in Mallorca at the end of December 1347 from which transportation by ship caused early contamination of commercial towns and cities on the Spanish mainland and the establishment of a southern Iberian plague front in the spring of 1348.

Bordeaux, the large commercial hub on the Atlantic coast in south-western France, was the other city that played a particularly important role in the distribution of the Black Death in Europe. In the spring of 1348, ships leaving Bordeaux sailed to some seaport near Santiago de Compostela in northern Spain, in all likelihood La Coruña, to Rouen in north-western France, and to Weymouth in southern England, events that caused the early establishment of second northern plague fronts in the Iberian Peninsula and in France, and introduced the Black Death to England. From Weymouth, where its presence was recognized shortly before 24 June, the Black Death spread by metastatic leaps westwards to Bristol, which was contaminated at the end of June, and eastwards to London, which appears to have been contaminated already by the early days of August.

From south-eastern England new metastatic leaps by ship transported the Black Death to south-eastern Norway, almost certainly at the end of 1348, and to Bergen on the western coast in July 1349, probably quite early in the month.

Norway too was then conquered by two plague fronts reflecting two independent introductions by metastatic leaps. From Bergen new metastatic leaps by ship took the Black Death as far north in Europe as it is possible to trace its movement through the extant sources, to the cathedral city of Nidaros (Trondheim), and as far north-westwards, to the Faroe Islands in the Norwegian Sea.

In the summer of 1349, plague was transported by ship from England or south-eastern Norway to Elbing in Prussia, whence the Black Death began to spread into north-eastern Germany, forming in a few months a northern German plague front that began moving south-westwards, eventually meeting the epidemic forces of the Black Death that spread northwards in Germany after having marched through northern Italy, Austria and Switzerland. In the late autumn of 1349, a number of Hanseatic cities and towns on the Baltic Sea were contaminated by the Black Death, obviously by metastatic leaps by ship. Lastly, the contamination of Elbing was to become of particular importance because the plague front that eventually conquered Russia moved out of this epidemic epicentre. Thus, the Black Death conquered its easternmost territories in 1353.

Metastatic leaps by ship also occurred along the large navigable rivers that are so numerous in Europe, and that were so central to the commercial networks. The Black Death leapt, for instance, along the R. Rhine from the Swiss border city of Basle via Mainz to Cologne in north-western Germany in 7.5 months, according to the datings of the outbreaks, corresponding to an average daily pace of 2.2 km along this stretch of 500 km, about three times as fast as the pace of spread over land. Plague contagion was also spread by metastatic leaps from the Hanseatic towns and cities on the North Sea and the Baltic Sea up the many large navigable rivers and tributaries in northern Germany in the late autumn of 1349 and the following winter.

English scholars underline the significance of river transport for the rapid spread of the Black Death.

Metastatic leaps occurred also by land, but over shorter distances. There are not many clear instances. Apparently, some metastatic leaps by land took place out of Arles via Montpellier, Béziers and Carcassonne, and somewhere between Carcassonne and Bordeaux. These were very important events in the Black Death's European campaign, because these middle-range metastatic leaps by land caused the early contamination of Bordeaux on the Atlantic coast that made it possible for the Black Death to contaminate ships waiting in Bordeaux's harbour for the beginning of the sailing season, and, therefore, to begin the spread of contagion over long distances already by the end of March.

Another series of middle-range metastatic leaps by land took place from the original Italian epicentre in Pisa to Modena, Bologna, Perugia and Orvieto.

Metastatic leaps by ship greatly hastened the Black Death's conquest of Europe, and, arguably, made the almost total success of the European campaign possible. This meant that the Black Death moved with such pace and in such an apparently fortuitous manner in the eyes of the contemporaries that the weak and rudimentary medieval administrations of countries, city states or municipal authorities had no chance to organize effective countermeasures, such as blocking harbours to ships coming from abroad. However, the profound religious outlook of medieval man would often prevent or hamper seriously rational administrative action.

Pace of spread along sea lanes and by road

The speed of ship transport in the first half of the fourteenth century is poorly studied. It is clear that the vicissitudes of weather caused considerable variation. Ship technology still had a long way to go before ships were sufficiently developed to allow regular commercial sailing on the open sea, or before ships could sail efficiently against the wind. Consequently, commercial ships usually sailed along the coast and had to break off sailing at night. In this book, it has been argued that average daily distance achieved by ship was about 40 km. The realism of this assumption is reflected in the fact that this norm does not conflict with the time frame of any of the significant number of metastatic leaps by sea that have been discussed in the preceding chapters, from Constantinople to Alexandria, from Constantinople to various destinations in Italy or France, from Bordeaux to La Coruña, Rouen or Weymouth, or from Bergen to Nidaros, and so on.

Plague's natural pace of spread by land, i.e. (mainly), without the agency of human beings, has been exemplified by the speed with which it has been spreading across the American continent, namely 25 km per year since 1900, corresponding to 0.065 km = 65 metres per day.[1] Infected people or people carrying infective rat fleas in their clothing or hand luggage would not get far if they went on foot. Horseback, pack horses and horse and cart were the usual means of transport by land, which

---

[1]   McNeill 1979: 145. See also above, p. 47.

would often involve goods that might be contaminated in the sense that infected rat fleas could be riding with them. There are, unfortunately, not many cases in which the date the outbreak was recognized (in the sense clarified above) is known in two or more interconnected places, which alone can make it possible to perform estimates of the pace of spread between them.

The Black Death should be expected to spread at a maximum average pace by land along the main roads for trade and travel in the areas that were particularly densely settled and comprised many cities and sizeable towns. On the road from Marseilles to Avignon the Black Death spread at an average daily pace of 2 km, and again from Avignon to Lyons, if we correct somewhat for wintry conditions. Correspondingly, the Black Death moved the 160 km from Pisa on the coast of Tuscany to Pistoia at an average daily pace of 1.78 km, a pace that must be assumed to have been slowed down by cool winter weather, and thus also indicating a maximum average daily pace at a distance of about 2 km.[2]

The pace along secondary lines of communication in southern France was much slower. From Avignon to Alés, 65 km north-west of Avignon, it moved at an average daily pace of about 0.75 km; from Avignon to Die, a route that comprised first quite a long distance along the main road before it branched off into the French countryside west of the R. Rhône, the average daily pace was about 1.15 km. More generally, the pace of movement can be seen to slow down north of Lyons: from Lyons to Givry (or Chalon, 12 km east of Givry) the Black Death advanced at an average daily pace of 1.2 km, while along the 120 km on the road from Chalon north-eastwards to Besançon the pace appears to have slowed slightly to c. 1.1 km per day. The pace continues to slow down as the Black Death moved further northwards, and from Besançon to Strasbourg the average daily pace was 0.9 km. This slowdown must mainly be owing to a much-reduced density of traffic on the main roads north of Lyons. Some of this slowdown was owing to a sharp seasonal diminution of pace caused by cool winter weather; on the stretch of the road between Besançon and Montbéliard the Black Death moved at an average daily pace of only 0.4 km.

Recent Swiss data support these estimates of diminishing pace of spread as we move away from the main arteries of trade and travel. The Black Death marched the 60 km down the road from Geneva to Lausanne at an average daily pace of c. 0.66 km, and the 150 km from Geneva to Sion at an average daily pace of 0.75 km; in the latter case, however, the pace may have been slowed down by cool or cold winter weather for about half the time on the road.

Thus, the data on the Black Death's pace by land at a distance indicates a maximum of about 2 km per day along heavily trafficked main roads in very densely

---

[2]   Biraben states that the Black Death moved from Florence to Orvieto via Arezzo at an average rate of 3.36 km per day. However, he provides no information on its arrival in Arezzo. Instead, he refers to the early outbreak in Perugia in April, which, in my view, represents one of a number of metastatic leaps in Tuscany and surrounding regions, and it is the metastatic leap to Perugia that is the cause of the early outbreak in Orvieto that was already recognized in May. These metastatic leaps should, as pointed out above, be seen as leaps out of Pisa. The recognized outbreak in Florence in March is contemporaneous with a number of other outbreaks in cities and towns at considerable distances beyond Florence in the same month.

Biraben also asserts that the Black Death moved from Basle to Frankfurt at an average rate of slightly above 4 km per day. However, this episode reflects another metastatic leap, this time by ship down the R. Rhine (and upstream on the R. Main). For obvious reasons, spread by river transport is generally much faster than by land.

settled areas, in southern France for instance. This average pace slows down strongly as the Black Death moves northwards, with a clear decrease of pace north of Lyons to slightly above 1 km per day. There is also a strong reduction in average daily pace when the Black Death branches off the main roads into secondary communication lines in the surrounding regions, or when it branches off into countries that are more peripheral to the main European road system, into Switzerland, for instance.

This analysis of the Black Death's characteristic pace of spread by land in various parts of Europe and under various seasonal circumstances contains clear evidence to the effect that the Black Death normally, although not necessarily always, operated in the mode of epidemic bubonic plague (which will ordinarily comprise a small incidence of cases of primary pneumonic plague). Epidemics of primary pneumonic plague disseminated by cross-infection would have spread at a much faster pace in order to preserve its epidemic momentum because the victims would be infectious for such an extraordinarily short time, namely on average only 0.8 day (see above), and they would, on average, have to infect at least one other person if the epidemic should not become extinguished.

Thus, the Black Death spread by land at a pace that was only a tiny fraction of the pace by ship, namely 0.5–2 km per day by land versus 40 km per day by ship.

Pace of territorial spread and the significance of population density

The question of pace of spread is really twofold. It comprises the question of pace along roads and sea lanes discussed above and the question of the time needed for the Black Death to blanket rural areas and regions with local townships and urban centres. In Part 2, on the Black Death's conquest of Europe, a number of observations have been made that bear on this second question. Interestingly, high population density can be seen to have increased the pace of spread along the communication lines, but to have slowed down the pace of conquest in the sense that it increased the time needed to blanket regions and complete the epidemic processes there. Much the same was the case (with)in urban centres.

In Norway and Sweden, population densities were particularly low, about 1 and 2.7 persons per sq. km, respectively. Although the populations were mostly settled within smaller areas with higher population density, the pivotal point remains that these two countries had very low population densities. Both countries comprise quite large territories. The Black Death's conquest of these two countries followed a closely similar pattern. Despite the quite large territories and dispersedly settled populations, both countries appear to have been invaded in the late autumn, in 1348 and 1349, respectively, and next, to be completely engulfed in one plague season, starting in the spring and ending at the turn of the year. In the case of Norway, this was owing to the establishment of two plague fronts, of which the earliest in Oslo started its formation and spread from the very beginning of the plague season in April, which gave it time to cover completely the Oslofjord area, Østlandet ('East Country') and Sørlandet ('South Country'). The western plague front started its spread at the end of July or around 1 August, which appears to have given it sufficient time to cover most of the western and northern parts of Norway, but also leaves open the possibility that some areas could have been spared because the epidemic was suppressed and extinguished by cold weather before it reached them.

In the case of Sweden, the Black Death presumably managed to cover the whole of Sweden in one plague season in 1350 because the contagion had been introduced into the westernmost areas in the autumn of the preceding year and probably at several more places than it has been possible to indicate on the basis of the very poor source material for the history of the Black Death in this country.

The size of Denmark's territory was only a small fraction of the territories of Norway or Sweden, but its population was much larger, quite likely nearly as large as the populations of the two other Scandinavian countries combined. It was as expected that the Black Death covered the whole country in one plague season in 1350 after having crossed the border into the country at several places in the south-west and in the opposite corner in the north-east the preceding autumn. Conspicuously, the Black Death needed as much time to finish its grisly work in Denmark as in the two other countries, which again shows the significance of population size and population density for the spread and duration of a disease with plague's specific properties.

Although the population densities of Switzerland and Germany at the time are poorly known, it is clear that they were considerably higher than in Norway or Sweden but modest compared to those in Italy, France or the Low Countries. Because it appears to fit into a pattern, it is interesting to note that the Black Death conquered Switzerland and Germany in about a year and a half.

Italy and France were among the most densely settled countries in Europe: on the eve of the Black Death they apparently had about 35 and 40 persons per sq. km, respectively. Italy was invaded at the end of 1347, and all Italian regions had been invaded by the Black Death by the autumn of 1348, but the Black Death did not manage to complete the conquest of Italy until 1350. The same pattern can be seen in France, which, one should keep in mind, had a much larger population within a much larger territory. Although Marseilles was invaded in September 1347 and the meta-static leap to Rouen opened a second plague front early the next summer and all main regions had been reached at the end of 1348, the process of engulfment was not completed before 1351, and there is also mention of an outbreak in 1352.

However, England, which had the same population density as France and Italy, appears to have been conquered according to a time schedule more similar to that of Switzerland and Germany; nor is there a corresponding tendency for the Black Death to linger for several years in the same region. Why the process of spread should be different in England remains an intriguing and unexplained question.

This tendency of increasing duration of the epidemic process with increasing population density is, as should be expected, most clearly seen in the Low Countries, both in 'Belgium' and 'the Netherlands', where population levels were much higher than in any other European countries, apparently around 80 persons per sq. km. In some regions, like Hainault, it was well above 100 persons per sq. km. Regions that were invaded in the summer or the autumn of 1349, like Ath or southern Hainault, still suffered heavy mortality in 1352. In the Netherlands, the Black Death first invaded Friesland in the late autumn of 1349, and had not finished its ravages until 1353. The very long duration of the Black Death in these small countries is a highly conspicuous feature.

Of course, in the case of diseases spread by cross-infection from diseased to healthy persons, increasing population density should be expected to increase their powers of spread by increasing the number of persons that each diseased person would, on average, infect, as in the cases of influenza or smallpox, for instance. The principal epidemiological cause of the Black Death's peculiar pattern of spread in time and space characterized by increasing slowness of the epidemiological processes with increasing population densities must be the fact that cross-infection plays only a minute role and that, instead, it is overwhelmingly transmitted from rats to human beings by the agency of rat fleas.

The more densely settled a rural area or region was, the higher number of houses the Black Death had to enter in relation to the size of the territory in order to blanket it. In each of these houses, the Black Death would trigger a rat epizootic that must have run its course before the rat fleas for lack of rat hosts turned on human beings in their immediate vicinity. This is an obviously time-consuming process compared with the mechanisms of cross-infection, and the more houses the more time was needed to engulf the area. This is the reason that the district of Ath in the very densely populated Duchy of Hainault, which was invaded in 1349, still suffered serious mortality in 1351–2. Also in the much more thinly settled rural districts of Norway the Black Death's tendency to linger can be observed, but in a shorter time perspective reflecting the much lower levels of population density than in Italy, France or the Low Countries. In the summer of 1349, the Black Death was in full swing in the neighbouring rural districts of Eiker and Sandsvær, 60–100 km south-west of Oslo, but appears not to have petered out until December, when the arrival of cold winter weather undoubtedly played a part. In the case of Sweden, a similar tendency can be discerned in the region of Småland.

Seasonality of epidemics and its epidemiological implications: Bubonic plague or primary pneumonic plague?

The seasonality of plague epidemics contains important clues as to the mechanisms of spread and may, therefore, serve to test once again the assumption that the Black Death was overwhelmingly an epidemic of bubonic plague and that epidemics of primary pneumonic plague and of mixed epidemics, in the sense that they comprised a substantial proportion of pneumonic cases, must have been rare. As pointed out above, the mode of plague has implications too for the likely order of magnitude of plague mortality, namely that it should be expected to be much higher in the case of bubonic plague. Pneumonic plague is characterized by low diffusibility, and epidemics rarely comprise over one hundred persons/victims (see above).

In the case of Southern Europe, the term winter relates predominantly to the months December–February, while in Northern Europe, in Norway, Sweden and large parts of Russia, for instance, winter comprises in addition the months November and March, and the temperatures tend to be much lower as well.

The seasonality of the Black Death exhibits a very clear pattern. In southern Europe, winter weather temporarily slowed down its pace of spread or stopped its territorial spread. This feature has been observed by several scholars in a national context, for instance by Henri Dubois in relation to the Black Death's spread in France: 'usually, it was stopped or slowed down by the winter'.[3]

---

[3]   Dubois 1988b: 316. My translation from French.

The exception was spread by metastatic leaps when infected rat fleas were spread at a distance by goods or luggage, triggering at the place of arrival a smouldering enzootic (see Glossary) in local rat colonies that is so characteristic for the unobtrusive winter process. In a moist and cool climate, fleas can survive for many weeks without drawing blood and can be transported at quite long distances; this environmental situation has much in common with sea transport. In the early spring, this aspect of the Black Death's epidemiology in cool and cold weather manifests itself in more or less contemporary outbreaks at considerable distances, which cannot be integrated in an orderly and systematic territorial progression of the plague epidemic. This special pattern is most clearly discernible in Tuscany and the adjacent Italian regions, in southern France, and in northern Germany.

Slowdown of the Black Death's pace of spread and epidemic intensity in cool winter weather can be observed, for instance, in Mallorca I. and in the Iberian Peninsula at the end of 1348. The Black Death's pace of spread can be seen to slow down out of Aix-en-Provence in the direction of Arles and Avignon and then in the direction of Lyons. It slowed further down when it moved into mountain areas, for instance on the road to the town of Die, where cold winter weather lasted longer than in the lowlands. A characteristic instance of slowdown can also be seen in north-eastern France, where the Black Death moved the distance of about 120 km from Chalon to Besançon at an average daily pace of c. 1.1 km, and the roughly 220 km from Besançon to Strasbourg at an average daily pace of 0.9 km. However, this small slowdown for the distance as a whole can be explained by the strong slowdown between Besançon and Montbéliard in winter weather, when the average daily pace fell to about 0.4 km.

In Central and Northern Europe the arrival of winter weather usually heralded a stop in the epidemic. In the late autumn of 1348, the Black Death was prevented from crossing over the mountain areas from Austria into Germany's south-eastern province of Bavaria by the advent of winter, while, at the same time, it continued to spread westwards across the Austrian lowlands into Switzerland. The onset of cold winter weather is also the probable reason the Black Death did not march on directly into Germany's south-western province of Baden-Württemberg from Constance on the Swiss–German border where it broke out in November. The invasion of Germany had to await the arrival of spring and milder weather. The same pattern can be seen in Switzerland, where the last case of the Black Death in Engelberg in the canton of Uri is observed on 6 January 1350, after having broken out in early September the preceding year.

A large area around the axis Nuremberg–Würzburg in the north-western half of Bavaria avoided being invaded by the Black Death in the autumn of 1349 by the arrival of cool or cold weather, but it was only a short respite; with the end of winter and the arrival of warmer weather the conquest of the area appears to have been completed.

In Germany, the territorial spread of the Black Death northwards was arrested in central Germany by cold weather in the late autumn of 1349. However, the pattern of outbreaks in the spring of 1350 shows that, in the late autumn of 1349, the Black Death had been widely disseminated among the Hanseatic cities and towns on the North Sea and the Baltic Sea. Although the outbreak in Lübeck is dated by the chronicler Detmar to mid-May 1350, other sources show that there was an outbreak in the late autumn that was stopped temporarily by winter weather. Arguably, the other outbreaks in May also reflect the same pattern. It can also be seen that during the winter the Black Death had been transported with goods from the commercial cities on the northern coasts far inland in northern Germany along the many large water-ways and main roads, a process that manifests itself in the contemporaneous outbreaks of the Black Death in a number of cities and towns in the spring in a pattern that in many cases rules out interconnected spread.

In Northern Europe the seasonal pattern is clear. In Norway, the Black Death was evidently introduced into Oslo in the late autumn of 1348, but was suppressed by the arrival of winter weather. It broke out in the following spring and had covered at least most of the southern half of the country and had severely depleted the rat popula-tions before it was extinguished by the onset of winter weather (a few cases are mentioned in December, the last plague case at the beginning of January 1350). The introduction of the Black Death in Bergen at the beginning of July 1349 unleashed the plague in western Norway whence it leapt by ship to Nidaros, the urban hub of central Norway, apparently engulfing those two regions. But again the plague disap-pears completely with the advent of winter weather. In my recent book on Norway's plague history from the Black Death to the last outbreaks in 1654 it has become clear that there never was a winter epidemic of plague in Norway: plague epidemics receded with chilly autumn weather and always disappeared in the face of winter cold.[4] In Sweden, it appears possible to discern the beginnings of outbreaks in the south-western region of Västergötland and in south-western Småland at the end of 1349, but they were suppressed by winter weather. As in Norway, the Black Death broke out in the spring, and it managed to spread all the way to the Baltic Sea and cover at least most of the country before it again was extinguished by the onset of winter weather.

Clearly, the Black Death drew strength from mild and warm weather all over Europe, and cool and cold weather impeded or prevented its spread. Also clearly, primary pneumonic plague that is disseminated by cross-infection through the agency of droplets containing plague bacteria coughed up by patients in an advanced stage of the disease's course of development, is not dependent on the season. As shown above, the spread of this mode of plague is primarily dependent on social mores and customs that encourage close physical proximity and intimacy between diseased and healthy persons. On the other hand, the powers of spread of bubonic plague, which is dependent on transmission by fleas, requires a climate with moderately warm temperatures that promote the procreation of fleas and the reproduction of the flea population. Cool or cold climates impede or prevent procreation, in which case the high natural mortality of fleas causes a rapid decline in flea populations. Cool or cold climates also impede or prevent the reproduction of plague bacteria in rats and in the guts of fleas, and, thus, also the formation of blockage in fleas. Thus, there can be no doubt that this seasonal pattern reflects that the Black Death was overwhelmingly an epidemic of bubonic plague. This does not rule out, however, the episodic occurrence of primary pneumonic plague.

---

[4] Benedictow 2002.

Did epidemics of primary pneumonic plague occur in the Black Death?

In a few instances, winter epidemics of plague are mentioned, and these instances have been interpreted as epidemics of primary pneumonic plague. The evidence most often referred to is the clinical description of the Black Death given by Gui de Chauliac, personal physician to Pope Clement VI and to the Papal Court at Avignon:

> The great death toll began in our case in the month of January [1348], and lasted for the space of seven months. It was of two kinds: the first lasted two months; with continuous fever and spitting of blood; and death occurred within three days. The second lasted for the whole of the remainder of the time, also with continuous fever, and with ulcers and boils in the extremities, principally under the arm-pits and in the groin; and death took place within five days. And [it] was of so great a contagion (especially when there was spitting of blood) that not only through living in the same house but merely through looking, one person caught it from the other.[5]

The French historian Emmanuel Le Roy Ladurie draws the immediate conclusion that the first type of plague was primary pneumonic plague. However, this inference is not obvious, as can readily be seen from the presentation of this form of plague above, on the basis of a total review of the medical and epidemiological research on the pneumonic forms of plague.[6] Cases of primary pneumonic plague have an average duration of 1.8 days, and it takes, on average, 24 hours from the onset of the disease until they develop into the phase characterized by a frequent cough with bloody expectoration; this second phase lasts, consequently, on average, 0.8 day or 19 hours. This normal duration of the illness corresponds poorly to Chauliac's clinical description, according to which the duration of the phase with cough and bloody expectoration could last 72 hours. It is very conspicuous that he focuses on the possible duration of illness, but does not mention the frightening extreme brevity and fulminant form of the usual course of illness, especially the few hours characterized by cough and bloody expectoration. One should also note that he gives a duration for bubonic plague that agrees with the normal time frame as indicated by modern medical research, i.e., 3–5 days; if the time horizon he gives on the duration of bloody expectoration is based on the same approach, the indicated duration does not fit with primary pneumonic plague, but could well agree with secondary pneumonic plague.

Of course, it is true that in ordinary cases of primary pneumonic plague a few patients would hold on to life for three days, but this would be very atypical. Instead, the considerable incidence of dramatic fulminant courses of illness in which diseased persons died within the day, even in a few hours, and before the characteristic bloody expectoration had time to develop, would make a great impression on physicians and chroniclers alike.

One should keep in mind that medieval physicians and chroniclers were fascinated by the dramatic features of plague, and their accounts often contain also imaginary and fantastic assertions. The fantastic element is very much in evidence also in

---

5 Le Roy Ladurie 1981: 45.
6 The review of pneumonic plague in this chapter and elsewhere in this book draws upon the complete review of all medical research on pneumonic plague presented in Benedictow 1993/1996a: 25–9, 214–27. See also the brief comments in the Glossary.

Chauliac's account where he asserts, for instance, that the disease cross-infected readily 'through looking'. This notion of extreme contagiousness 'through looking' is also linked directly to cases characterized by the 'spitting of blood'. However, in the standard medical works on plague, including on primary pneumonic plague, it is stressed that neither primary nor secondary pneumonic plague cross-infect easily: 'respiratory transmission occurs most frequently to medical personnel or household contacts who are directly involved with the care of the patient', and 'an overwhelming majority of cases receive infection through being in the direct range of a cough'.[7] This aspect of primary and secondary pneumonic plague and its medical explanation is precisely the main reason that these forms of plague play a peripheral role in the dynamics of plague epidemics in general and in the Black Death as well, and that primary pneumonic plague only very rarely and under exceptional circumstances such as in Manchuria develops into largish epidemics. In addition, as mentioned several times, the power of spread of primary pneumonic plague is much reduced by the fact that a substantial proportion of persons that contract primary pneumonic plague die without developing cough with bloody expectoration, and thus without having become contagious at all. Le Roy Ladurie is definitely in error when he assumes that the great mortality in the Black Death in Provence was due to it being mainly an epidemic of primary pneumonic plague. It will be shown below that the mortality in Provence was no higher than elsewhere.

If the plague epidemic in Avignon had really been pneumonic plague, Chauliac would, in my opinion, in all likelihood have focused on the very dramatic facts that most people died on the same day as the 'spitting of blood' began, and that it was quite usual for patients to die a few hours after the sudden onset of fulminating fever without exhibiting any cough at all (because the patient died too soon for the coughs to develop). In this perspective, it is hard to envisage that he would take much interest in a few cases he might have observed of a somewhat longer course of illness.

Instead, Chauliac's account conforms quite closely to the modern medical descriptions of secondary pneumonic plague that have been set out and explained above and in the Glossary. This form of plague arises from cases of ordinary bubonic plague in which the plague bacteria introduced by a blocked flea overwhelm the lymphatic system and soon pass on from the swollen lymph nodes into the bloodstream. In these cases, plague bacteria are transported to the lungs where they may consolidate and cause the development of ulcers that provoke a frequent cough with bloody expectoration; this condition is called secondary pneumonic plague because it is secondary to the primary infection of buboes. After the usual incubation period, the further course of this version of plague disease is characterized by the sudden onset of fulminating fever and the development of bubo(es), progresses with the invasion of plague bacteria into the bloodstream (secondary bacteraemia), and, after a day, the development of a cough with bloody expectoration that will often last for a day or two before the patient almost invariably dies. This means that the time horizon of secondary pneumonic plague is quite similar to the duration of illness indicated by

---

[7] See above, pp. 27–31 and the references given there.

Chauliac; it corresponds in practice also to the criterion of certain death (the very rare instances of survivors will only be registered by modern medical statistics).[8]

However, because secondary pneumonic plague is a normal feature of bubonic plague epidemics, comprising 10–25 per cent of all cases,[9] Chauliac's division of the epidemic into two distinct phases becomes intriguing at best, and rather unrealistic: there cannot have been any phase of the Black Death that did not also include quite a sizeable proportion of patients that were 'spitting blood'. Perhaps we would understand Chauliac's epidemiological description better and be able to identify an empirical element reflecting real observation if we do not presuppose a modern scholarly level of emphasis on observation and accuracy but, instead, assume that he, as a typical representative of humanistically educated scholars, was prone to make his case in the classical rhetorical form of gross exaggeration and juxtaposition of extreme contrasts. This approach makes it possible to suggest an epidemiological interpretation to the effect that the Black Death in Avignon (and adjacent areas?) may have comprised an initial phase where it took on the character of a *mixed epidemic* according to a pattern best known from the plague epidemics in Madagascar and Upper Egypt in the first half of the twentieth century, in which 20 per cent and 30 per cent, respectively, of all cases were cases of primary pneumonic plague; in Java I. (in Indonesia), the incidence of pneumonic cases was smaller, 4–8 per cent, but a consistent feature.[10]

One should note that Madagascar, Egypt and Java, where the regular incidences of pneumonic cases within bubonic epidemics were so high that they inspired the development of the concept of mixed epidemics of plague, are areas with temperate or hot climates. On the other hand, the medical studies of pneumonic plague have not been able to establish a positive connection between cold weather and a high incidence of

---

[8] The clinical interrelationship between buboes, bloody expectoration and sharp pangs of pain was observed and described by a number of physicians in connection with the Black Death. The Icelandic *Lawman's Annal* contains, for instance, the following description of the clinical symptoms of the Black Death in Bergen:

> the disease was such that men did not live for more than a day or two with sharp pangs of pain, then they began to vomit blood, and then they expired.

In a typically somewhat confused fashion and with a characteristic fascination with the bloody cough, this clinical description refers to some central aspects of an epidemic of bubonic plague with cases of secondary pneumonic plague (which is normal). It starts with the bubonic phase, which lasts 1–2 days and is characterized by the development of intensely painful buboes; next follows the secondary pneumonic phase characterized by a frequent cough with bloody expectoration, and then the patient (almost) invariably dies. Modern physicians doing research on plague patients will easily recognize the real reference of the expression, 'sharp pangs of pain'. It refers to the extreme painfulness of buboes. In the words of modern plague researchers, buboes are 'painful and exquisitely tender', or characterized by 'extreme tenderness'. Reed, Palmer, Williams et al. 1970: 479; Welty, Grabman, Kompare et al. 1985: 641–3; Butler 1983: 73–4. Cf. Simpson 1905: 263, 274.

Michael Platiensis observed the Black Death's arrival in Sicily in 1347. He relates that the characteristic symptomatic features were outbreak of buboes and swollen glands simultaneously with profuse bloody expectoration, with death occurring after three days.

In Piacenza, Gabriel de Mussis noted that the patients were first attacked by chills and shivers, and they felt pricking spikes as if they were pierced by arrows; then they were hit cruelly in the axillas or in the groin where buboes began to develop, and, after some time, the patients also began to spew blood. Sticker 1908: 47, 52–3.

[9] Benedictow 1993/1996a: 25, and the medical works referred to there.

[10] Benedictow 1993/1996a: 28–9.

pneumonic plague. Historians' strong tendency to emphasize the significance of cold weather ought either to be strongly reduced or preferably to be discarded.[11]

This means that culturally conditioned behavioural features relating to disease and death should be assigned far more weight. According to modern medical studies performed early in the twentieth century, quite high frequencies of primary pneumonic plague within the framework of epidemics of bubonic plague are caused by culturally and climatically induced behaviour favouring this type of spread, especially behaviour leading to close physical contact between diseased and healthy persons. Hypothetically, such behavioural patterns could also have been practised in parts of medieval Europe. The group of researchers who studied plague in Upper Egypt in the years 1899–1913 report:

> In Egypt the ignorance of the people and their habit of clinging to traditional customs and prejudices encourage direct transference of the infection. The practice of crowding round and kissing the sick, the assemblage of men and women at funeral ceremonies, and the attempts that are made to conceal deaths and to evade the measures for controlling the disease, add greatly to the difficulties of the Sanitary Administration.[12]

The emphasis on behavioural factors for explaining the relative incidence of pneumonic cases in plague epidemics lends the Egyptian scenario a broader relevance as a model for analysis. Certainly, Le Roy Ladurie argues energetically to the effect that great intensity of social contact and intimacy between diseased and sound persons was the case in Provence.[13]

One should note that the characteristic weak powers of spread of primary pneumonic plague have also been observed in relation to mixed epidemics. The scholars studying the mixed plague epidemic in Upper Egypt state tersely, for instance:

> Viewing the outbreaks as a whole we find that the number of cases in each is small, and that the majority remained isolated. When the escape of contacts from the primary outbreak led to the introduction of the disease into neighbouring villages, there were seldom more than three or four secondary offshoots. It is clear then that, although in the affected districts foci are apt to flare up, the outbreaks that follow are characterized by low diffusibility.[14]

Seen in conjunction with a substantial proportion of secondary pneumonic cases that could quite realistically have comprised 20–25 percent of all bubonic cases,[15] this means that 40–55 per cent of all cases could theoretically have exhibited the dramatic clinical manifestation of 'blood spitting', which conceivably could suffice to produce the impression in Chauliac, according to the workings of his medieval humanistic mentality that 'blood spitting' was a normal or usual feature of the course of illness. If an element of primary pneumonic plague of the indicated order of magnitude disappeared after a couple of months, the medieval scholarly mind could easily have

---

[11] Cf. Meyer 1961: 253.
[12] Petrie, Todd, Skander et al. 1924: 143.
[13] Le Roy Ladurie 1981: 47–51.
[14] Petrie, Todd, Skander et al. 1924: 143.
[15] Benedictow 1993/1996a: 34.

ignored the continuing occurrence of a much smaller incidence of cases characterized by cough with bloody expectoration. This, then, is only an explanatory hypothesis.

The Black Death in Novgorod is the second episode of the Black Death that is quite often assumed to have been an epidemic of primary pneumonic plague.[16] This assumption is based on a combination of the fact that the epidemic is said to have lasted through the winter of (1352–)1353 and clinical descriptions in *The Chronicle of Novogorod I* and *The Chronicle of Nikon*:

> Innumerable good people died in this time [15 August–Easter]. The characteristic features of this mortal disease were the following: people have a bloody cough, and this goes on for three days until they die. This was the case not only in Novgorod, this punishment spread all over the country. And the persons God called, died, and the persons that God preserved, He chastened with this punishment so that they should live their remaining days virtuously and innocent to God.[17]

This description of the clinical symptoms to the effect that the duration of the phase with a cough producing bloody expectoration lasted 72 hours does not correspond at all to the modern medical clinical descriptions of the duration of this phase in primary pneumonic plague, which lasts, as mentioned, on average, for only 19 hours. Instead, the chroniclers' clinical descriptions agree nicely with the third phase of the development pattern of secondary pneumonic plague as presented and explained in modern medical research.

Furthermore, primary and secondary pneumonic forms of plague are for all practical purposes a hundred per cent fatal. However, the chronicler mentions survivors as a quite normal phenomenon. This is an indirect reference to bubonic plague, the ordinary form of plague that is survived by about 20 per cent of those who contract it.

Because a cough with bloody expectoration is such a dramatic feature of the illness, and because the patients almost invariably die, the quite frequent incidence of this symptom will dominate the observers' perception of the disease. At the time of the Black Death, physicians who had studied classical Greek medicine at the medical faculty in Salerno or in other medical faculties of universities were present in significant numbers only in Italy and France, and in most of Europe such medical specialists were extremely rare or even non-existent. This was also the case in Russia at the time, which means that treatment was religious and not medical, and that plague patients were not examined physically for diagnostic and clinical features, especially not in such a sensitive region as the groin where buboes most often develop. It is, therefore, quite usual that descriptions of plague cases do not mention buboes, although other features of the description such as, for instance, duration of the illness, make it clear that the epidemic is bubonic plague with an incidence of pneumonic variants that is characteristic and normal for this disease.

The epidemic lasted until Easter, but the intensity of the winter epidemic as compared with the autumnal phase is not indicated. Conceivably, it could have been characterized by an endemic incidence of cases, a type of development that can be

---

[16] Dörbeck 1906: 14; Sticker 1908: 72.
[17] My translation of the Russian text.

studied in detail in the instance of the plague epidemic in Bergen in 1565–6.[18] According to the chroniclers, the Black Death in the town of Pskov ended with the arrival of winter. One may wonder why the Black Death should have taken on a very different character in Novgorod than in Pskov.

The fact that the Black Death could last through the winter until Easter without having taken on the character of primary pneumonic plague can be illustrated by another case relating to the countship of Bigorre in south-western France close to the Pyrenees, more specifically in the valley of Barèges. In a notarial document, it is stated that the Black Death first appeared in the town of Luz on 29 June 1348 and lasted until Easter the following year; in other words that it lasted through the winter. In addition, we are also told more generally that it was a glandular epidemic in Barèges, which unequivocally identifies the epidemic as bubonic.[19]

---

[18] Benedictow 2002: 196–198.
[19] Berthe 1976: 51, 198.

Part Four
Mortality in the Black Death

26

The Medieval Demographic System

Introduction

It has generally been agreed that the Black Death inflicted horrible mortality upon Europe's populations. This event is important to historians because it affected social and economic structures and the existential and cultural outlook of people in profound ways. It heralded an historical period in which new waves of plague continued to cause great mortality and deepen the effects on societies and people. Together with more long-running trends, the Black Death and ensuing plague epidemics moulded the *social formation* that constituted the last period of the Middle Ages, namely the Late Middle Ages, and gave dynamic input to the profound transitional societal changes leading from medieval to early modern society.

However, for a long time almost no valid data on the mortality caused by the Black Death were available, i.e., mortality data that were the products of demographic and statistical study of suitable sources. Only the outcomes of such studies could constitute a sound empirical basis for concrete and reasonably accurate synthesis and inference as to the real level of mortality. The assertions of historians of great mortality were impressionistic, based on the horrified assertions of chroniclers, a few physicians, clerics and literary authors like Petrarch and Boccaccio. But were Boccaccio's assertion that 100,000 persons perished in the Black Death in Florence true? What was the basis for this assertion? Did Florence really contain as many as 100,000 people on the eve of the Black Death? The Icelandic chronicler who asserted that two-thirds of Norway's population perished in the Black Death, should he be believed? What was the material basis for this assertion, if any? Could he be credible at all, given that immediately before this assertion he maintains that only fourteen people survived in London? The historians' accounts used to be fraught with such problems.

True, the assertions of chroniclers and contemporary authors on population mortality are useless or highly problematic. They are usually written in the medieval version of classical humanistic rhetorical scholarship. They are not intended to be accurate and are with a few exceptions not based on collection and processing of numerical data. They are literary rhetorical statements intended to convey the drama and shock of having lived through an incomprehensible epidemic disaster. This has been illustrated above in the form of assertions by chroniclers to the effect that all persons in a town or district died in the Black Death, or that more people died in some town or city than we know on the basis of modern demographic studies actually lived there.

However, from 1920 in Norway, 1935 in Germany and 1950 in England, pioneering studies were published by S. Hasund, W. Abel and M. Postan, respectively, that heralded a new phase in the study of the economic and demographic history of the Late Middle Ages. The horrified assertions of contemporaries on the Black Death and subsequent plague epidemics could be shown to be supported by reflections of greatly reduced populations in manorial studies and other types of local-settlement studies. These studies often uncovered a high incidence of deserted holdings and strongly falling rents and fines that had to reflect a huge or at least substantial deficit of tenants and, thus, a strongly diminished population. Studies on the development of prices and wages showed strongly falling grain prices and briskly increasing real wages both in the countryside and in the towns, which similarly had to imply a large deficit of workers relative to unused or underused productive resources. However, these studies mostly had a long-term character, covering large parts of the Late Medieval period, and, thus, included the effects of a number of subsequent plague epidemics, also with uncertain mortality effects, although clearly not so severe. The mortality caused by the Black Death itself remained veiled and continued to be related to in an impressionistic fashion by historians.

Thus, there remained a certain tension between the long-term late-medieval trends uncovered by these studies and the fragile empirical basis for assessing the specific demographic impact of the Black Death. Did it have an impact of epoch-making or period-forming significance? Or were the effects of the mortality it caused only of passing significance?

Early assumptions on mortality in the Black Death given by historians for local societies, towns, cities, regions, countries, parts of Europe or all Europe are generally high and dramatic, but also conspicuously rounded off in a manner revealing a high level of uncertainty and a low input of demographically valid data, usually assuming quite arbitrarily that a quarter or one-third of the population in question may have perished.

A new phase in the demographic study of the Black Death started in the early 1960s. A considerable number of demographically valid studies on the mortality in the Black Death were published in the last four decades of the twentieth century. For some reason, they have largely been ignored or neglected, perhaps because they often are published in local journals or local histories that tend to be out of the sight of university historians; perhaps also because they tend to indicate mortality levels that within the narrow horizon of the individual local study may seem either incredible or to be a fortuitous, unrepresentative local and singular case. The fragmentation of their publication, localization and representativeness appears to have marginalized these studies and to have concealed their consistency and collective evidential powers. For the first time they will be collected, examined and synthesized into general data in this book.

General principles

Mortality in the Black Death must be discussed in the general perspective of normal medieval death rates and the medieval demographic system or regime. Normal death rates in any society are not fortuitous or accidental phenomena, but are always closely associated with the societal system, also called *social formation*, in this case with the *medieval societal system*. Societal systems are characterized by the specificity of their main structures, i.e., their economic, technological, political, social-class, cultural and mental structures, and, of course, the demographic structure. Such structures are societal subsystems, generally referred to as the economic system, the political system, and so on. In the case of the Middle Ages, these subsystems were represented, for instance, by the feudal manorial system, or the feudal political system, and, consequently, there was also a corresponding specific medieval demographic system. The systemic character of societal structures ensures structural specificity and stability; and in the case of the demographic structure characteristic normal levels of mortality and life expectancy that also comprise specific and quite stable patterns of age distribution and gender distribution of mortality and life expectancy. Basic medieval demographic data from various countries and regions should be expected to be quite closely related, and, as we shall see, they are indeed.

Thus, demographic history did not begin with transitional processes around 1750 associated with the mature Early Modern period and the Industrial Revolution, as is astonishingly often arbitrarily assumed. On the contrary, demographic history, like the other main disciplines of history such as economic history, political history, history of culture, religion and mentality, and so on, is closely associated with the specific social formations that constitute historical periods. Historical periods are not fortuitous or arbitrary divisions of historical time, but are identified on the basis of the specificity of their social formations as they are formed by the specific character of their economic, technological, social, demographic, political, cultural, religious and mental structures, and by the specific way these social structures interacted dynamically in the production of the grand historical process of societal change.[1] Thus, to the concepts of modern European history, early modern history or medieval history, there are corresponding specific notions of qualitative differences between these historical periods' social formations as moulded by the specificity of the main social structures of these periods and the way these structures interacted.

In this perspective, the feudal or semi-feudal structure of medieval societies constitutes a very distinct social formation when compared to early modern societies, even more when compared to modern societies. Social formations are phenomena *sui generis*, of their own peculiar and unique kind, confronting human beings as objective realities, easily frustrating modern political radicals' endeavours at creating new societies according to their ideologies. Social formations change in a grand and majestic fashion, slowly but inexorably, having long transitional periods characterized by a mixture of the old and new structural elements before reaching a mature form of the historical period; next, this is followed by new transitional processes, leading eventually to the establishment of a new historical period in its early form or phase. Thus, historical periods contain long or longish phases reflecting transitional processes when pre-period structural elements are phased out and the new structural elements are phased in and develop into a mature phase, to be followed by a transitional final phase when the constitutive structural features of the subsequent historical period emerge or take on a new, increasingly dominant character that progressively translates into qualitative societal differentiation. The Middle Ages, for instance, are divided into the early, high and late phases. Likewise, the Renaissance, for instance, is a concept of historical periodization referring to the transitional phase of European society/civilization straddling the Late Middle Ages and the Early Modern period that was also characterized by dynamic cultural innovation and development. For some strange reason, it tends to be overlooked that the Early Modern

---

[1]   See also Part 5 below.

period has obvious phases that could be designated early, high and late, or by other suitable synonyms.

Even if for no other reason, the clearly recognized qualitative specificity of a social formation's other societal structures would affect populations in correspondingly specific ways; consequently, the demographic structure would also inevitably have a period-specific character. In reality, of course, the demographic structure interacted with the other structures and affected them more or less as much as it was affected itself.

All social formations contain a specific demographic regime or system that it is important to identify for two main reasons: firstly, because the specificity of the demographic system reflects the dynamic formative powers of the other social structures and is, as such, a platform for the study of more comprehensive social processes; and secondly, because the demographic system exerts dynamic social formative powers of its own, which also must be understood in order to acquire a broad understanding of the social processes that shaped people's lives, produced social formations and societal change, the superordinate historical processes. These are the reasons that make historical demography an important historical discipline.

It is a fallacy of the methodology of the social sciences to assume, as some scholars do, that demographic structures of some historical period can be projected across the dividing lines of other historical periods, from the Early Modern period into the Middle Ages, for instance, or across the societal dividing lines between civilizations. This does not mean that there cannot be some similarity across these dividing lines, only that it cannot be assumed to be the case. There is no alternative to period-specific or civilization-specific evidence. If no medieval sources were extant that could indicate the main outline of a medieval demographic regime, historians would have to admit that nothing of substance was known of medieval demography, and that this case was closed. Fortunately, not least with respect to this book, that is not the case.

Medieval sources used for demographic studies present both source-critical and technical problems, in the latter case because they contain incomplete registrations of populations: usually, they do not register children, often do not register adolescents and only rarely record women, except the few that were heads of households. In the scholarly endeavours to identify and develop knowledge on the medieval demographic system, *model life tables* are useful analytical tools that have proved their value, as we shall see below in the discussion of mortality rates in various contexts. As mentioned rather simplistically in the Glossary, model life tables contain series of age-specific death rates for each gender and show, thus, the probabilities of dying within particular age intervals according to various life expectancies at birth. Or, if focusing on the probabilities of surviving, life tables show life expectancies at each age level according to the various life expectancies at birth of different societies in time and spatial localization. The ages are organized according to five-year intervals (quinquennia), excepting ages 0–4, which are divided into the first year of life (infants) and the subsequent four years (young children), because of the very high mortality in these age categories that used to obtain in developing countries and were such a regular feature of old-time Europe. Several works containing life tables are available, and here we use the second edition of Coale and Demeny's widely recognized work *Regional Model Life Tables and Stable Populations*. Life tables are constructed in four regional variants, called North, West, South and East, according to observations relating to roughly corresponding parts of Europe and developing countries. An example of such a model life table can be seen in Table 10.

Table 10. Life expectancy and mortality at various ages in a population of males with life expectancy at birth (e_0)[a] of 25 years, and the number of deaths at each age level and the number alive at the start of each age level out of an original population of 100,000 persons, according to Model West, life table, level 4

Age(s)	Deaths per thousand	Number of deaths	Number alive	Life expectancy	Age(s)
0	322.57	32257	100000	25.26	0
1	195.23	13226	67743	36.13	1
5	51.41	2803	54517	40.57	5
10	36.97	1912	51714	37.65	10
15	50.17	2498	49803	33.99	15
20	71.10	3364	47304	30.65	20
25	79.51	3494	43941	27.79	25
30	91.75	3711	40447	24.97	30
35	107.09	3934	36736	22.23	35
40	128.38	4211	32802	19.59	40
45	147.54	4218	28591	17.09	45
50	183.83	4481	24373	14.59	50
55	220.24	4381	19892	12.29	55
60	290.59	4507	15511	10.03	60
65	371.25	4085	11004	8.08	65
70	480.85	3327	6919	6.31	70
75	623.98	2241	3592	4.75	75
80	744.08	1005	1351	3.49	80
85	869.24	300	346	2.51	85
90	952.01	43	45	1.77	90
95	1000	2	2	1.24	95

[a] e_0 is a standard abbreviation in demography meaning life expectancy at birth, *e* being an abbreviation of the Latin word *etas* meaning age, *o* referring to age at birth. Life expectancy at other ages, at age 15, for instance, will correspondingly be written e_{15}.

'The immediate purpose' of the two demographers who calculated these model life tables was to 'estimate birth rates, death rates, and approximate age distributions in research on populations for which there were only incomplete or inaccurate data'.[2] Although these scholars had in mind problems demographers met with in relation to developing countries, their work serves the study of historical populations as well, supplementing incomplete or inaccurate early modern or medieval demographic data, putting them into a more holistic demographic perspective, bridging lacunae in the age dimension of a population, usually with respect to infants and children, showing the proportion of a population at a specific age in a society with a usefully known demographic regime, the proportion of males in the age cohort 50–54, for instance.

[2] Coale and Demeny 1983: 31–4.

For the time being, the available medieval data on life expectancy and mortality are relatively few and confined to a few countries. However, they have conspicuous consistency, are conspicuously different from those of the mature Early Modern period, and constitute a coherent and specific demographic regime or system. They are also obtained from independent types of sources, from various types of documentary evidence created in several countries as well as osteological studies of skeletal populations in medieval cemeteries that provide closely similar demographic data. When studies of independent types of evidence on a subject provide similar outcomes, evidential synergy effects arise. Therefore, taken together, these data permit inference at a substantial level of validity to the main aspects of the medieval demographic system.

One should keep in mind that old-time European demography had much in common with the demography of developing countries in the first half of the twentieth century. Relating to the Indian censuses of 1911, Coale and Demeny consider that 'a maximum estimate of 22–24 for e_0 [life expectancy at birth] is warranted' 'in spite of obvious uncertainties'.[3] Average life expectancy at birth in France around 1700, for instance, was 25 years, while at the time of the French Revolution it had increased significantly to 29 years.[4] Similarly, in eighteenth-century Italy, life expectancy 'oscillated' 'between twenty and twenty-five years, and reached only rarely the limit of thirty years',[5] which shows that the medieval demographic regime lasted even longer in Italy, presumably because of the regressive economic and social developments in the Early Modern period. T. Bøhm has studied the records containing the Norwegian censuses of all males taken in the 1660s and has shown that life expectancy at birth, according to the crude data contained in the records, was 26 years;[6] if it is taken into account that there is a significant underregistration of infants and young children and a conspicuous rounding upwards of ages[7] (high age was prestigious in those days, and in some age cohorts it would also serve to rule out eligibility for conscription), it becomes clear that life expectancy cannot have been more than 25 years, and may well have been lower. In the mid-1700s, average life expectancy in Norway had increased to around 35 years.

Thus, it can clearly be seen that life expectancy rose significantly and even substantially in the mature Early Modern social formation of Europe, both in the north and in the west of the continent. Actually, Bøhm has been able to show that in Norway transitional demographic processes leading from the medieval demographic system to the Early Modern demographic system started in the 1640s. Recently, L.T. Palm, the Swedish historical demographer, has argued vigorously to the same effect in the case of Sweden.[8]

Summing up the sprinkling of French data on medieval life expectancy based on studies both of skeletal and documentary materials, J.-N. Biraben states cautiously:

[3] 1983: 33.
[4] Fourastié 1972: 30.
[5] Belletini 1973: 491, 494. My translation from Italian.
[6] Bøhm 1999: 40–6.
[7] Havstad 1875: 46–7; Benedictow 1996b: 201.
[8] Palm 1999a: 64–90; Palm 2000: 49–81, and 129–30 in English.

life expectancy at birth appears to have been of the order of magnitude of 25 years, probably a little more in the case of the privileged (excepting the noblemen because of premature deaths in combat) and a little lower in the case of the peasants and the poor. Likewise, in prosperous periods, it could have reached 26 or 27 years, but in the periods of the great crises, especially in the 9th and 10th centuries and from the middle of the 14th century until the middle of the 15th century, it may not, perhaps, have even reached 22 or 23 years [. . .] one should not forget that this figure is an average, and that although a quarter or one-third of all infants died before their first birthday, there were also old people and even the rare centenarians in the Middle Ages.[9]

There is a small logical dissonance at the beginning of this citation, because the privileged classes constituted such a small proportion of the population and male noblemen (including gentry) had to be excepted, and the social category of people that could have had an average life expectancy at birth of a little more than twenty-five years constituted hardly more than 5 per cent of the population, while the peasants and the poor who had a somewhat lower life expectancy at birth than twenty-five years constituted probably 80–85 per cent of the population. The urban populations must be assumed to have had even higher mortality and shorter life expectancy. The logic of this constellation of facts is that average life expectancy at birth of the medieval French population was lower than twenty-five years, probably around twenty-four years. In this context, one should keep in mind that the first half of the fourteenth century was characterized by serious population pressures, and those were really hard times that inevitably must have caused mortality to inch upwards and life expectancy to sag.

   English medievalists have produced more medieval demographic data based on documentary evidence than scholars in any other country. These data are in complete accordance with the data from other countries. Demographic studies based on pre-plague medieval documentary evidence show consistently much higher mortality rates and correspondingly shorter survival rates and life expectancies among adult men in all cohorts above ages 11, 14 or 19 than studies based on early modern evidence, corresponding to a life expectancy at age 20 of 20–30 years, much shorter than in the Early Modern period. A larger number of studies provide similar mortality and life-expectancy estimates for the period c. 1390–1540, which, perhaps, should be expected since the medieval social system was the general societal framework and the population was more or less stationary or declining slightly. These mortality rates are compatible with Model West life tables for populations with life expectancy at birth of 20–28 years, and especially with life tables for populations with life expectancy at birth of 20–25 years, corresponding to mortality rates of 4–5 per cent.[10] The statistical chance that all these studies should fortuitously have found

[9]   Biraben 1988: 425. My translation from French.
[10] Postan and Titow 1958–9, and Russell 1948, both revised by Ohlin 1966: 70–7, 84–9; Dyer 1980: 229–30; Razi 1980: 43–5; Ecclestone 1999; Hatcher 1986: 19–38; B. Harvey 1993: 114–29; V. Davis 1998: 115–16 (above).
   Ohlin's pioneering discussion of the relevant English studies published by the 1960s, those of Russell 1948 and Postan and Titow 1958–9, is extraordinarily valuable and also constitutes the basis of Miller and Hatcher's statement on medieval life expectancy in England, 1978: viii. Later studies have consistently

material reflecting extreme cases of mortality is illusory. Instead, they identify a medieval demographic system.

In 1993, the American scholars D. Loschky and B.D. Childers published a study of all the available English medieval demographic data, using life-table techniques in innovative and highly competent ways. They concluded that there was a strong fall in mortality in the second half of the fifteenth century that heralded a transition to the demographic system of the Early Modern period, and furthermore, there was a change in the demographic parameters, from patterns of mortality and life expectancy that fitted best to Model West to a clearly distinguishable new pattern in the early modern period that fitted best to life tables of Model North.[11] They point out that the English medieval demographic data systematically show patterns closely related to Model West life tables, levels 1–4, corresponding to a general mortality of 40–55 per thousand and a life expectancy at birth of 20–25 years. Life expectancy at age 20 for the generation born between 1276 and 1300 was 25.19 years, corresponding to Model West life table, male level 2, of life expectancy at birth of twenty years. They also point out that 'mortality studies for years before 1348 (Ohlin, Razi, and Russell) all suggested crude death rates in the range of fifty per thousand' with a correspondingly low average life expectancy at birth.[12] In a concrete and decisive manner, they also show that Wrigley's and Schofield's reconstructions of demographic parameters of the Early Modern period could not be used for inference to the medieval demographic system. Thus, Loschky and Childers confirmed empirically and analytically the rather obvious truisms predicted by historical sociology. In doing so they also exposed the use of Early Modern demographic data as representative of medieval demography or the mixing of such data with medieval demographic data as fallacies of the methodology of history and the social sciences.[13]

The fit with Model West life tables had already been pointed out by Hatcher, who indicates that his data are close to level 3, corresponding to a life expectancy at birth of less than twenty-three years,[14] while Loschky and Childers consider that his data fit level 4 best, corresponding to a mortality rate of forty per thousand and life expectancy at birth of twenty-five years for this cohort of socially 'privileged' men. Since then, two other studies based on other types of sources have produced data for the

---

supported Ohlin's conclusions to the effect that life expectancy at birth was in the range of 20–28 years, and quite likely around 25 years or lower (Razi, Dyer, Ecclestone, Hatcher, B. Harvey). Hatcher points out that his study of the mortality among the monastic community at Christ Church, Canterbury, suggests a life expectancy at birth of 21–23 years, according to model life tables and normal assumptions with respect to infant and young-child mortality. B. Harvey's study of the mortality of the monastic community at Westminster Abbey shows remarkably similar mortality rates. The mortality rates and survival rates of the members of these male monastic communities are consistent and systematically different from comparable Early Modern mortality rates in the same ages, but they are easily compatible with other medieval data. It is highly unlikely, indeed, that this should be fortuitous. I cannot accept that R.M. Smith's discussion of this problem, 1991: 57–60, is fair to the real substance of the works of Ohlin, Postan and Titow or Miller and Hatcher.

[11] Loschky and Childers 1993: 91–5.

[12] Loschky and Childers 1993: 94–5.

[13] See, e.g., Poos 1991: 115–19; Poos 1986: 16–20. Poos commences with medieval tithing data (see below) but with quite heavy infusions of data from the Early Modern period, and makes choices of life tables in accordance with his arbitrary assumptions to the effect that medieval and Early Modern demography were basically identical or similar. This makes, of course, for circular argument. As should be expected, this circular approach produces the predictable outcome.

[14] Hatcher 1986: 32.

pre-plague period that show the same peculiar features with respect to mortality and life expectancy and the same similarity to Model West life tables level 2–3 for the age categories covered by the sources.[15]

Interestingly, Coale and Demeny 'suggest using the "West" family in the usual circumstances of underdeveloped countries where there is no reliable guide to the age pattern of mortality that prevails'.[16] The same appears to hold good also for the Middle Ages. They also point out, as mentioned, that the immediate purpose of the demographers who calculated model life tables was to 'estimate birth rates, death rates, and approximate age distributions in research on populations for which there were only incomplete or inaccurate data'. The study of medieval demography meets with related types of deficient data that trouble modern demographic studies of developing countries and that inspired the construction of model life tables.

Usually, medieval documentary material provides mortality and life-expectancy data starting at ages 12, 15 or 20. This means that the pattern of mortality for these ages and for older cohorts constitutes the basis for selection of life tables. By implication, mortality data for younger ages are usually interpolations taken from life tables, and these interpolations are included in inferences to general mortality based on life tables. Loschky and Childers correctly point out that medieval demographic data consistently exhibit considerably higher mortality rates at age 20 and older ages than early modern data, which also leads to selection of life tables with correspondingly higher mortality rates for cohorts below age 20.

In this connection, it becomes a point of some significance that various demographic studies have uncovered the fact that the relationship between mortality and life expectancy at age 20 and older and mortality and life expectancy for infants and young children comprise a significant range of variation that may potentially affect estimation of mortality or life expectancy significantly because of the high mortality among persons of the youngest ages. In relation to this subject, it is important to keep in mind that life tables are based on the normal correlations, in other words on central values, what should be expected or likely.[17] In the careful phrasing of Coale and Demeny: 'the separate families of model life tables provide estimates that in our judgement are quite reliable when utilized judiciously for populations within the areas upon which each family of model tables is based'.[18] Use of the normal values provides outcomes at levels of validity that can be designated likely or at least plausible; extreme values are inherently rare and will lead to extreme outcomes with correspondingly peripheral or marginal levels of validity and relevance. All premises or assumptions that are based on empirical observation provide valid outcomes, but results based on normal observations or correlations will always have precedence or priority. It is a methodological misconception that a small incidence of correlations that deviate significantly from the main pattern of observations falsifies or destroys the usability and clear precedence of central values based on normal occurrence: it all relates to the concept of level of validity.

In view of the fact that all English medieval studies of mortality among males

---

[15] Ecclestone 1999: 22–4; V. Davis 1998: 115–16.
[16] 1983: 25.
[17] Loschky and Childers 1993: 86.
[18] 1983: 24.

above ages 11, 14 or 19 show consistently much higher mortality rates for all cohorts than studies of the same cohorts of males in Early Modern society, it is hard to understand on what grounds such reflections of grossly unhealthy environments should fail to cause at least correspondingly higher mortality also among the most vulnerable and susceptible persons in society, namely infants and young children. In fact, there are as a rule quite close interconnections, a strong systematic co-variation, between the shape of mortality in cohorts of adolescents and adults on the one hand and among infants and young children on the other hand in the same society, because they are exposed to the same nexus of causal factors created by the workings of the social system. In short, the mortality rates among adolescents and adults will usually or normally give good indications as to the mortality rates among children and infants. This is also the pivotal point made by Coale and Demeny, which, in their opinion, justifies the use of life tables for interpolation when certain precautions are observed.

Clearly, the use of life tables is not unproblematic and deserves further discussion. It should also take into consideration that the medieval mortality rates among all known cohorts of adolescents and adults are so high that even interpolation of considerably lower infant mortality rates than indicated by the life tables selected on the basis of mortality among adolescents and adults, 250 per thousand instead of 325 per thousand, for instance, will still produce much lower life expectancies at birth than typical of Early Modern society, typically around 25 years. Instead, rampant disease, squalid housing, widespread malnutrition and undernourishment, grossly unhygienic environments both indoors and outdoors, and unsanitary sources of drinking water contaminated by seepage from latrines, manure and animal droppings, and so forth, could be expected to lead to relatively higher mortality levels among infants and young children than indicated by the mortality of adolescents and adults who had survived the brutal immunological selection processes that were in operation.[19] Thus, use of life tables should be expected rather to lead to underestimation of the mortality among infants and young children in medieval society than to exaggeration. Recurrent grave epidemics of exanthematic typhus, which causes slight case fatality rates among children and adolescents and disastrous case fatality rates among adults, have the potential for skewing the age-pattern of mortality in a society, but, of course, at the time of the Black Death this disease had not yet arrived in Europe. Occasionally, use of life tables for interpolation is rejected, however, without addressing these questions.[20]

In the opinion of this author, it is, therefore, justified to accept the values of infant mortality found in life tables of the order of magnitude of 300–350 per thousand associated with model life tables, Model West, levels 2–4. Actually, all over continental Europe, from Southern Europe to the Nordic countries, infant mortality rates of around 250 per thousand were prevalent or usual much later, around 1750, when, as we have seen, life expectancy had improved considerably and was in the process of continuing improvement. Biraben is on safe ground when he asserts that 'a quarter or one-third of all infants died before their first birthday' (see above). His view is in full

---

[19] Cf. Benedictow 1996b: 77–88; Benedictow 1996c: 165–74.
[20] Ecclestone 1999: 21–2.

accordance with Ohlin's, who considers that the medieval demographic data available at the time (1966) indicated a minimum infant mortality rate of 250 per thousand and concludes that average life expectancy at birth was 'in the neighbourhood of 25 years', that it is 'likely to have fallen within the range of perhaps 22–28 years, and it might well have been lower'.[21] In a cautious way, then, Ohlin suggests that infant mortality quite likely could have been higher than 250 per thousand and average life expectancy at birth could quite likely have been identical with the conclusion drawn by Loschky and Childers a generation later.

Studies of skeletal populations in Nordic medieval cemeteries have uncovered similar life expectancies that lie in the range of 20–25 years, the average quite likely being in the middle of that range.[22] If infant mortality rates at the level that obtained in the Nordic countries and continental Europe at the middle of the eighteenth century are applied, life expectancy at birth in this case also hovers around 25 years.[23] However, in four Nordic medieval cemeteries, the soil has permitted the preservation of such high proportions of the skeletal remains of infants and young children that they constitute evidence of both a specific medieval age-structure and corroborate the assumptions of life tables with respect to these cohorts.[24]

The fact that mortality in Western and Northern Europe was substantially higher in the Middle Ages than in post-transitional Early Modern societies implies that fertility must have been sufficiently higher to compensate for the higher losses. All known societies have normative systems securing a level of fertility that prevents their populations from dying out, in other words, that secure the survival of their populations and their continuation as societies. This general observation arises from the inherent behavioural patterns of the individual persons who constitute populations and form societies, aimed (in accordance with evolutionary theory) at making it likely that they will, under the general social circumstances moulding their lives, succeed in passing on their genetic material and securing the continuity of their basic social network of descent group and local society. The medieval demographic system would have to reflect these endeavours. Higher mortality and higher fertility, in other words higher rates of inflows and outflows of members of populations and societies (turnover rates), were structural features that distinguished the medieval demographic system from the demographic system of the subsequent historical period. In short, the medieval mortality data predict significantly lower age at marriage, especially for women who have a relatively short fertile period, and fewer that remained unmarried (celibates) in the Middle Ages than in the Early Modern period.

Corroborative empirical evidence has been adduced, coming from various European countries ranging from Italy in the south to England in the west and Iceland and Sweden in the north.[25] This evidence shows that medieval women usually married at

---

[21] Ohlin 1966: 76–7.
[22] Benedictow 1996b: 36–41; Benedictow 1996c: 156–65.
[23] Benedictow 1996b: 230–7; Benedictow 1996c: 159.
[24] Benedictow 1996b: 29–36. Cf. Palm 2000: 77–8.
[25] Herlihy and Klapisch-Zuber 1978: 207, cf. 399; Dubois 1988b: 348, 351; Hollingsworth 1969: 383–5; Razi 1980: 63, 135–7; Hanawalt 1986: 96; Bennett 1987: 72; Thrupp 1962: 171; Palm 1999a: 55–90; Palm 1999b: 78–84; Palm 2000: 49–81; Myrdal 1994: 5–7; Sigurðsson 1995: 321; Lindal 1976: 495, Jochens 1985: 100. Sadly, in a recent paper I. Øye maintains that Jochens in her book *Women in Old Norse Society* of 1995 states that 'information in the sagas indicate that both men and women got married in their twenties'. Øye

ages 14–20, which contrasts with the high average age at marriage of around twenty-five years characteristic of Early Modern society. This evidence, which is based on documentary material, is supported by studies of skeletal populations in Hungary, Normandy and medieval Denmark (present-day south-western Sweden) showing a sudden increase in female mortality at ages 15–20, which must be assumed to reflect the onset of reproduction-related maternal mortality.[26]

Lower age at marriage for women and higher fertility mean more pregnancies with reduced immunity to contagious disease and other health hazards, more parturitions with their own hazards and more frequent post-parturition exposure to infections. Thus, lower age at marriage and higher reproduction rates for women imply higher mortality for women relative to men. This interesting subject of reproduction-related supermortality cannot be further discussed and specified here.[27] However, it indicates that women presumably did not live longer lives than men in pre-modern Europe, but rather somewhat shorter lives. In Italy, official population statistics for the period 1899–1902 still show female supermortality in relation to men in all ages from age 1 to age 49.[28] This inference is corroborated by studies on skeletal materials obtained from cemeteries containing pre-modern populations.[29] In our context, this means that the life tables for men and women for practical purposes in most cases are largely interchangeable at the levels of mortality and life expectancy indicated above.

This brief presentation of the main features of the medieval demographic system is the backcloth against which the discussion of the mortality caused by the Black Death must be seen.

1999: 29. However, Jochens' book contains nothing to this effect, but, instead, three incidental references to female age at marriage at ages 13–14/15. Jochens 1995: 47, 52–3. Jochens has published her opinion on the matter in an earlier work, stating that age 18 was the usual age at marriage for women in the Icelandic family sagas. Jochens 1985: 100. The opinions of male Icelandic scholars on the matter that I have referred to here and in several other works are tacitly ignored.

The term 'family sagas' is unfortunate, because the word translated as 'family' has the meaning of descent or kin group, and is much closer in meaning to clan than to family. Frank 1973: 475, asserts, in complete accordance with the previous discussion, that 'the lack of spinsters in these sagas [the Icelandic family sagas] has to do with the importance which thirteenth-century Iceland attached to marriage, family connections, and procreation, an emphasis that made any female figure of interest to the saga-authors either married or about-to-be'.

[26] See discussion and references in Benedictow 1996b: 52, 55–6.
[27] See Benedictow 1996b: 62–8.
[28] Delille 1974: 434–8
[29] Benedictow 1996b: 56–75.

27

Problems of Source Criticism, Methodology and Demography

The best source material and the best estimates of mortality in the Black Death relate to Spain, Italy, France and England. North Africa, the Near East, the Middle East and Central and Northern Europe have little or nothing to offer in the form of demographically valid estimates of mortality. Dols has made a heroic but, unfortunately, unsuccessful attempt at producing an estimate of the mortality in Egypt and Syria.[1] In the case of these countries and regions, we are dependent on the chroniclers, who regularly claim high, but also highly varying mortality rates. This provides a sort of flimsy and impressionistic notion of high or dramatic mortality. It is also clear that the recurrence of plague epidemics reduced the populations throughout these regions still further, according to a pattern that in an impressionistic manner suggests considerable similarity to the demographic developments in Europe.

Only data based on registrations of populations living in the same area before and after the Black Death can come into consideration for mortality estimates. The concept of population is here used in the demographic meaning of any category of people living within a defined area. It can refer to total or general populations, for instance, national populations, regional populations, diocesan or parochial populations, urban populations or rural populations. It can also refer to special social segments of people living within a defined area, nobility, gentry, upper classes, peasants, children, women, bishops, parish priests, town councillors, burghers, artisans or subgroups under that concept such as bakers or smiths, and so on. (It may even refer to animals, in our case rat populations or flea populations.) Differential mortality according to age, gender or social class can reveal information on the Black Death's epidemiology and on the social structures that conditioned the social behaviour of various social groups or segments. Dramatic mortality in the upper classes may affect the mentality of the time and its artistic, cultural and religious expressions with particular social impact.

Mortality data showing the mortality rates in ordinary populations are the most useful to historians: it is primarily the total mortality level that affects social and economic structures and people's religious and cultural outlook in ways that can cause

---

[1] Dols 1977.

societal change and the formation of the type of society or social system characteristic of a historical period or subperiod, in this case more specifically the last phase of the Middle Ages. In the eyes of the historian and the demographer, great mortality takes on the impersonal shape of social causation, formative dynamic powers that make history by shaping societies and peoples lives. Within this frame of reference, estimates of national or regional populations are the most valuable and important data both from the perspective of social science and from the national and ethnic perspectives that finance universities, organize academic communities and shape the usual national scope of scholarly studies and readerships.

In most European countries and regions, 85–95 per cent of the total populations lived in the countryside, making their living from primary agricultural activities. Italy, France and the Low Countries were the countries with the highest degrees of urbanization; they contained regions where a quarter or one-third of the populations lived in towns and cities, making their livelihoods mostly from non-agrarian activities. Nonetheless, clearly, estimates of the mortality among the peasantry are generally far more important and useful than studies of any other social category. Studies comprising peasant populations are a necessary requirement for generalization to national or regional mortality rates in the Black Death.

In order to obtain first-class mortality data, we should be able to follow the same households and their individual constituent members through the epidemic period, but such advanced statistical material was rarely produced in the Middle Ages. No general censuses of national or regional populations were taken shortly before and after the Black Death anywhere in the vast area that was conquered by the epidemic.

However, in a number of European countries or regions quite numerous, comprehensive registrations of the populations for the purpose of collecting taxes, rents or fines were produced at the time. Because fiscal and manorial records were produced without any intention of usefulness as demographic sources, they are characterized by a number of deficiencies in this respect. Taxes and rents were almost always payable by household, which was entered in the registers as hearth (feu, fuego, fuocho) according to the name of the head of the household, i.e., the householder; the registers rarely, therefore, contain information on the composition and size of the households. In addition, they often leave out some groups or categories of people, those who at the time were considered too poor or destitute to pay, and the clergy and the noble classes (= nobility plus gentry), which normally enjoyed tax exemption. Fortunately, a number of registrations of populations are extant that aim at producing a complete registration, also recording all poor and destitute households and, thus, provide essential information. There are only a few cases of censuses or registrations that also record the individual members of the households and, thus, provide vital information on the social composition and size of the households. Nonetheless, the fact remains that populations can rarely be broken down into their constituent social categories according to age, gender and social and economic status that alone permit first-rate estimates of population mortality. Thus, the study of medieval mortality rates must for a number of reasons normally be considered in the light of significant or substantial margins of uncertainty.

Generally, the individual members of populations had strong motives for evading censuses or tax lists because such registrations were normally produced for the obvious purposes of taxation or military recruitment. Tax evasion is a notorious problem that consistently dogs the reliability and usability of tax records as demographic sources.[2] Even in the advanced well-administered countries of Western Europe of today it is generally agreed that tax evasion is a significant problem. However, when making this comparison one must also take into account the vastly greater complexity of modern western society. It is in the nature of this problem that it is hard to get at and even harder to quantify.

As mentioned, in some cases it is the intention of the authorities to register also the poor and destitute households in tax-related records in order to gain a complete picture of the social and economic scene and the potential tax base. Nonetheless, social classes that are too poor to bear any tax assessment such as sharecroppers, sub-tenants, cottagers, day labourers, migrant seasonal workers or industrial proletarians will tend to be passed over by tax registrars. This is so because it serves no useful fiscal purpose to put effort into recording them; and because they constitute such fleeting classes living on casual labour, seasonal work or short-term work contracts they would tend to slip through the administrative net that is cast over them. Fortunately, there are a few exceptions: on the manors of Glastonbury Abbey the resident males of age 12 and over of the landless classes were recorded each year because they were liable to pay an annual head tax to the lord of the manor, and these records survive for the years around the Black Death. On some manors of the bishopric of Winchester, the landless classes were liable to pay death duties in the form of small money payments called *heriots* in order to obtain the right to transfer the disposal of cottages and tiny plots of land to inheritors. These heriot registers appear to be complete from 1270 up to and through the time of the Black Death.[3] In three parishes near Chambéry in the County of Savoy in south-eastern France, the mortality in the Black Death has been studied on the basis of records registering small money payments by the households for permission to collect firewood.[4] These lists appear to record also the landless classes who also needed firewood for cooking and heating. New lists of these rural householders were produced each year, and they thus reflect directly the impact of the Black Death. These types of sources do not, of course, provide full registration of the poor and destitute social classes – paupers, the disabled, and other social categories of persons would for various reasons be exempted or passed over – but there can be no doubt that they provide valuable demographic and social insights on the poor classes, not least in relation to their mortality in the Black Death.

Tax lists and censuses as sources for historical and demographic studies must be subjected to source-criticism according to Benjamin's principle: the stronger the general popular hostility towards a government taking a census, or the stronger the popular hostility towards the purpose(s) of a census, and the more people know why they are to be counted, the worse the result will be.[5] The tax lists of the English poll tax of 1377 were intended to record all inhabitants of age 15 or older and are considered to be of a high standard for their time. J. Cox Russell assumed that it was sufficient to add 5 per cent in order to compensate for tax evasion and underenumeration

---

[2] Cf., e.g., Carrasco Perez 1973: 146.
[3] Ecclestone 1999; Postan and Titow 1958–9: 408; Ohlin 1966: 84–9.
[4] Brondy 1988: 88.
[5] Benjamin 1955: 288–93.

of the genuine destitutes.[6] Professor Michael Postan rejected this out of hand, pointing out that economists assume that tax evasion in modern societies amounts to 5 per cent, and asserting that the deficit in the poll tax registers quite likely could have been 25 per cent.[7] In its turn, this estimate has been criticized as being too high, while it is agreed that 5 per cent is too low: J.Z. Titow calls it 'quite unacceptable', and John Hatcher describes an allowance of 'five per cent for evasion and fraud, for destitutes who were legally exempt from taxation, and for the inevitable inefficiencies in the collection' as 'derisory'.[8] Thomas Hollingsworth considers the assumption of a deficit of 5 per cent 'sanguine', and argues instead that the adult population could quite likely have been underenumerated by 15 per cent.[9] However, also this estimate is quite likely too high.[10]

There were also registrations of populations that must be assumed to be quite complete censuses, especially registrations implemented by governments of Tuscan communes aimed at ascertaining the need for provision of grain and flour to the population in times of dearth. In such cases, the whole population would have a strong interest in being recorded, especially the poor and destitute who were normally neglected or ignored by authorities and registrars alike. The registrations contained in ordinary tax lists cannot be directly compared to such sources for the purpose of estimating mortality without compensatory additions aimed at establishing comparability.

Another problem arises from the fact that the proportion of the poor and destitute that were unable to pay taxes or rents was dramatically reduced in the wake of the Black Death. In the small city of Albi in southern France, the recorded proportion of the population that was too poor to pay taxes diminished from 42 per cent in 1343 to 28 per cent in 1357; much the same appears to have been the case for the small city of Millau in the same region.[11] Correspondingly, in the fertile Ribera area of the merindad of Estella in north-eastern Spain (Kingdom of Navarre), the proportion of poor and destitute households fell from at least 38 per cent in 1330, more probably of the order of magnitude of 40–50 per cent, to 23 per cent in 1350.[12] Similar findings relate to the pre-plague and post-plague social composition of English manors (see below).

This strong diminution of the proportion of the poor and destitute poses problems for the use of tax records in producing estimates of mortality in the Black Death, because it reduces the comparability of pre-plague and post-plague tax records. In order to resolve this problem in a satisfactory fashion that will permit re-establishment of useful comparability, the main social mechanisms and the extent of social mobility in this context must be reasonably well determined.

When tenant households were swept away in great numbers, or were ravaged so severely by the Black Death that they lost their ability to run a good tenement, numerous tenements were left vacant and reverted into the hands of the landlords. In

---

[6] Russell 1948: 145.
[7] Postan 1966: 561–2; Postan 1972: 29.
[8] Titow 1969: 68; Hatcher 1977: 14.
[9] Hollingsworth 1968: 122–3.
[10] Cf. Poos 1991: 104–5.
[11] Prat 1952: 18; Wolff 1957: 501–2.
[12] Carrasco Perez 1973: 146–8; Berthe 1984: 157; and Ch. 28 below, on Spain.

this situation, many of the surviving rural proletarians were quickly recruited into the vacant tenements because it was in the interest of the lords of the manors to maintain the incomes from their land.

Local migration would also tend to be triggered immediately, during the epidemic and in the immediate aftermath as survivors scrambled to acquire the best vacant tenements that were up for grabs. Both territorial and social mobility are triggered by severe epidemic crises and occasion quite rapid changes in the size and social composition of the post-crisis population that will distort and veil the real epidemic impact as reflected in fiscal sources.

The realism and significance of these comments with respect to these economic and social processes can be illustrated from many sources, but comments by an Icelandic chronicler will do:

> Great pestilence and plague over the whole of Iceland, except in the Vestfjords [. . .] wide areas were desolated [. . .] Then, poor, common people came from the Vestfjords, married men with wives and children, because they knew that there were deserted holdings in the north of the country. They could choose the land on which they would settle, and many northerners are descended from them.[13]

Thus, the landless classes were depleted twice, first by plague mortality, next by social mobility into the peasant classes in the aftermath of the epidemic onslaught. Consequently, their proportional decline will be much stronger than that of other social categories. Registrations of peasant households and tenements in operation in the wake of the Black Death will not reflect the full extent of the mortality, because the real impact of the Black Death has been veiled by a great burst of upwards social mobility by the landless classes whose numerical depletion would usually remain unknown, and often also unrecognized as a demographic problem by many scholars.

Moreover, when a grave mortality crisis swept away a large part of the population, survivors of no or modest means frequently inherited significant or substantial values in the form of land, goods or valuables that elevated them into the taxpaying and/or rentpaying social categories. Also for this reason, the number of households registered in tax records will often not reflect the real impact of a plague epidemic. Again, a terse comment by an Icelandic chronicler can illustrate the point:

> [. . .] Much property then came in the hands of many, almost everybody received inheritance from relatives, third cousins or closer relatives [. . .][14]

Thus, the poor and destitute classes will be proportionally far more reduced than the upper classes, partly by (super)mortality, partly by social mobility, and to some degree through inheritance. All these factors present difficulties and uncertainties in the scholarly endeavours to identify or reconstruct the size and composition of a

---

[13] See next note. My translation from Old Norse.
[14] Excerpts of these chroniclers' accounts of the second plague epidemic in Iceland are rendered in English translation in Benedictow 1993/1996a: 212–13. My translation from Old Norse. Plague reached Iceland only twice, at the very beginning and end of the fifteenth century.

population on the morrow of the Black Death. All these factors tend to lead to under-estimation of the mortality in the Black Death.

The strong decrease in the proportion of the poor and destitute in the post-Black Death populations also has another effect that must be taken into account when tax records are used for estimates of mortality in the Black Death. It means that there were proportionally far fewer poor people that the registrars would tend to pass over in post-plague society than in pre-plague society. Tax lists produced after the Black Death should be expected to be appreciably less flawed by underregistration than before, because the social-class reasons that induced such flaws had been substantially reduced. For this reason, using the same supplementary addition to fiscal registra-tions of populations before and after the Black Death in order to compensate for underregistration will tend to veil some of the impact of the plague epidemic and to affect mortality estimates in the direction of underestimation. This point will cautiously be taken into account in population estimates by assuming as a standard assumption a deficit in registrations of pre-plague populations of households of 7.5 per cent and in the post-plague registers of 6 per cent.

The fact that the basis of most estimates of mortality caused by the Black Death is sources recording taxpaying or rentpaying householders requires further method-ological and source-critical discussion. In this context, problems arise from the fact that this social segment is unrepresentative in three important respects: (1) because they have at their disposal economic resources that in various ways are assets also in the face of epidemic disease; (2) because they are adults; (3) because they are male adults. The first of these three points implies that the taxpaying and rentpaying householders as a section of the population, albeit a large section, will have lower mortality than the poor householders of the population and, for this reason, will exhibit lower mortality rates than obtained among the general population of which they were part. Some concrete notions are needed as to the proportion of the pre-plague populations that was too poor and destitute to bear tax assessment, and with respect to the supermortality among these social classes, in order to reconstruct general populations and approach the question of general population mortality. For this purpose, the supermortality of the poor must be identified and proportionally distributed.

In the case of plague, there are two central reasons for supermortality among the poor and destitute social classes. Firstly, poor people lived in far more unhygienic environments both indoors and outdoors than the better-off social classes, which increased their exposure to rat fleas; secondly, in pre-plague society, many poor and destitute people may have had their physiological resistance to disease (immunity) significantly impaired or weakened by long-term undernutrition or malnutrition.

The most important reason for supermortality among the poor and destitute in the case of plague is probably much greater susceptibility to secondary catastrophe effects. Many viral diseases produce good and lasting immunity in survivors, such diseases taking on the character of children's diseases because adolescents, parents and other adults had acquired immunity after having survived them in childhood. This means that economic activities, nursing care of diseased and care for children will function quite normally in times of serious outbreaks of viral epidemic disease. This is not the case with bacterial diseases like plague that generally confer only weak and transient immunity in survivors. There are even registered quite a number of persons who contracted plague twice in the same epidemic.[15] The Black Death was the first plague epidemic in Europe for many hundred years: consequently the question of immunity is without interest.

Thus, in relation to the Black Death the whole population and all members of its constituent social entities, namely households, were equally susceptible. In this situation, two important factors would tend to produce substantial and even strong supermortality, especially among common people. Firstly, nursing care tended to break down, because adults and children contracted the disease at much the same time, namely when blocked rat fleas in great numbers left house rats at the time of their death at the end of the rat epizootic and could not find alternative rat hosts. The breakdown or weakening of the social functions of a large proportion of families meant that many persons died from 'neglect' who would have survived the disease if they had received proper nursing care. This phenomenon is observed by contemporary chroniclers, for instance by the Florentine Marchionne di Coppo Stefani who refers to the fact that 'many died by themselves and many died of hunger'.[16]

Many children, especially in the age brackets up to about 10–12 years, would succumb for lack of nourishment and normal care, even if they were not infected. In his study of a plague epidemic in the provincial English town of Colyton in 1645–6, R. Schofield succeeds in showing that if the father survived and the mother died, nine out of ten children died; if the mother survived and the father died, nine out of thirteen children died; if both parents survived, eleven out of forty-seven children died, corresponding to mortality rates of 90, 70 and 23 per cent, respectively.[17] B. Bennassar found high supermortality of children in the great plague epidemics in northern Spain in the 1590s.[18] Supermortality among children in the plague epidemics of the late fourteenth and early fifteenth centuries in Tuscany is analysed by Herlihy and Klapisch-Zuber.[19] R. Cazelles has adduced valuable evidence to the effect that there was a substantial supermortality of children in the Black Death in north-western France, although not on the basis of sources that allow quantification.[20]

Secondly, when all adults were susceptible and contracted the disease in great numbers within a short period of time, economic activities broke down both in town and countryside. With this breakdown vanished the trickle of income from elementary production of goods, casual manual work and services upon which most of the poor and destitute households were dependent for their livelihood with small margins to undernutrition and hunger.[21] This means that plague was often followed by widespread undernutrition, hunger or starvation both in the countryside and in the urban centres. In the case of the Black Death, it is reported from the city state of Siena, for instance, that 'fields were neglected and animals left untended, as men were scarcely able to care for their own ill',[22] a statement that also hints at the breakdown of the familial functions of nursing care.

---

[15] See an exhaustive review of the medical and historical studies on this question in Benedictow 1993/1996a: 126–45.
[16] Cited after Henderson 1992: 145.
[17] Schofield 1977: 118–19. See also, for instance, Hirst 1938: 690.
[18] Bennassar 1969: 18, 50.
[19] 1978: 370–80.
[20] Cazelles 1962: 303–5.
[21] See, for instance, Baratier 1961: 33.
[22] Bowsky 1964: 23.

The secondary catastrophe effects of epidemic onslaughts are a normal feature of plague epidemics that systematically increases the death toll substantially above the mortality caused by the infective microbiological agent alone. Also the middling classes of rural and urban society suffered substantial supermortality for these reasons. However, for obvious reasons the mortality effects increased with increasing poverty, because the poor were highly vulnerable to the detrimental effects of loss of income and because their households were smaller and did not contain living-in servants or maids, which would increase the likelihood that at least some adolescent or adult person was able to perform the exceedingly important functions of nursing care. The supermortality of the poor and destitute in plague epidemics is often mentioned by chroniclers and other contemporary commentators.[23] The Scottish chronicler John of Fordun, for instance, stated in his chronicle that the Black Death in Scotland 'everywhere attacked the meaner sort and common people [. . .] seldom the magnates'.[24]

In the plague epidemics that raged in India and China at the end of the nineteenth century and in the first decades of the twentieth century, it was noted that Europeans had much lower case fatality rates than natives, namely 40–50 per as compared with about 80 per cent. Because no medication was available, the only explanation was much better nursing care in combination with better levels of nutrition and hygiene.[25] This reduced level of mortality in cases of untreated bubonic plague that are well-nourished and enjoy the benefits of a good level of nursing care has been confirmed by recent American experience.[26] The potential extent of social inequality in the face of plague is, therefore, very large, and was much in evidence also in connection with the Black Death and later plague epidemics. This perspective is, for instance, much in focus in the discussion below of the relative levels of mortality in the Black Death of the English beneficed parish clergy and among the English population in general.

Studies of plague epidemics show that social elites and upper classes living in stone buildings, and to some extent also in half-timbered houses, which are less suited to the lifestyle of rats, also for this reason have substantially lower mortality rates than the lower classes.[27]

Thus, the upper classes in any society should be expected to have significantly lower mortality rates in any epidemic disease, and markedly so in plague epidemics, than the lower classes, because they were better housed, fed, clad and nursed, and because they were much less exposed to economic secondary catastrophe effects.

Although scholars have found interesting impressionistic material on the characteristic supermortality of the poor in the Black Death, lack of precision precludes any demographic usefulness in most cases. Fortunately, it has been possible to quantify this supermortality in some cases and, thus, to acquire a more concrete and operational notion. Three rural parishes near the town of Chambéry in the County of

---

[23] See, e.g., Cipolla 1973: 107–8; Cipolla 1974: 280–3; Cipolla and Zanetti 1972: 198–202; Cazelles 1962: 300–1; Biraben 1974: 505–8.

[24] Dodgshon 1981: 13.

[25] Simpson 1905: 173; Hirst 1938: 690; Hirst 1953: 145; Pollitzer 1954: 418, 509; Benedictow 1993/1996a: 146–56.

[26] Reed, Palmer, Williams et al. 1970: 483.

[27] See Benedictow 1993/1996a: 136–7.

Savoy are covered by registers that record money payments by the households for permission to collect firewood and, therefore, also include the poor and destitute classes. These registrations were made each year and are extant for both 1348 and 1349 (see below). The mortality rate in the Black Death estimated on the basis of these registers was about 2.5 per cent higher than in other localities in the Savoy that are covered by fiscal registers recording the taxpaying or rentpaying better-off social classes, for instance in the castellany of Ugine, the parish of Sallanches or in eight parishes in the nearby castellany of Montmélian (see Table 24, below).

The registration of the lower classes for the right to collect firewood was undoubt-edly not entirely complete, for some destitute households would have had difficulties in paying, sub-tenants could probably avail themselves of the permission purchased by the peasant householder, and so on. For this reason, it seems reasonable to assume that the registration of the poor and destitute social classes was less complete than of the better-off social classes and that the real supermortality rate was slightly higher than indicated by this material, around 3 per cent.

Seventeen manors of Glastonbury Abbey in the south-western county of Somerset in England contain records of an annual head tax payable by a specific category of males called 'garciones', comprising all males attached to the manor, aged 12 and older, who did not hold property and did not pay rent, and, thus, constituted the landless classes of cottars, day labourers, sub-tenants, and so on. The mortality among this landless class of males appears to have been about 5 percentage points higher than among the customary tenantry, which held land in amounts sufficient for subsis-tence farming (see below).

The significance of these findings for mortality estimates can only be determined on the basis of knowledge on the proportion of the poor and destitute classes in the population as a whole. In 1343, the city council of the small city of Albi in southern France decided to acquire a fresh oversight over the tax potential of the population. New tax records were produced that should comprise the whole population according to householders and that were based on careful evaluations of all the households' assets and income. The poor and destitute households that could bear no tax assess-ment were recorded in the form of names of householders without valuations of assets or tax contribution. In 1343, this was the case with 42 per cent of the house-holders; much the same appears to have been the case for the small city of Millau in the same region.[28] In both cases, there was undoubtedly some underregistration of the poor and destitute, because registration served no fiscal purpose, which invited insouciance by the registrars, and because the poor and destitute classes tend to be quite fleeting, with high turnover rates in their localities.

The tax records of the so-called 'monedaje' levied by the Kingdom of Navarre in north-eastern Spain in 1330 are extant for the fertile Ribera area of the merindad of Estella, and show a proportion of poor and destitute households of at least 38 per cent, more probably of the order of magnitude of 40–50 per cent. Similar or some-what higher proportions of poor and destitute households appear to have been usual in the merindad of Sangüesa.[29] Professor Michael Postan, who studied the social

[28] Prat 1952: 18; Wolff 1957: 501–2.
[29] Carrasco Perez 1973: 146–8; Berthe 1984: 145–7, 157; Ch. 28 below, on Spain.

composition of 104 English manors in the thirteenth century, concluded that 'tenants with ten acres or less formed more than one-half of the population on all estates except those of St Peter's, Gloucester, where manorial sources conceal from our view large numbers of tenants' sub-tenants'.[30] Another study has shown that the landless classes were as numerous as the customary tenants.[31] Much the same picture emerges from in-depth parish studies on settlement and economy in pre-plague Norway.[32]

As can readily be seen from these instances, the proportion of the poor and destitute that did not pay taxes or rents in pre-plague society appears usually to have been of the order of magnitude of 45–55 per cent. Other data referred to below consistently support these findings, which may then appear to represent a fairly consistent feature of medieval society at the time. Seen in the perspective afforded by the data of the County of Savoy and the 'garciones' on the manors of Glastonbury Abbey, this distribution of the social classes in medieval society indicates that the mortality among the poor and destitute was 5–6 percentage points higher than the mortality among the better-off social classes. This difference constitutes the supermortality of the poor. The evidential underpinning of this estimate is obviously weak, and generalization on such a weak basis is open to criticism and caution is, of course, recommended. However, this represents the available knowledge on the matter today and seems *a priori* to be a rather moderate estimate that will tend to keep estimates of total or general population mortality on the low side.

When the estimates of the mortality among the taxpaying or rentpaying householders who represent the usual basic data are linked with the findings on the supermortality of the poor and destitute classes and the relative proportions of these social categories in the population, it appears that an addition to the mortality rate estimated for the taxpaying or rentpaying households of 2.5 per cent will provide a useful cautious estimate of the total mortality among all householders in a population.

The overriding objective of this book is to reach good estimates on general population mortality. In order to convert the pre-plague and post-plague numbers of householders within specified localities into pre-plague and post-plague population estimates that will reveal general population mortality, concrete notions of the average size of the households on the eve and on the morrow of the Black Death are required. Again we must start with source criticism. As mentioned, the sources used for the study of mortality in the Black Death consist mainly of registers of taxpaying or rentpaying householders who overwhelmingly were male adults. This activates again the significance of the supermortality among children and women that was discussed above in connection with secondary catastrophe effects. Obviously, supermortality among women and children affected the size and composition of the households in ways that make estimates of plague mortality among male householders correspondingly unrepresentative of the mortality among the population contained in their households. Three central causal factors have been identified in the discussion of these aspects of secondary catastrophe effects. Children and women were liable to contract the disease more often than men because they stayed more indoors and closer to the blocked rat fleas that transmitted the contagion, and thus had a higher risk of exposure. Women's central and varied activities

---

[30] Postan 1966: 622.
[31] Ecclestone 1999: 14.
[32] See, e.g., Benedictow 1996b: 166–7.

in relation to preservation, storage and cooking of food increased further their exposure to rats and their fleas relative to that of men. Children were also far more vulnerable than adults to the detrimental effects of the breakdown of nursing care.

In addition, there are physiological factors. First, pregnant women who contract plague invariably give birth and die. This is not only a modern medical observation, but was also noted repeatedly in the past.[33] In the plague epidemic of 1630 in Pisa, about a thousand pregnant women were admitted to the plague hospital, all of them had confinements, none of them survived, and only three of the infants they gave birth to, survived.[34] Women were often pregnant in those pre-contraceptive times when matrimonial life was associated with natural fertility. Breast-feeding peasant women seems to have had, on average, birth intervals of c. 29 months, and were, thus, pregnant over 30 per cent of the time.[35]

The characteristic supermortality of women in plague epidemics surfaces in most research on suitable sources. Accurate differentiation of mortality between genders requires good sources, and the best studies on this subject tend, therefore, to relate to the last waves of plague epidemics in Europe. In this book, the point can only be made with a few illustrative examples. Because knowledge on rural populations is particularly important, gender-specific rural data are preferred. In 14 parishes in the diocese of Sant' Agata de Goti in the region of Salerno south of Naples in Italy, women had a supermortality of 15 per cent in the great plague epidemic of 1656.[36] In two rural parishes outside Copenhagen (Amager) with a normal annual mortality of 85 persons in the first decade of the eighteenth century, 1,207 persons perished in the plague epidemic of 1711; 1,175 of these 1,207 persons can be identified, and 638 of them or 54.3 per cent were females.[37] In the great plague epidemics in India that broke out in 1896 and lasted for several decades, supermortality of women was a consistent feature in the countryside where 'the incidence of females was considerably higher than of males'. The main reason for female supermortality in plague could be studied in almost pure form in Kurdistan in the 1960s. Almost all plague deaths were women or children who stayed at home, because, in the plague season, the menfolk were with the large cattle herds and slept in the fields.[38]

Secondly, modern medical research has shown that plague tends to have a particularly fulminant course in children and adolescents who, consequently, will have higher case fatality rates and, thus, fewer survivors from the disease than adults – in short, supermortality.[39] Much historical and modern medical research shows that the supermortality of children and youngsters is a characteristic feature of plague epidemics.[40] Chalin de Vinario who, like Guy de Chauliac, was a personal physician to

---

[33] Pollitzer 1954: 418; L.-T. Wu 1926: 263–4; Hirst 1938: 690; Biraben 1975: 2/29; Benedictow 2002: 207–8. Cf. Dols 1977: 186.

[34] Feroci 1892: 137.

[35] Benedictow 1985a: 32–8; Benedictow 1988: 200–5.

[36] Delille 1974: 428–31.

[37] Mansa 1840: 415.

[38] Indian Plague Research Commission. Reports on Plague Investigations in India. XXV. 1907: 921, 959–73; Baltazard, Bahmanyar, Mostachfi et al. 1960: 152.

[39] Burkle 1973: 296; Butler 1972: 274.

[40] Hirst 1938: 690; Reed, Palmer, Williams et al. 1970: 470, 472–7; Riley 1982: 753. This feature of plague epidemics has been uncovered in many historical studies: see, e.g., Cazelles 1962: 293–305; Herlihy and Klapisch-Zuber 1978: 195–8; Bradley 1977: 73; Schofield 1977: 109–19; Bucher 1979: 33–5, 37.

the pope, observed during the Black Death in Avignon that sudden death was a common occurrence in children and adolescents.[41] The burial register of Givry, the only extant (almost) complete parish register that records the mortality of a population in the Black Death (see above), shows that the Black Death 'above all struck the children'.[42] Thus, summing up this line of argument, the mortality among householders must be assumed to be significantly smaller than among the population constituted by the households that they fronted.

Any hypothesis on the social structure of the epidemic processes at work will include assumptions to the effect that there must have been a significant incidence of plague fatalities within the households of surviving householders. The households of surviving householders must be assumed to have lost members that had been infected in extraneous contexts and circumstances, contracting the disease at work, at play, when socializing, at gatherings of relatives and inheritors and of neighbours and friends for commemoration of deceased persons, at wakes, funerals, and so on. Empirical support for this assumption is provided by the Danish scholar Michael Gelting. Gelting found material in the governmental archives of the counts of Savoy in Chambéry that enabled him to study the fate of most of the constituent members of the 11 taxpaying peasant households contained in the mountain hamlet of Grenis in Maurienne, and has presented them in the form of 'mini-biographies'. After having deleted a female householder in order to ascertain comparability with other material consisting of male householders, this material consists of a miniature cohort of ten male householders. These biographies show that not a single household escaped unscathed from the Black Death, as can be seen from Table 11

Table 11. Mortality in the taxpaying households of Grenis in the Black Death

1. Johannes de Greniaco and his brothers died, probably without legitimate progeny.
2. Jacobus Coste probably died, perhaps without legitimate progeny; his wife survived.
3. The late Johannes Loymant had two children, Johannes and Johanna; Johanna died in the plague, her brother survived.
4. Aymo de Molario survived, but lost his nephew or grandson ('nepos') Aynardus de Molario.
5. Aymo de Furno died, leaving two daughters, one of whom died later in the plague.
6. Johannes de Furno died, leaving his widow with minor children.
7. (Another) Johannes de Furno died in 1346, leaving three minor daughters. None of the girls seems to be mentioned after the Black Death.
8. Ansermus Castelli had two boys, Michael and Petrus. Petrus and their mother Agnessona died in the plague, Michael survived.
9. Stephanus de Griniaco died, leaving at least three children who survived.
10. Johannes Amedei survived, but lost his wife.

---

[41] Sticker 1908: 58.
[42] Gras 1939: 307.

Another type of data can be taken to support or confirm the impression of a considerable intra-household mortality. In some cases, the number of households in a locality falls sharply only after the next visitation of plague. In the Piedmont in northern Italy, for instance, the village of Sant'Antonino in the vicinity of the town of Susa had 50 (registered) hearths/households in 1335, 40 in 1356 (after having had time to recuperate somewhat from the effects of the Black Death), a number that suddenly fell sharply to only 24 in 1367 after a much smaller second visitation of plague.[43] Similarly, in nine parishes in Normandy (diocese of Lisieux), the number of (registered) hearths declined by 23 per cent in the period 1326–55, and by 36 per cent in the period 1355–65 that included the mortality of the much smaller second plague epidemic of 1362.[44] Such data can be taken to indicate that many households had been so seriously reduced by the Black Death that they collapsed when they lost a member in the next epidemic.

On the other hand, the surviving householders must be assumed to have taken in the odd surviving relative or child from ravaged households for charitable reasons, and this inter-familial movement must be assumed to have been concurrent with the epidemic itself. Statistically, this inter-familial movement will tend to counteract the losses suffered by the households with surviving householders; the average size of households on the morning of the epidemic will be the outcome of both these demographic tendencies.

This discussion has prepared the ground for a more direct analysis and discussion of the available basic data on household size in the decades around the Black Death. These data are in the main Italian, provided by censuses of good quality produced in Tuscany and the Piedmont, and are rendered in Table 16 below. The main problem is that they are few, but the remarkable consistency of the outcomes of studies on these entirely independent sources strengthens their trustworthiness substantially. As they stand, these data indicate an average pre-plague rural household size of 4.3 persons, which was reduced to about 3.8 persons a couple of years after the Black Death, and that the pre-plague size was restored around 15–20 years later. Censuses taken for the purpose of providing local political authorities with good information on the population's need for supplementary grain and flour in the time of dearth must be assumed to be quite complete, because it was the objective to record the poor and destitute, and because the whole population would see their interest being served by being registered. Perhaps, nonetheless, some tiny element of underregistration is unavoidable; in that case these data could be said to indicate that the normal pre-plague household size was 4.5 and 4 persons in the countryside and towns, respectively, and had been reduced to 4 and 3.5 persons, respectively, on the morrow of the Black Death.

These Italian data are conspicuously similar to a sprinkling of other European data on average household size in pre-plague Europe, ranging from H.E. Hallam's study of three censuses of the bondmen of the Benedictine priory at Spalding in the county of Lincolnshire (eastern England)[45] to Norwegian estimates based on three different

---

[43] Rotelli 1973: 87.
[44] Fournée 1978: 21.
[45] Hallam 1957–8: 340–61. Hallam's study shows an average household size of 4.68 persons, but this slightly higher figure is assumed to reflect that in the area where the Benedictine priory of Spalding was situated, namely the Lincolnshire Fenlands, there was relatively brisk population population growth at the time

approaches.[46] Presumably, this conspicuous cross-European similarity of average household size identifies another structure of the medieval demographic system.

Thus the Italian household data indicate that the surviving households, in most cases households with surviving householders, had, on average, been reduced by 0.5 person in the epidemic. This factor covers both the supermortality of women and children, the losses suffered by households of surviving householders, and the taking in of surviving relatives from households ravaged by the Black Death. This implies that the mortality among the population constituted by the households would be 11–12.5 per cent higher than among the recorded householders. The significance of this factor can be usefully illustrated: for instance, in the case of registers of a rural locality containing 4,000 householders on the eve of the Black Death and 2,000 householders on the morrow of the epidemic, the populations contained in the households represented by the householders would amount to 18,000 and 8,000 persons, respectively; thus, while the mortality among householders was 50 per cent, the population mortality was 55.5 per cent.

Even if the intra-household mortality in Grenis for some unknown reason(s) may have been extraordinarily high, the suspicion remains that a standard assumption of an average decrease of the surviving households of 0.5 person is somewhat too small. However, caution must be the guiding principle. Since only the Italian data are based on accurate registrations of quite large populations in the decades around the Black Death, these data should, therefore, prevail and function as standard assumptions on developments in household size related to the demographic effects of the Black Death.

The basic tendency of pre-plague population developments all over Europe was stationarity; in most countries and regions population size had reached the maximum that could be maintained with the prevailing agricultural technology, and hovered at

owing to the opportunities offered by land reclamation. This attracted young adult immigrants and allowed local young adults to get married at an earlier age, which gave them higher fertility than was usual at the time in England or most of Europe. Cf. Miller and Hatcher 1978: 31. Hanawalt 1977: 23–4, and Dewindt 1972: 171, have attempted to estimate average household size in pre-plague England on less suitable types of sources than censuses, with outcomes in the range of 3.5–3.8 persons. The somewhat lower estimates in these cases presumably reflect weaknesses of the sources that let more persons slip away. On source-critical grounds, they can, therefore, be taken to suggest or to support an average household size that is quite similar to the averages indicated by Hallam's study, the Italian data and the Nordic data (see below).

[46] Benedictow 1996b: 155–72; Benedictow 2002: 86–8. Average household size has been estimated in three independent ways. One estimate is based on the fairly numerous demographic data obtained from osteological studies of medieval churchyard populations. Secondly, average household size has been estimated on the basis of the size of production on tenements and holdings of a local society (Eidsvoll) and how many persons this production could nourish. In both cases an average household size of 4.5 persons is indicated The third approach is based on the censuses of all Norwegian males that were taken in the 1660s, which show an average size of the individual settlement population of c. 6 persons distributed on 57,000 settlements. However, in the first half of the seventeenth century, a new social class of 'undersettlers' (sub-tenants) had arisen for special economic and technological reasons, and this social development represented an additional 17,000 households within the areas of tenements and holdings held by other householders. If this new social class is subtracted, an average settlement population of 4.7 persons will emerge. However, in the mid-seventeenth century the Norwegian population was growing at quite a brisk pace, which for this reason would give a somewhat larger average number of persons on each individual settlement than in pre-plague society when the population was fairly stationary. Thus, in this case too, an average of about 4.5 persons, or slightly less, is indicated. This agrees well with similar data from other parts of medieval Europe (see above). It is important to keep in mind that average household size and average size of the individual settlement population are two different concepts, which in the latter case may also comprise living-in households and sub-tenant households.

the Malthusian 'ceiling'. The fact that many of the pre-plague registrations of house-holders were made some years earlier does not present serious difficulties in reaching realistic assessments of the size of these populations on the eve of the Black Death. Most of the registrations of householders used for estimates of the post-plague popu-lation size were not produced on the morrow of the Black Death, but some years later, mainly in the period 1350–7. This means that the information contained in these records must be corrected as much as possible for post-plague demographic and social developments that affected the number of householders and household size. This will make it possible to identify as closely as possible the surviving population on the morrow of the Black Death that alone can be realistically compared with pre-plague registrations for the purpose of estimation of mortality.

Among the important factors that must be taken into account in this connection is the development in the marriage market for young adults. The great population pres-sure that was a general hard fact of life for European populations in the decades preceding the Black Death meant that many young adults had difficulties in finding employment and income that would make marriage possible. In the aftermath of the Black Death, plenty of vacant jobs and tenements were suddenly available. The social functions of this new social scene created by the carnage caused by the Black Death are exhibited with full clarity in the only extant marriage register from the time of the Black Death, that of Givry in Burgundy where the Black Death broke out in mid-July 1348 and raged for four months (see above). In the period 1336–41, an average of 17.5 couples got married in this small town each year. In 1349, 86 marriages were entered in the register, 42 of them already in the first period after the end of the epi-demic when it was permitted by the Church to marry, namely from 14 January to 24 February 1349. In the following two years, there were 33 and 22 new marriages, respectively; it was a more normal annual incidence of new marriages that reflected the sharply reduced population and the much easier economic conditions for marriage that appear to be established in 1355–7.[47] Documentary evidence that exhibits a great increase in new marriages in the wake of the Black Death has also been uncovered for the town of Orange in western Provence (20 km north of the city of Avignon), and in England within a manorial context.[48] This social function of the great mortality is also noted by contemporary chroniclers, for instance by the French chronicler Jean de Venette, who described it as a general European feature:

> After the end of the epidemic [. . .] the men and women who stayed alive did everything to get married.

The same pattern of events in the marriage market has also repeatedly been uncov-ered in studies of later plague epidemics in other countries.[49]

Importantly, the surge in new households in the wake of the Black Death will tend to veil the real impact of the Black Death in estimates using the number of recorded households at some point in the following years. The effects of this surge must be deducted in order to reconstruct a number of surviving households on the morrow of

---

[47] The estimates are based on data provided by Gras 1939: 303.
[48] Gaspari 1970: 217; Razi 1980: 132–5; T. Lomas 1984: 260.
[49] See, for instance, Greslou 1973: 159–60; Bucher 1979: 37–9.

the Black Death that can serve as a base for realistic estimates of the mortality when compared to a pre-plague registration of households. A cautiously realistic standard assumption could be an annual net increase of the number of households owing to the formation of new marriages at a rate of 0.5 per cent in the towns and of 0.75 per cent in the countryside. The surge would be strongest in the immediate aftermath of the Black Death when the pool of marriageable young people who had not succeeded in acquiring the economic basis for getting married under the difficult pre-plague circumstances was tapped, and would taper off gradually into a more normal inci-dence according to the pattern of Givry. This dynamic pattern should be taken into account in the case of tax lists redacted according to households a few years after the Black Death.

Most of the young adults who got married in the immediate wake of the Black Death must be assumed to have lived in parental households. When many young men and women suddenly moved out of their families of origin in order to form new families, the number of households and their social composition and structure changed appreciably. The number of households in the community will, as mentioned, increase relatively rapidly, but the average number of persons consti-tuting households would be concomitantly reduced for a number of years until the loss was replaced by the offspring of the newly wed couples. And this was a diminu-tion that came in addition to the reduction caused by the significant loss of household members in the households that survived the epidemic. Some of this erosion of the households' 'manpower' would be offset by remarriages of bereaved spouses with or without children. All these factors would affect the sociological structures and demo-graphic dynamics of the population and give it a specific post-Black Death transitional form. These considerations underscore the importance of source criticism based on demographic and social insights in the opposite processes of population pressure and population deficit in relation to the social and economic conditions constituting marriage opportunities.

Wills reflect more the fear of death than death itself. A large proportion of those who made wills in the face of an immediate epidemic threat to their lives would be alive at the end of the day. Abrupt changes in the number of wills relate to crisis mortality in an impressionistic and flimsy fashion, and the correlation between changes in the incidence of wills and death rates is not quantifiable.

28

Spain

Some good estimates of mortality in the Black Death come from the Kingdom of Navarre in north-eastern Spain. They are based on two types of registers of royal income organized according to the main administrative divisions of Navarre into four so-called 'merindads' (and, in addition, the so-called 'lands of Ultrapuertos').

One type of register records the special tax called 'monedaje', a name that refers to the fact that it was levied to finance the emission of new coinage when a new king had acceded to the throne. These registers are particularly valuable because, with the usual reservation in respect of underenumeration, they comprise also the poor and destitute classes, both those who paid reduced amounts and those who were too destitute to pay anything at all. 'Monedajes' were levied both in 1330 and 1350, but, unfortunately, the records of the 'monedaje' of 1330 are extant only for the Ribera area of the merindad of Estella. For this reason, comparison of the registers in order to estimate the mortality caused by the Black Death can be carried out only for this area.

The other type of register that can be used for demographic analysis records the annual collection of rents from the royal estates in Navarre, and is basically a cadastral type of material. The royal system of rent collection had two main forms, but only the one called 'pechas capitales', which was collected according to households ('pechas') and registered according to the name of the householders ('capitales') can be considered for possible demographic usefulness. The system of 'pechas capitales' was mostly used in the highlands in the Pyrenean regions, in the merindads of Pamplona (Montañas) and Sangüesa. The use of these cadastral registers in demographic studies is problematic because they register only the households in the villages that held royal land in the form of tenancies, whether large or small, and paid rents accordingly. They leave out the large segments of the rural population that cultivated the lands of other seigneurs; they leave out the exempted class of gentry ('hidalgoes') and the freeholders ('francos') who did not owe rents; and most seriously, unlike the 'monedajes', they leave out the countryside's proletarian classes, those who did not pay rent because they held no or insignificant amounts of land.

According to the 'monedaje' of 1350, the proletarian classes constituted 23 per cent of the population of the Ribera area of the merindad of Estella, and 22 per cent of the populations of the merindad of Sangüesa and the merindad of Pamplona

(Montañas).[1] However, it is a central feature of the post-plague situation all over Europe that poor and destitute households moved into good tenancies vacated by the Black Death in the countryside. As this discussion of mortality moves through Europe, the sources repeatedly provide the opportunity to uncover the importance of this process. This means that the real impact of the epidemic on a peasant population will tend to be substantially underregistered in tax lists or manorial cadasters redacted even a few years after the plague. It also means that the proletarian classes will be relatively more depleted than the upper classes, because their numbers were reduced twice, by death from plague and by upwards social mobility in the wake of the plague.

There cannot be any doubt that the proportion of poor and destitute households was substantially higher also in pre-plague Navarre than in the aftermath of the Black Death. It could be that this is reflected in a peculiar way in the records of the 'monedaje' of 1330 that, as mentioned, are extant only for the Ribera area in the merindad of Estella: the percentage of designated poor households is a minuscule and incredible 2 per cent, while the proportion of households headed by women amounts to an incredible or rather impossible 36 per cent. It is tempting to suspect that poor male householders kept away from their households when the collectors visited in order to ensure the lowest possible tax assessment for their households, and households headed by women were as a rule for good reasons considered very poor. Thus, this 'monedaje' indicates a pre-plague proportion of poor and destitute households of 40 per cent or, if proper account is taken of the likely larger underenumeration of these social classes than of the upper classes, of 40–50 per cent.

It is, as mentioned, only possible to compare the records of the 'monedajes' of 1330 and 1350 for the southern part of the merindad of Estella, the Ribera area, which stretches from the rivers Arga and Aragon to the R. Ebro on the border of Old Castile. The area was densely populated, fertile lowlands. In 1330 it contained 6,538 households, which in 1350 were reduced to 2,408, a diminution of 63 per cent.[2]

This figure cannot be accepted at face value as a true reflection of the effects of the Black Death unless the developments in population size between 1330 and 1350 can be satisfactorily determined. However, fairly broad evidence on developments in population size do not relate to the Ribera area, but to the two Pyrenean merindads. These data are based on the 'pechas capitales' that register payment of rents from peasants holding tenements of the royal estates in the villages, which raises questions of representativeness with respect to general demographic developments. We cannot be certain that the social structure of this category of peasant households was sufficiently similar to the social composition of peasant society as a whole to be really representative.

In addition, the developments are not estimated on the basis of the demographic status in 1330 but according to status in 1333. The reason for this is that long-term population growth reached its preliminary peak in 1333, then, in the next three years, followed a series of bad harvests that caused noticeable supermortality. On the basis of the 'pechas capitales', the number of households in the merindad of Pamplona has

---

[1] Carrasco Perez 1973: 146–8.
[2] Zabalo Zabalegui 1968: 83; Carrasco Perez 1973: 120.

been estimated to be 5.5 per cent lower in 1346 than in 1333, but as the population had been growing quite briskly in the years 1331–3, the difference between 1330 and 1346 must have been quite negligible. In the merindad of Sangüesa, there are clear differences between the 50 villages where the peasants holding royal land paid their rents in money and the 49 villages where such peasants paid in grain. In the first category of villages, the number of households increased by 12 per cent in the years 1334–46, while in the second category there was no change. In view of the fact that the population generally grew quite briskly in the period 1321–33, it must be assumed that both categories of villages had more households in 1346 than in 1330, quite likely something in the order of magnitude of 15 per cent and 3 per cent, respectively.[3]

Then, in 1347, Navarre went through the severest famine of the Late Middle Ages. The number of peasant households holding royal tenancies in the merindad of Pamplona was reduced by 17 per cent, while the number of such households in the merindad of Sangüesa fell by 7 per cent. Unfortunately, the relevance of these data relating to the Pyrenean regions for inference to the similar events in the fertile lowlands of the Ribera area in the merindad of Estella is also problematic.

The few data on the famine's impact on the population of peasant households holding land of the royal estates in the merindad of Estella show a quite high level of decline in the north, but much smaller in the south near the Ribera area, in the order of magnitude of 5–9 per cent.[4] This may cautiously be taken as an indication that the demographic effects of the famine in the Ribera area were of the same order of magnitude as in the merindad of Sangüesa, and that, if the peasant population holding land from the royal estates was reasonably representative of the general peasant population, general population size at the end of 1347 was of about the same size or slightly higher than in 1330. In that case, the possible changes in the population size between 1330 and 1350 do not affect the estimate of the decline in the numbers of householders in the Black Death of 63 per cent, at least not in a significant way.

However, it must be assumed that poor and destitute classes of rural society, the landless or all-but-landless social classes, were particularly harshly hit by a severe famine and suffered some supermortality as compared to the peasant classes. These rural proletarians are assumed to have constituted 40–50 per cent of the population, and supermortality in a section of the population of this order of magnitude may represent a concealed further reduction of the population in the famine than registered by the 'pechas capitales'. This factor warrants an adjustment of the estimated decline in the number of households caused by the Black Death in the Ribera area downwards to about 60 per cent. (The diminution in the number of householders in the merindad of Pamplona in 1347 represents a worst-case scenario that, if applied to the 'monedaje'-material for the Ribera area, implies an unadjusted minimum mortality rate in the Black Death of c. 55 per cent among this social category, and an adjusted minimum mortality rate of c. 52 per cent.)

The diminution of the population constituted by the households was larger than the mortality rate among the householders. Even if the householder survived,

[3] Berthe 1984: 245–6.
[4] Berthe 1984: 285–99.

chances were that not all the other members of the household would live through the ordeal, because, as mentioned above, especially children but also women suffer supermortality in plague epidemics, and some members of households would contract the disease elsewhere in various extraneous circumstances.[5] The standard assumption is that the average size of households diminished from 4.5 persons to 4 persons in the countryside and from 4 persons to 3.5 persons in urban centres.[6] This means that the 'monedajes' indicate a general population mortality of c. 65 per cent. This should be considered a central estimate. (Use of the mortality rate for the house-holders of the merindad of Pamplona in 1347 gives a minimum mortality estimate of 57 per cent.)

The weakening of the surviving households by loss of members and their vulnera-bility to further demographic strain is reflected also in the dramatic further diminu-tion of their numbers in the following plague epidemic in 1362–3. In the Ribera area of the merindad of Estella. where the number of households had fallen from 6,538 to 2,408 in the Black Death, the number of households had declined further to 1,458, or by 40 per cent, according to the 'monedaje' of 1366.[7] These data indicate that the French scholar M. Berthe's assumption on the decline of household size is nearer the mark than the standard assumption of this book, which, however, is intentionally low and cautious. The two plague epidemics appear to have reduced the Ribera area's population by around 75 per cent.

The registers of 'pechas capitales' show that the Black Death invaded 200 of the 215 communities that in the merindads of Pamplona and Sangüesa contained peasant households holding royal lands, and only a few hamlets escaped unscathed. This shows another aspect of the tremendous mortality caused by the Black Death, namely plague's overwhelming ability to blanket rural areas. Only 7 per cent of all settle-ments escaped its visitation, mostly small peripheral hamlets that, consequently, contained an even smaller proportion of the population involved. At the end of 1350, these 200 communities show a diminution in the number of households holding royal tenancies, 'pechas', of 44 per cent compared to the number at the start of 1348 in the merindad of Pamplona, and a diminution of 42 per cent in the merindad of Sangüesa. In all 215 communities taken together, 1,141 householders out of 2,933 had disappeared, a diminution of 39 per cent. It has been possible to show that a substan-tial proportion of the households of the surviving householders had lost members, in other words that average household size had diminished significantly. This fact induced Berthe to conclude, perhaps somewhat arbitrarily, that 'no doubt' almost 50 per cent of the individuals living in these households on the eve of the Black Death had lost their lives.[8] Applying the standard assumption on the usual development of

5   Cf. Berthe 1983: 306; Berthe 1984: 310.
6   See the general discussion on mortality above, and the discussion of Italian data below in connection with the mortality in Florence.
7   Zabalo Zabalegui 1968: 85.
8   Berthe 1984: 310; Berthe 1983: 306. The earliest sources showing the composition and size of households in Navarre are from around 1430. In 1430, the population had been reduced to a small fraction of its pre-plague size. The numerous landless people working for minimal wages, which was such a prominent feature of pre-plague society, were swept away by the winds of change, by plague and by social mobility, the survivors joining the class of solid tenants. Because extra hands were few and expensive, it was quite usual for the major tenants to pool their labour by forming joint or multiple households (see below), and 20–30 percent of the households appear to have been of this type around 1430, contributing to a quite high average

household size through the ravages of the Black Death, the mortality rate of this special population segment, the peasant population that held land of the royal estates, will be somewhat lower according to my estimates than suggested by Berthe, namely 47 per cent.

At this point, the serious shortcomings of the registers of 'pechas capitales' must be taken into account. They record only a minor part of the rural population, those who held land of the royal estates, and as such, the registered households as a whole constituted a better-off segment of the peasant population that was clearly unrepresentative of the general rural population. The majority of the tenantry that held land of other landlords is not registered, and, even more importantly, they do not include the landless classes. Equally, the scholar does not take into account the problem of social mobility, that many 'pechas' that had been obliterated by the Black Death could have been substituted by households recruited from the landless classes or dissatisfied peasants on non-royal manors wishing to take advantage of their good luck as survivors. In short, much could have happened in the two years from the Black Death to the redaction of the registers of 'pechas capitales' that would serve to conceal a considerable part of the mortality. The extent of this development cannot be measured in any accurate or concrete way, but it certainly represents an argument to the effect that the real loss of population must have been significantly and probably substantially higher than the c. 50 per cent suggested by Berthe. Perhaps 55–60 per cent could be a cautious suggestion in the light of other data from other countries and regions (the Piedmont, the Savoy, England).

No doubt, the source material represented by the 'monedajes' must be preferred over the 'pechas capitales' because, in principle, they should register the whole population, with the exception only of the exempted classes, including the proletarian classes of the population. They must be assumed to contain a fairly representative registration of the population, with the reservation that the poor and destitute would, no doubt, have been passed over more frequently than members of other social classes despite the efforts of the taxable social classes to evade taxation. One should also note the point made above to the effect that the registration must be assumed to have been somewhat better after the plague than before. Encouragingly, the disparity between the mortality rates indicated by the 'monedajes' and the 'pechas capitales' must be considered modest and, in view of the narrow social basis of the 'pechas capitales', it serves to confirm the trustworthiness of the mortality rate indicated by the 'monedajes'. Everything considered, caution may, perhaps, favour an indication of general population mortality in the Kingdom of Navarre in the range of 60–65 per cent, but it is not difficult to argue for a somewhat higher mortality rate of around 65 per cent.

This remarkable loss of population, which to modern man suggests the effects of atomic warfare, occurred to a population that was overwhelmingly rural. Although about 30 per cent of the population lived in communities that according to formal

household size of around 5 persons. The motive for forming such households was much weaker in pre-plague society, but because labour was cheap, well-off households would quite likely contain more living-in servants. (The terms joint family/household refers to the co-habitation of biologically related families, whether horizontally or laterally organized in a generational perspective; if cohabitating families are not biologically related, this social constellation is called a multiple family/household.)

demographic criteria (population size) could be defined as urban, almost half of the
population of the urban centres were actually peasants or agricultural labourers; in
other words, only 15 per cent of Navarre's population was genuinely urban on the
eve of the Black Death.[9]

Studies of mortality in the Black Death at the other end of Spain, in the south-eastern
region of Catalonia, show similar levels of mortality. Two studies have been
performed on rural communities in the Plain of Vich (Plana de Vich), situated about
65 km north-east of Barcelona and 50 km west of Girona. In the parish of St Ándreu
in the district of Gurb, there were 160 hearths before the Black Death and only 41 in
operation in 1352, a diminution of 74 per cent; in Taradell, there were 111 hearths
before the Black Death and 38 in 1352, a diminution of 66 per cent.[10] The same reservations apply to these estimates with respect to the demographic significance of the
lack of information on the social segments that were too poor to pay hearth tax, the
'impotentes' in the terminology of the time and place. Furthermore, many surviving
households having lost members, average household size must have declined appreciably. In short, ordinary demographic considerations suggest that in reality the
general mortality rates were even higher.

   Gyug's study of the mortality among clerics who held benefices in the diocese of
Barcelona can be said to be based on a sort of mass material.[11] The diocesan registers
show that over 616 clerics held benefices in Barcelona in 1344 and that the number
was about the same in 1350. The first clerics died from plague in May 1348, the last in
May 1349. In this period, 380 provisions were made to benefices vacant through
death, giving a gross death rate among the beneficed clergy of 61.7 per cent. The
normal annual death rate of clerical holders of benefices appears to have been 3–3.5
per cent.[12] This is lower than in the general population, which probably had a normal
annual mortality rate of 4–4.5 per cent, corresponding to an average life expectancy at
birth of 25–22.5 years. Some of the clerics who died from plague in this period would
have died anyway, but, because they died from plague, they must be included in
plague mortality; probably at least half of those that would have died anyway died
from plague instead. Plague-specific mortality appears to have been around 60 per

---

[9]   Berthe 1984: 310.
[10] Pladevall 1963: 364–5.
[11] Gyug 1983: 385–95.
[12] This estimate is based on Gyug's figures for clerical mortality by month in 1347, but the assumed normal
level has been adjusted downwards. The number of clerical deaths in 1347 was 25, or 4 per cent, but 1347
was a year of serious dearth that unleashed hunger-related epidemics, which also caused clerical
supermortality. According to Gyug's figures, a supermortality of about five clerics is suggested in May and
November. This indicates that normal annual clerical mortality was more likely 20 than 25 persons, and that
the ordinary annual mortality rate was more likely 3–3.5 per cent. Emery has estimated the mortality of
scribes and legists in Perpignan in the period 1317–37 and found a median annual loss of 3.25 per cent.
Emery 1967: 615. These two professional categories would have age composition and social-class characteristics comparable to those of the clerics of Barcelona.
   A normal annual mortality rate of 3–3.5 per cent reveals quite a high average age for the clerics of Barcelona. The life table for populations with an average life expectancy at birth of 25 years shows that this death
rate sets in around age 50. This means that Malthusian pressures were very much active in this professional
category, and lots of men with clerical education had to wait for many years of dutiful work until they
obtained a benefice. This fact is reflected in another way: the diocesan administration replaced the enormous
number of deceased clerics without any difficulty. These observations correspond closely to those pertaining
to English beneficed clerics (see below).

cent, and about 1.7 per cent died from other causes. Of these clerical benefice holders, 374 died in the twelve months May 1348–April 1349, implying that the mortality rate in the plague year was 15–20 times higher than in a normal year. A total of 237 of these ecclesiastical deaths took place in the four months June–September 1348 when the Black Death crested, which means that 40 per cent of all clerics in Barcelona died in this short period, 104 in July alone.

The mortality rate among the beneficed clergy in the Black Death in Barcelona is strikingly similar to the mortality rates obtained for the general population in areas in the Kingdom of Navarre and in the Plain of Vich, but cannot be accepted without further analysis and discussion. Although many individual parish priests and vicars had quite meagre livings, as a social category the secular clergy was far better fed, clad and housed than the average population; in the case of disease, they would also have much better nursing care. On the other hand, to the extent that they visited the homes of parishioners dying from plague in order to administer the last rites, they would have a particularly high degree of exposure to dangerous rat fleas in their professional role; but, to the extent that they lived in stone houses and the rooms had better standards of cleanliness and sanitation, their exposure would be considerably smaller than the average in their spare time at home and at night (see above).

In the general discussion above of problems relating to the mortality in the Black Death, it was underscored that the social classes of the poor and destitute, the age categories of children and adolescents, and women, all generally suffered mortality rates above the average in plague epidemics. One should also note that no social category of people attained high average age at death in the Middle Ages whatever their social circumstances, and not even the clergy had a high average age at death according to modern standards; as a social category, their physiological and immunological competence were presumably not seriously impaired by age. The question of a possible clerical supermortality in the Black Death cannot be usefully discussed in the light of possible marginally higher case fatality rates (it is, on average, 80 per cent), but must be discussed in the perspective of possible superexposure to infection. In this discussion the numerous social advantages of the clerics in the face of epidemics must be considered as well.[13]

The clerics were sufficiently numerous to constitute a valid statistical basis for estimates with relevance for more general perspectives on mortality; clerical personnel lived all over the city, and their territorial distribution in the city would not be expected to affect the death rates of clerics in a substantially different way from that of the general population.

Summing up, it is not clear that the beneficed clerics of Barcelona should be expected to have a significantly higher level of mortality in the Black Death than the ordinary population. In other words, the death rate of these clerics should rather be quite suggestive of the order of magnitude of the general population's death rate. It appears reasonable to conclude that the clerical mortality rate in Barcelona is indicative of general population mortality in the city. This conclusion can be usefully compared to the mortality rates of the English parish priests in four cathedral cities,

---

[13] This subject is discussed more thoroughly below in connection with the English beneficed parish clergy.

which are substantially higher than for the rural beneficed clergy and more in the line with general population mortality.

The usability of mortality rates in social or professional elites for approaching the question of general mortality is limited at best, often marginal, but as a general rule social elites and the upper classes should be expected to have substantially lower mortality rates than the lower classes or the general population for reasons that have been discussed above. Four out of Barcelona's five councillors and almost all members of the governing Council of One Hundred died.[14] It is not known that these two samples of persons recruited from the city's ruling classes engaged in types of behaviour that would give them superexposure to infective rat fleas, and, privately, they lived in circumstances that would give lower exposure to disease than the general population and far better nursing care in the case of disease with consequent lower case mortality.

The paucity of data on mortality in the Black Death in Catalonia calls for caution, but they show consistently very high rates of mortality, in the range of 50–70 per cent. Consistency strengthens their credibility, both their internal consistency in the form of a systematic level of mortality, and their external consistency in the form of similarity to the Navarrese data.

Demographic studies of fourteenth-century tax lists organized according to households have been produced also for Mallorca, the largest of the Balearic Isles. In Mallorca, a tax called 'morabati' was levied each seven years on (the heads of) households that had possessions worth more than ten pounds (in the silver currency of the time) and were not exempt (mostly clerics and gentry).[15] The 'morabati' was levied in 1343 and in 1350. The registers of these two years are extant and have been used for the study of the population developments in the intervening years, which are taken to be indicative of mortality in the Black Death.

The estimates performed on the basis of a comparison of these two sets of hearth-tax records are intriguing, but are also methodologically problematic in many respects because they 'refer only to isolated phenomena of limited duration'.[16] They show a decrease of the population of only 4 per cent in the city of Palma de Mallorca where, according to the 'morabati', c. 37 per cent of the households were resident in 1343, while the demographic regression in the countryside amounts to 23 per cent. The scholar does not conceal his surprise at the discrepancy between urban and rural mortality rates, but characterizes it as anomalous and incongruent.

However, the scholar does not refer to the exceptionally low mortality rate in the Black Death of only 16 per cent for the island's population as a whole.[17] According to the 'morabati', it is, actually, quite similar in size to the reduction in the number of

---

14 Capmany y de Montpalau 1962: 987.

15 Sevillano Colom 1974: 234–9, 242.

16 Sobrequés Callicó 1966: 83. My translation from Spanish.

17 Santamaría Arández 1969: 119–23; Santamaría Arández 1970–1: 187. According to Santamaría Arández, the total number of households in the island was reduced from 11,258 in 1343 to 9,461 in 1350, i.e. by 16 per cent. According to Sevillano Colom 1976: 247, the total number of 'morabati'-paying households in the island was reduced from 11,305 in 1343 to 9,161 in 1350, i.e., by 19 per cent. The reason for this discrepancy is not explained.

taxpaying households in the period 1329–43.[18] If this should be proven correct, the comparable demographic diminution of the population in the two decades preceding the Black Death and from the Black Death would be unique in contemporary European history. In that case, the history of the Black Death in the island would not be interesting in a synthetical perspective. Instead focus would be directed to the grounds for the uniqueness, but so far no scholar has come up with any epidemiologically relevant reason(s). In this connection, it is also intriguing to put it mildly, that a comparison of the 'morabati' of 1329 and 1343 show a diminution in the island's urban population of 23 per cent, while the rural population actually increased by 2 per cent, almost an inversion of the distribution of the mortality in the Black Death.[19] These Mallorcan data are, therefore, infested with major problems of demography, sociology and source criticism both with respect to the level of total mortality and to the distribution of mortality between town and countryside. Depressingly, the reduction in the number of recorded households in the city and the slight increase in the countryside could be explained by a hypothesis of increasing tax evasion by a population that with increasing tax-experience learned how to deal with the tax-recording and tax-collecting administration, and, no doubt, burghers would be better at it than peasants.

Strangely, the number of Jewish households in the city had not declined at all; on the contrary, it had increased greatly from 333 in 1343 to 516 in 1350, by 55 per cent, although, as the scholar underscores, the plague ravaged the Jews as violently as the Christians.[20] The scholar's explanation, based on migration of Jewish families into the city, appears problematic for several reasons: there appears to be no information on the number of Jewish households living elsewhere on the island; at least no such information is provided by the scholar. The economic activities of Jews would normally contain strong incentives for them to settle in urban centres. It would, therefore, be anomalous and incongruent if so many Jewish households lived in the villages and townships in the countryside that the survivors could not only substitute for the losses suffered by Jewish households in the city, but also could bring about a large increase of more than 50 per cent in the Jewish community there. One should consider that the Jews who had managed to carve out a living in the countryside would be tied down by their local economic assets in properties, homes, securities for loans, debtors, developed circles of customers, and so on.

Alternatively, one could take interest in several instances of known persecutions of Jews on the mainland: in Barcelona, Cervera and Tarrega, Jews were killed and their ghettos looted, because frightened Christians regarded them as 'plague-spreaders'; similar events are reported from Lérida and Girona.[21] Many of the survivors, and also Jews in other towns and cities in Catalonia, would, no doubt, have liked to pack up whatever valuables they could take with them and leave the seething and murderous hatreds behind them and go to places where they could feel safer, and, then, Palma de Mallorca could be an attractive alternative. In short, Jews elsewhere could have special motives for resettlement, and this permits hypothesizing that the great

---

[18] Santamaría Arández 1970–1: 185.
[19] Santamaría Arández 1970–1: 185; Sevillano Colom 1974: 247.
[20] Santamaría Arández 1969: 121. Cf. Carreras Panchón, Mitre Fernandez and Valdeón 1980: 62.
[21] Sobrequés Callicó 1966: 80; Shirk 1981: 363.

increase in the number of Jewish households in the city of Palma de Mallorca was due not so much to inter-local migration on the island as to immigration from abroad.

This highlights more generally the issue of possible lively immigration from the mainland to this lovely island by people who would like to take up work opportunities or land that had been left vacant by the Black Death.

Nor does the scholar discuss the possible significance of the fact that the 'morabati' registered only those who possessed sufficient means to bear tax assessment. As mentioned above, the crude data of the 'monedaje' of 1330 for the Ribera area in Navarre, which aimed at registering the non-taxpaying poor and destitute social classes, indicate that they constituted at least about 40 per cent, and probably rather 40–50 per cent of the population. This illustrates the order of magnitude of the problem of mobility. In addition to the problem of immigration to the island, this problem includes both territorial and social mobility within the island of large population segments seeing the opportunity for entering good tenements, or finding full employment in well-paid jobs or small businesses left vacant by the ravages of the Black Death whether in the countryside or in the city. Many of these enterprising households would rise in the social hierarchy and enter the taxpaying classes. This would also tend to occur for a very different reason: when people die in great numbers, many of the survivors would receive inheritance and enter the taxpaying classes on this basis. And, of course, all of these social phenomena could happen to the same household. These types of social developments were illustrated by Icelandic material above, i.e., by material relating to another island society, albeit at the other end of Europe.

In short, the 'morabati' tax records give too little information about the social scene to be useful for estimating mortality in the Black Death. In addition, the problem of tax evasion seems particularly intractable in this case.

Little is known of the effects of the Black Death in Castile. A study on the subject has been carried out in the bishopric of Palencia in north-central Old Castile.[22] The scholar compared ecclesiastical cadasters redacted in 1345 and 1353 that allowed him to identify the settled villages within the diocese in those two years. It appeared that 82 of the 420 villages in 1345 had become completely desolated by 1353, i.e., 19.5 per cent.[23] This registration of deserted villages gives, of course, only a suggestive and frustrating inkling of the real magnitude of the mortality caused by the Black Death. The fact that over 19 per cent of the villages were completely deserted does not at all indicate that this was the level of general mortality. The larger villages that contained most of the population could live on with only a small fraction of the houses inhabited and the tenements in operation; partial desertion would be the usual reflection of great mortality, and this feature would not be registered or reflected in these sources. Furthermore, the effects of the famine year of 1347 cannot be identified and subtracted.

The completely deserted villages were mostly small and marginal settlements colonized on the plain in the High Middle Ages under the impact of steadily growing

---

[22] Cabrillana 1968: 245–58. Palencia borders on the provinces of Santander, Burgos, Valladolid and Léon.
[23] Cabrillana 1968: 256–7.

population pressures. The fact that they became desolate does not necessarily reflect that they were more severely ravaged by the Black Death than the larger, anciently settled villages. Instead, it could reflect the fact that the old-settled villages remained more attractive and that survivors in the former villages and hamlets happily moved into vacant better tenements there. Much resettlement could have taken place in the five years between the onslaught of the Black Death and the time the second register was made in 1353. Typically, the districts that were distinguished by the highest degree of juridical and social liberties for the peasantry had most immigration and did best under the circumstances: mountain villages colonized more or less outside the economic and political control of the ruling classes did better than the villages on the plain.

Consequently, the demographic effects of the Black Death in Old Castile cannot be identified with any accuracy, although it is possible to discern clear indications of a serious population contraction at the end of the 1340s. This is the last Spanish study that uses mass materials to identify the demographic effects of the Black Death on the ordinary population, particularly the peasantry.

R.W. Emery's study of the mortality in certain upper-class categories of professionals in Perpignan may also be of some interest insofar as it comprises a largish group of scribes and legists, mostly notaries, lawyers and judges, mentioned in 1346–7, in all 125 persons. He found that a minimum of 58 per cent and a maximum of 68 per cent died in the Black Death.[24] Although many of these professionals would visit homes of dying people much like parish priests did, in order to draw up wills and charters of endowments, it is not clear that their social behaviour as a whole exposed them more to the plague than the common population. They would for most of their time relate to environments that would be less infested with rats, and when contracting the disease, they would have better chances of surviving because they would be better fed and nursed.

In Girona, the number of notaries was halved by the Black Death, otherwise the ruling elites and upper classes appear to have been less severely depleted than in Barcelona.[25] These affluent classes of people could easily have moved into the countryside and have moved further on when the Black Death approached, and they could have learned lessons from the events in Barcelona.

The usability of the mortality rates in these special urban social and professional categories for inference to the mortality in the general population is, as mentioned, not clear. However, the mortality rates estimated for the beneficed clergy of Barcelona and the scribes and legists of Perpignan are conspicuously similar to the mortality data obtained for the general population.

Summing up, the available evidence on the mortality in the Black Death in Spain is insufficient in volume and has too narrow a territorial distribution to allow general-ization at any substantial level of validity. This means that generalizations on the present evidential basis can be changed or modified by a number of new studies that

---

[24] Emery 1967: 614–27.
[25] Guilleré 1984: 26–36.

show substantially lower mortality rates in other regions. However, as stated before, for obvious statistical reasons one should expect to encounter the normal exactly because it is usual; extreme or unusual events are by definition rare or unusual. The probability that so many scholars working on materials with great territorial distance and produced by different administrative systems should fortuitously pick this number of unusual or extreme events and without exception miss the normal or usual is so tiny that it can be equated to winning big money on the pools or a jackpot in the great lotteries. Certainly it must be clear that the present mortality data do not at all confirm the usual unsubstantiated assertions to the effect that a quarter or one-third of the population died.

As can be seen from Table 12, taken together, the available Spanish data suggest the staggering mortality rate of 60–65 per cent. The interesting data on the mortality of the beneficed clergy in Barcelona does not fit into the table, but is indicated in the parenthesis under the heading of General population for Catalonia with its mortality rate of 60 per cent, which, according to the comparative sociological and epidemiological discussion, was assumed to be suggestive also of general population mortality in the city of Barcelona. If the tentative estimate of the populations of the Spanish kingdoms at 6 million on the eve of the Black Death is correct,[26] it was reduced to 2–2.5 million inhabitants.

Table 12. Mortality in the Black Death in Spain according to region %

Region and country	Tax- and rentpaying householders	Tax- and rentpaying population	General population
Kingdom of Navarre	55–60	60–65	60–65
Catalonia	(71)	(74)	(60–70)
'Spain'	55–60	60–65	60–65

It is a basic tenet of epidemiology that the powers of spread of any disease increase with increasing density of the susceptible population. An interesting general observation made by several scholars is that, in Spain, the Black Death ravaged the countryside even more severely than the towns.[27] This observation conforms to the general studies of the territorial distribution of plague mortality. The fact that the Black Death as an epidemic tends to exhibit stronger powers of spread in the relatively thinly settled countryside than in the towns shows that it was overwhelmingly an epidemic of bubonic plague: it is a unique feature of this disease that the densities of rats and rat fleas overrule the effects of the density of the susceptible human population that is the decisive factor for the dynamics of epidemic spread in the case of all diseases that spread directly between human beings by cross-infection (see above).

[26] Ballesteros Rodriguez 1982: 38. The Kingdom of Granada is assumed to have had a pre-plague population of 1.5 million.
[27] Vilar 1962: 464; Shirk 1981: 365; Berthe 1984: 314.

29

Italy

The available data on mortality rates in the Black Death in Italy relate only to the highly developed northern third of the peninsula. There can be no doubt that Italy went through an unimaginable catastrophe. In Florence, Marchionne di Coppo Stefani described the social scene in this way:

> All the citizens did little else except to carry dead bodies to be buried; many died who did not confess or receive the last rites; and many died by themselves and many died of hunger [. . .] At every church they dug deep pits down to the water-table; and thus those who were poor who died during the night were bundled up quickly and thrown into the pit. In the morning when a large number of bodies were found in the pit, they took some earth and shovelled it down on top of them; and later others were placed on top of them and then another layer of earth, just as one makes lasagne with layers of pasta and cheese.[1]

The most frightening feature of this enormous demographic disaster in the author's mind is, according to the religious beliefs and mentality of the time, that people died without confession and without receiving the last rites, and, thus, in the moment of death faced perdition and eternal punishment. Observation of secondary catastrophe effects, that many people died from lack of nursing care, and even from starvation, also had made strong impressions on the author.

Actually, good mortality data come from the city of Florence itself and from the surrounding region of Tuscany, which, consequently, will constitute the territorial centrepiece of the discussion of mortality from the Black Death in Italy. Population estimates show that Tuscany must have had over two million inhabitants on the eve of the Black Death,[2] a substantial portion of Italy's population. Politically and administratively, Tuscany was divided into a number of city states and local communes, the largest city state by far being Florence, which had already conquered and subjugated a number of previously independent city states and communes.

In the case of the city of Florence, the question discussed most eagerly relates to the size of the pre-plague population. According to the exceptionally reliable contem-

---

[1] Cited after Henderson 1992: 145.
[2] Fiumi 1962: 290.

porary chronicler Giovanni Villani, Florence's population in April 1347 amounted to
at least 94,000 persons, an estimate that he insists was based on good data collected by
the city authorities and also included the poor. He also relates that 4,000 inhabitants
succumbed in a serious dearth in that year. Reviewing the discussion, Falsini
concluded in 1971 that Florence contained probably somewhat more than 90,000
persons on the eve of the Black Death, but less than 50,000 persons in 1352.[3] A few
years later, Herlihy and Klapisch-Zuber concluded that the city probably contained
around 120,000 inhabitants on the eve of the Black Death, which was reduced to
about 42,000 inhabitants by the epidemic. The two scholars reached this result
primarily by discussing some additional data given by Giovanni Villani that they
claim indicate a substantially larger population.[4] It is an important point that
Giovanni Villani considers his pre-plague population figure to be a minimum estimate, but it may appear that the figure of 120,000 inhabitants arrived at by Herlihy
and Klapisch-Zuber is the result of overemphasizing a few arguments supporting a
higher estimate. Thus, according to the present status of research, Florence contained
between 120,000 persons and about 92,000 persons on the eve of the Black Death.

Because Giovanni Villani's diverse pieces of demographic information relating to
population size with a few exceptions tend to be consistent and reasonable, and
because he himself considered the estimate he gives as to April 1347 a minimum
figure, one could reasonably conclude that the population size at the time probably
was around 96,000 persons, but obviously could have been even somewhat larger.
According to Villani, 4,000 persons succumbed from the dearth of that year, and this
dearth was immediately followed by the Black Death, so that the population could
not have recuperated significantly. This means that Falsini's analysis appears reasonable to the present author, who concurs that Florence's population on the eve of the
Black Death probably amounted to c. 92,000 persons. The fact that this still must be
considered quite close to a minimum figure means that the subsequent estimate of
Florence's population loss in the Black Death will be realistic and probably on the
low side.

The lists of a tax levied in 1352 recorded 9,955 households in Florence.[5] The medieval Tuscan tax lists, tax surveys and censuses have not been discussed thoroughly and
comprehensively from a source-critical point of view in order to establish the degree
of completeness with which the populations were recorded. Such records were
normally redacted with considerable intervals so that there is also little independent
material available with which the completeness and accuracy of the records can be
tested. It appears to be a usual opinion among historians and demographers who
have worked with these sources that they are quite reliable for their time, but because
this opinion is more based on impression than systematic and exhaustive source-
critical analysis it stands on quite shaky foundations so far. One important reason for
the formation of this opinion is that the non-paying classes of the poor and destitute
are normally quite well registered; at least they are entered in impressive numbers.
The numbers of households or persons entered in these registers are therefore taken

---

[3]   1971: 425–36.
[4]   1978: 173–7. Cf. Falsini 1971: 428. The fact that Giovanni Villani is exceptionally reliable does not, of
course, imply that he cannot be mistaken or provide erroneous information.
[5]   Barbadoro 1931: 615, 619.

to represent such complete registrations of the populations that they are used without additions for underregistration or underenumeration. However, as pointed out above and underscored by Carrasco Perez, Postan and Hollingsworth, even good registrations of populations are subject to significant evasion and underenumeration, and an assumption of a deficit of 5 per cent must be considered sanguine, of 15 per cent not obviously exaggerated.

In Tuscan society, the urban centres contained quite a large fleeting class of proto-industrial proletarians who bore no tax assessment and often moved between casual labour in the various wards and quarters of the urban centres and between the urban centres and the countryside and, therefore, at least to some extent, would avoid registration or be passed over by the registrars. In the countryside, a large part of the population consisted of sharecroppers, sub-tenants, cotters and day labourers who bore no tax assessment when registered and who likewise constituted quite fleeting social classes whose members would tend to drift to the urban centres or to migrate to other parts of the Tuscan region in search for work and livelihood, and for these reasons they would at least to some extent would avoid registration or be passed over by the registrars. Registration of these social classes of have-nots (the 'nullatenentes' or 'popolo minuto') would also tend to be imperfect because the bailiffs and scribes who redacted the registers would not have any real motive for putting much effort into an accurate and complete registration of social classes that at the end of the day would not make any tax contribution. In the words of Herlihy and Klapisch-Zuber, poverty constituted a 'justification for an implicit exemption', namely by non-registration in tax records.[6] The problem of underregistration was discussed in a more general and thorough fashion above, and it was decided to assume a general deficit of 7.5 per cent in fiscal registrations of pre-plague populations that were intended to cover the total population, unless special reasons warrant otherwise. It was also pointed out that for various reasons underregistration would tend to be significantly lower after the Black Death than before, and that, for this reason, use of the same addition would tend to veil somewhat the real impact of plague and to affect mortality estimates in the direction of minima.[7] In order to take this factor at least partly into account, the standard addition to post-plague fiscal registers that were intended to cover the whole population will be 6 per cent. The urgent need for further discussion of this problem must be stressed.

An assumption to the effect that the tax records of 1352 missed a number of households representing 6 per cent of the real number of households implies that the Florentine population really comprised 10,552 households at the time.

However, for two main reasons there were more households in Florence in 1352 than on the morrow of the Black Death, namely because many new households had been formed in the ensuing years and because of immigration from the 'contado'. As was pointed out above in the general comments to this section on mortality, and was illustrated by the marriage registers of Givry, great mortality triggered an immediate

[6] Herlihy and Klapisch-Zuber 1978: 161. Cf. Bowsky 1964: 9.
[7] Fiumi has argued in favour of a very high addition to the number of households entered in the tax lists of 1352 and 1355, corresponding to an increase of 50 per cent. This has not been accepted by subsequent research, e.g., Herlihy and Klapisch-Zuber 1978: 177, and Falsini 1971: 431–2. These scholars prefer to make no additions at all, which also is a problematic approach.

marked surge in the number of marriages as young people suddenly found them-selves in a situation with many good employment opportunities in a very favourable housing market. Many of them would also have improved their prospects after having received inheritance(s). It was argued in favour of a standard assumption to the effect that this post-plague surge in marriages caused a net increase in the number of households at an annual rate of 0.5 per cent in urban centres and of 0.75 per cent in rural areas. However, the huge industrial labour market in Florence would provide young adult men and women with much easier access to the basic incomes needed for entering into matrimony than in the countryside in pre-plague society.

In short, the situation in Florence could have had much in common with what happened in England in the Industrial Revolution, when the new manufacturing industries created vast numbers of new employment opportunities that allowed young adults to marry at will. As a result fertility in England sky-rocketed and the population began to grow so tremendously and unprecedentedly that Robert Malthus was startled into formulating the basic tenets of Malthusianism and modern demog-raphy.

In the specific case of Florence, therefore, it appears prudent to use the standard assumption of 0.75 per cent for an urban centre. This implies that formation of new households in the three years that had followed the Black Death had caused a net increase of 2.5 per cent in the number of Florentine households since the Black Death, an increase that must be deducted in order to approach an adequate estimate of the size of the Florentine population in the immediate aftermath of the Black Death. This deduction will give 10,320 households as the outcome.

However, this deduction does not produce a realistic estimate of the number of households or size of the Florentine population in the immediate aftermath of the Black Death, because it still contains households formed on the basis of immigration. Because the immigrants would contain a highly unrepresentative proportion of soli-tary and small newly wed conjugal households, this category of persons must be deducted not in the form of a number of households, but as a population element expressed as a number of inhabitants. This means that the preliminary estimate of the number of households must be converted into a preliminary estimate of the post-plague Florentine population. For this a household multiplier is needed.

On the basis of Florentine records of 1380 that registered both the households and their constituent members, these households are also generally assumed to contain, on average, 4.2 persons in 1352,[8] implying a population of almost 42,000 persons. However, surviving households would often have suffered the loss of one or more members. The relevance of this point is, for instance, corroborated by Gelting's study of the individual fates of the constituent members of the 11 peasant households contained in the mountain hamlet of Grenis in the Maurienne (see above). Other social developments also contributed to diminish the average household size. The great surge in new marriages has already been mentioned. This stream of young adult men and, according to the findings of Herlihy and Klapisch-Zuber, often adolescent women, out of their families of origin would, at the same time, reduce the average size of the surviving established households and cause a substantial increase in newly

8   Battara 1935: 352.

formed small families. It has been argued above that the huge (proto-)industrial labour market in Florence made it easier for young adults to find work that could form the economic basis for entering marriage. The huge industrial labour market also attracted immigrants from the countryside and, in this context, immigration is significant because it caused an increased incidence of small households, solitaries or newly wed couples that contributed further to the reduction of average household size.

For these three reasons, average household size should be expected to have declined noticeably during the epidemic and in the aftermath of the disaster, and be markedly lower than the 4.2 persons recorded in 1380. The pre-disaster demographic household structure, its size and composition would be largely restored only after 15–20 years. Quite likely, the average household size in 1380 is representative also of the average pre-plague household size. However, one could also suspect that the average size of the Florentine households in 1380 reflected to some extent not only the great surge of new marriages after the Black Death, but also smaller but significant surges after the quite serious plague epidemic of the early 1360s and another plague epidemic a decade later: in other words, these households may have contained a somewhat higher incidence of children than in a normal population that had not been ravaged by such extreme disasters.

This line of argument is supported by Enrico Fiumi's study of the census taken of the population in the Tuscan town of San Gimignano and the surrounding rural districts under its domination, its 'contado' in 1350. Children under the age of seven were left out of the census. Fiumi asserts that, when this omission is corrected for, the average household size cannot have exceeded 3.5 persons in the town or four persons in the rural districts, a wording indicating that the scholar actually presumes that the average household size in the town was of the order of magnitude of 3–3.5 persons and in the countryside of the order of magnitude of 3.5–4 persons.[9] A census taken of the rural population of the Commune of Prato in 1339, which probably is extraordinarily good, shows that the households contained on average 4.3 persons (see below). Similarly, a census of the population of the small commune of Moncalieri near the city of Turin taken in 1374 reveals that the 834 households contained on average 4.32 persons.

Table 13. Average household size in four Italian localities 1339–80

Locality	Year	Rural data	Urban data
Prato	1339	4.3	
San Gimignano	1350	4.0	3.5
Moncalieri	1374	4.3	
Florence	1380		4.2

The data contained in Table 13 can be used to form standard assumptions with respect to average pre-plague and post-plague household sizes, the so-called household multipliers. The similarity, and even consistency, of these disparate pieces of in-

---

[9] Fiumi 1962: 280.

formation on average household size in the decades around the Black Death, and their compatibility with the data from San Gimignano produced briefly after the epidemic, are astonishing and make them credible and suitable for use in population estimates. It will be assumed that the figures for San Gimignano reflect a reduction of the average household size in the town from 4 persons in the pre-plague population and a corresponding reduction in the countryside from 4.5 persons caused by the Black Death. Gelting's material attests to the cautious, even unrealistically cautious nature, of this assumption. For these reasons, it should be reasonable to reduce the average Florentine household multiplier by at least 0.5 person to 3.7 in 1352, instead of 4.2. The fact that this multiplier is probably on the high side makes it likely that the estimated population size will tend to be on the high side, and the estimated mortality rate on the low side.

We can now revert to the preliminary estimate of households in Florence in the immediate aftermath of the Black Death in 1349, which was designated preliminary because it contained also persons and households that had entered the city in the following three years. Applying a household multiplier of 3.7 to the reconstructed total of households, namely 10,320, gives a preliminary artificially high population estimate of 38,183 persons.

Lastly, there is the question of immigration. Unfortunately, there are no Florentine records that can give a clue as to the extent of immigration. Nonetheless, some useful notion of this problem could possibly be taken from the city of Bologna, where records of adult males in the ages 18–70 in 1357 show an incidence of immigration in relation to similar records of 1349 amounting to 5.5 per cent of the population of men of these ages.[10] Taking into consideration that some immigration had probably occurred between the end of the Black Death and the time the records of 1349 were produced, this immigration figure should probably be rounded upwards to at least 6 per cent, corresponding to an annual average increase of about 0.66 per cent in these years. The rate of immigration would probably be highest in the first post-plague years when the best vacant positions in the urban social structures were up for grabs, and would then tend to taper off. For this reason, it may appear reasonable to use a guestimate of an annual rate of immigration corresponding to an increase of roughly 0.8 per cent of the adult male population in the three years 1349–52, corresponding to an increase of 2.4 per cent of the adult male population. Medieval cities provided large numbers of jobs for women, mainly in the households of the affluent burghers. In Florence, the supply of jobs was even very much greater because of the huge wool industry, which required female workers for washing of wool, spinning, and so on. Presumably, as many women as men immigrated into the city. Of course, in addition many families of weavers and artisans would move into Florence from the townships and towns of the 'contado' and into the huge employment gap caused by the plague. No doubt, the dynamics of a precociously modern capitalistic industrial city like Florence would tend to be even greater than in Bologna, so that an immigration rate corresponding to an increase of 2.5 per cent in the three first post-plague years must be deemed cautious or conservative.

Deducting an assumed immigration into Florence in the three first post-plague

---

10   Pini and Greci 1976: 380.

years corresponding to a population increase of 2.5 per cent from the preliminary estimate produces an estimate of Florence's population size in the immediate after-math of the Black Death of 37,250 persons.

Summing up, these estimates of pre-plague and post-plague population size indicate that Florence's population fell from about 92,000 persons on the eve of the Black Death to around 37,250 persons on the morrow of the epidemic, a diminution of 59.5 per cent. Interestingly, Giovanni Villani's brother Matteo, who survived the Black Death and continued his chronicle, states that, in Florence, three of five inhabitants died in the Black Death, in other words, 60 per cent.

Taking into account the significant margins of uncertainty inherent in the premises of the estimate, not least with respect to the size of the plague-stricken population, it would be more correct to assume that Florence lost 55–65 per cent of its population in the Black Death. The realism of the indicated maximum is underlined by the fact that it is similar to the mortality rate if Herlihy's and Klapisch-Zuber's pre-plague population estimate of 120,000 is correct (65 per cent).[11] Although Boccaccio's awe-stricken assertion in the Introduction to the *Decameron* that 100,000 persons died in the Black Death in Florence can be shown to be much exaggerated, modern scholarship has also made it more comprehensible, the microbiological slaying of 55,000 fellow townspeople by this disease in the course of a few months within the confines of the city of Florence could easily have boggled anybody's mind.

This estimate of the carnage caused by the Black Death in Florence finds some independent support in two studies of special segments of the Florentine population. A demographic study of the Florentine noble class in the first half of the fourteenth century up to the Black Death has shown that there were, on average, slightly below three deaths each year. In the plague year of 1348, 68 deaths were registered, twenty-four times the annual average.[12] Unfortunately, nothing is said on the age composition of these deaths. However, a registered average annual mortality of under three persons in this social elite is so low that it cannot comprise child mortality; generally, deaths among infants and young children were so usual that they were often not entered in records relating to any social class. According to the estimate of Herlihy and Klapisch-Zuber, the mortality rate of propertied adult Florentine men in the years 1425–7 was 1.5–1.9 per cent.[13] Assuming that deceased children were not registered in these special records, this suggests that the adult noble-class population at risk in the Black Death had a death rate of 36–46 per cent. In view of the substantial supermortality of children, the mortality rate in this social elite as a whole must have been significantly higher, probably in the range of 40–50 per cent, and quite likely in

---

[11] Fiume 1950: 103–13, suggests a population size of 80,000 persons on the eve of the Black Death. After having argued for comprehensive additions to the tax records of 1352, he concludes that this population had been reduced to 63,000 persons in that year, implying a mortality rate in the Black Death of 21 per cent. His arguments and estimates have not been accepted by subsequent research. Herlihy and Klapisch-Zuber 1978: 176–7, assume, as mentioned, that Florence's population on the eve of the Black Death was about 120,000 persons, which was reduced to 42,000 persons 'in the years following the Black Death', implying a mortality rate of 65 per cent. These two studies represent the extremities of the scholarly discussion of this problem in the second half of the twentieth century. Falsini's estimates of pre-plague and post-plague populations (above) imply a plague mortality rate of slightly below 50 per cent.

[12] Livi Bacchi 1978: 42, 101; Del Panta 1980: 115.

[13] 1978: 459–60.

the higher reaches of that range. As should be expected, it would still be significantly lower than in the general population.

Lists recording persons that were interred with the habit of the Dominican friars in the church of Santa Maria Novella in Florence provides another interesting glimpse of the level of mortality. In the seven years preceding the Black Death, 18.3 persons were, on average, buried in this way each year. During the plague, the recording breaks down; the crucial point is, therefore, that in the following seven years the annual average fell to 8.3 interments, i.e., to 45 per cent of the pre-plague level.[14] These burials were performed with some pomp, the dramatic fall in their number reflecting primarily the mortality among the upper classes. The connection between the fall in the incidence of this type of burials and the plague mortality rate among the upper-class population at risk is quite likely quite close. If this numerical reflection of upper-class mortality is distorted in some way, it would rather be on the low side than on the high side because so many survivors would have become enriched after having received inheritance(s). Thus, the proportion of people who could afford such a burial should have increased and cause a corresponding relative increase in the incidence of this type of burial that would tend to veil some of the impact of the plague. The implied mortality rate of 55 per cent, or rather, perhaps, of 55–60 per cent, corresponds to the minimum estimate for the general population, but is, as should be expected, significantly higher than for the aristocratic population. Upper classes and social elites would be expected to suffer mortality rates more below the average. These glimpses of dramatic mortality in special upper-class social segments support the chilling estimate of general population mortality in Florence.

This estimate is further supported by the extreme mortality rates suffered by special religious communities. Undoubtedly to his great chagrin, the Florentine humanist Boccaccio (1313–75) became famous not for his good humanistic work, but rather infamous as the author of the *Decameron*, a frame story about young men and women who fled from the Black Death in Florence to a manor in the countryside where they whiled away the time by telling bawdy stories. In the Introduction, Boccaccio relates in some quite concrete detail the horrors of the Black Death that induced the 'merry company' to flee from the city, and that they met in the shadows of the Dominican monastery of Santa Maria Novella. The choice of meeting place was hardly fortuitous, but chosen to make the blood run cold in many of the readers who would have heard about the carnage in the monastery. The obituary of Santa Maria Novella shows that of the 130 members of the convent, 80 friars, three monks and three priests died, a mortality rate of 66 per cent. Only seven of 28 members of the Camaldolesian monastery of Angeli survived the Black Death's onslaught, representing a mortality rate of 75 per cent, which indicates a morbidity rate of almost 100 per cent. The great Guild of Chiavaioli lost three out of four masters ('consoli') of the guild in the plague.[15] This means that all special groups or communities within the city for which trustworthy mortality data are available, exhibit without exception even higher mortality rates than estimated here for the general population.

*

---

[14] Livi Bacchi 1978: 14.
[15] Falsini 1971: 434–5.

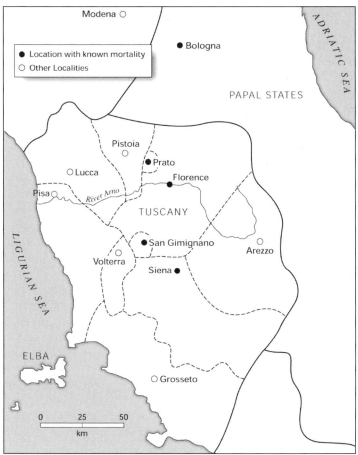

Map 3. Localities with known mortality in the Black Death in Tuscany

Good data on the size of the population before and after the Black Death are available for the Tuscan Commune of San Gimignano consisting of the town of San Gimignano and its 'contado', the rural districts under its domination. There are extant records from a general tax levied in 1332 and from a sort of census of the population taken in 1350. The census was taken in order to levy a special sort of tax called 'salt per mouth': all inhabitants excepting children below the age of seven had to purchase a certain amount of salt at a fixed price from the local government, which exercised a salt monopoly. This monopoly reflects that salt was a necessity of life in order to preserve food in a society without refrigerators or freezers. In practice, the records were also in this case redacted according to hearths, but the individual members of the households were identified (excepting children under the age of seven).

These two registrations of the population of 1332 and 1350 are not directly comparable: while nobody would consider it a necessity of life to pay taxes and tax evasion was rational behaviour at the individual level, salt was a necessity and the population would therefore have a vital interest in being registered with some significant exceptions and reservations. Day labourers who purchased all or most of their food for their wages would have only marginal interest in being registered, and this could possibly also to some extent have been the case for sub-tenants. All households with children would have a certain interest in claiming that as many as possible of their children were below the age of seven or to keep some of their children out of the registrars' way. Urban households that produced none or little of the food they consumed themselves would have a good motive for avoiding registration; when they wished to buy cheap seasonal food and cure it themselves for later consumption they would quite likely be able to buy at a nice price some of the surplus forced on other households. Urban households and rural households alike would undoubtedly frequently have reason to assume that their need for salt would be served also if they attempted to minimize the number of household members, concealing living-in servants or maids, lodgers, number of children above the age of six, and so on. Summing up, it is unrealistic and naïve to assume that the 'salt per mouth' census of 1350 was unaffected by evasion, although it can be accepted that it provides a more accurate registration of the population than the tax lists of 1332. Although an assumption of a deficit of 5 per cent is sanguine for ordinary tax records, this is not obviously the case with a census in relation to which the majority of the population would consider it vital to be registered. In relation to the tax records of 1332, the standard assumption of a deficit of 7.5 per cent will be applied. According to the tax records of 1332, the town and the rural districts contained 1,687 and 852 registered households, respectively, which, when corrected for an assumed underregistration of 7.5 per cent, correspond to estimated reconstructed totals of 1,824 and 921 households, in all 2,745 households.

According to the 'salt per mouth' tax of 1350, the town and rural districts contained 695 and 469 households, respectively.[16] When these registrations are corrected for an assumed underregistration of 5 per cent, these figures correspond to estimated reconstructed totals of 730 and 492 in the town and countryside, respectively. These numbers of households contain increases caused by marriages and immigration since the plague that must be deducted. According to the standard assumption on the surge in new marriages in the wake of the plague, the number of households will have increased by roughly 1.25 per cent in the town and 1.5 per cent in the countryside in the roughly 1.5 years from the end of the plague to the recording of the tax lists. Again the Bologna data on immigration must be used, which implies that the number of households in the town grew by about 1 per cent annually from this social development and from marriages contracted by young immigrants whether solitary or newly wed. This means that the countryside presumably lost almost the whole natural population increase through migration to the town, and that the reconstructed figure for 1350 for all practical considerations can be left unchanged. This implies that, on the morrow of the Black Death, there were 714 households in the town and 492 households in the countryside, in all 1,206 households.

Consequently, in the period 1332–50, the number of households in the town had diminished from 2,745 to 714 or by 61 per cent, the number in the countryside had declined from 921 households to 492 or by 46.5 per cent. In the whole commune of San Gimignano the number of households had declined from 2,745 to 1,206 or by 56 per cent.

16 Fiumi 1961: 166, 171.

The next problem is the question of average household size. In connection with the discussion of the same question in the general introductory comments, and, then, in relation to Florence, it was argued on various grounds that average household size must have been significantly smaller in the aftermath of the Black Death than before or a decade later. Table 13 above renders a number of Italian data on average household size in the decades around the Black Death. These data also comprise evidence from San Gimignano provided by the 'salt per mouth' census of 1350, which, according to Fiumi, shows that average household size cannot have exceeded 3.5 persons in the town and 4 persons in the surrounding rural districts, and was, thus, more likely in the order of magnitude of 3–3.5 persons in the town and 3.5–4 persons in the 'contado'.[17] The various problems of registration and evasion presented above indicate that the 'salt per mouth' tax was hardly as complete as assumed by Fiumi, and that his estimates of maximum household size should possibly rather be considered realistic central estimates. Because Fiumi does not reveal the premises of his estimates, nothing more can be said. This analysis is also, as mentioned, corroborated by Gelting's study of the individual fates of the constituent members of the 11 peasant households contained in the mountain hamlet of Grenis in Maurienne where not a single household escaped without loss of one or more members. On the basis of the Italian evidence contained in Table 13 above, it will be assumed that these figures for San Gimignano reflect that the Black Death had reduced the average household size in the town and in the countryside from 4 and 4.5 persons, respectively, in the pre-plague population to 3.5 and 4 persons on the morrow of the plague. The post-plague averages are considered maximum data by Fiumi, and Gelting's material also attests to the cautious nature of the assumption on the size of the decline in household size, i.e., by 0.5 person, which must be considered a minimum assumption. Use of these averages will tend to ensure that the mortality estimates will be on the low side.

When the reconstructed household estimates are multiplied with the estimated average household sizes in the town and the countryside, the following population estimates are produced (Table 14): in 1332, the town of San Gimignano contained 7,296 inhabitants, in the late autumn of 1348 there were only 2,500 inhabitants left, corresponding to a decline of the urban population of 66 per cent in the intervening years. The countryside had 4,145 inhabitants in 1332; this population had been reduced to 1,968 persons after the ravages of the Black Death, corresponding to a decline in the rural population of 52.5 per cent in the same period. The total population of the town of San Gimignano and the countryside under its domination was reduced from 11,441 inhabitants in 1332 to 4,467 inhabitants on the morrow of the epidemic, a diminution of 61 per cent for this Tuscan commune as a whole.

It cannot be concluded that the whole decline was due to the ravages of the Black Death. It must first be shown that the population had not declined in the years following the redaction of the tax records of 1332 up to the eve of the Black Death. The commune's population had been growing up to 1332, and because there are no indications of dearth in Tuscan sources, it may be assumed to have continued to grow in the following years. Probably the population of San Gimignano, like the populations elsewhere in Tuscany, suffered significant losses in the grave crisis of 1340, and

[17] Fiumi 1962: 280.

Table 14. Estimates of population, San Gimignano 1332 and 1349

San Gimignano	1332	1349	% Decline
Contado	4145	1968	52.5
Town	7296	2500	66
Commune	11441	4467	61

also some supermortality in the dearth of 1347. Presumably, it was easier to meet the needs of the relatively small population of San Gimignano with its own surrounding countryside than the population of the giant city of Florence with its huge industrial proletariat. For this reason, the relative population losses in the two crises in San Gimignano were quite likely less severe than reported by Giovanni Villani for Florence. Because the population had presumably been growing in the period 1332–9, it is not clear that the population was smaller in 1341 than a decade earlier. Also, the population of San Gimignano could have recuperated much of the loss in 1340 before the new crisis in 1347. Against this backcloth, it appears reasonable to infer that San Gimignano's population was not smaller on the eve of the Black Death than in 1332, and, if there was a reduction, it was quite slight. It appears, therefore, reasonable to conclude that the Black Death killed 60 per cent of San Gimignano's population, conspicuously, the same mortality rate as estimated for Florence. It is noteworthy that, in this case, the mortality was substantially higher in the town than in the 'contado'.

There are also interesting data available for another Tuscan area, the commune of Prato situated around 20 km north-west of Florence.[18] In 1339, a thorough census was taken of the population for the purpose of securing the provisioning of grain and flour for the population in a situation characterized by increasing dearth that would develop into a serious famine accompanied by epidemic hunger-related diseases in Tuscany in the following year. This was a census in which the population had strong motives to be recorded, especially the poor and the destitute who would hope that the commune would provide succour in a time of increasing need. It is, therefore, realistic to accept that the census is fairly complete. However, it is not perfect: for example, the mountain hamlet Popigliano, entered with 10 hearths in the tax lists of 1352, has fallen out of the census lists.[19] Because the number of hearths in this part of the mountains had declined by 43 per cent in the meantime, this hamlet may on statistical grounds be assumed to have contained 16 hearths with a population of 73 persons in 1339. According to the census, the city of Prato contained 10,559 persons and just crossed the sociological dividing line between towns and cities (see above). The countryside contained 7,763 persons (when the missing 73 have been added), and altogether the commune contained 18,419 inhabitants in 1339.

The earliest post-plague population registers that can be compared to the 1339 census are tax records organized according to households relating to one of the city's wards in 1351, namely the ward of Porta Fuia, and this is the only extant source

---

[18] Fiumi 1968: 71–88.
[19] Popigliano also appears in the tax lists of 1372. Fiumi 1968: 87, 73–5, 89–90.

material that can be used for estimating the mortality of the Black Death in the city. In 1339, this ward had 349 households containing, on average, only 3.56 members, corresponding to a total population of 1,243 persons. The lists of 1351 record 222 households.[20] According to the relevant standard assumptions, this figure must be assumed to represent an underregistration of 6 per cent, and to contain a post-plague increase of 3 per cent owing to the surge in new marriages and immigration that must be deducted, and to conceal a decline in the average household size by 0.5 persons to three members. This means that the population of the ward had declined from 1,242 persons in 1339 to 685 persons in the aftermath of the Black Death, a decline of 45 per cent. Taking into consideration the local government's well-organized programme for providing the population with grain and flour within a territory with control over a largish countryside, one would tend to assume that the losses in the crises of the 1340s were considerably smaller than Giovanni Villani indicates in the case of the huge industrial city of Florence, and that the city of Prato had largely recuperated from the losses in the larger crisis of 1340 by the time the milder crisis came in 1347. Probably, in the year of the Black Death the mortality in this ward was 42.5–45 per cent.

Fortunately, the records of a tax survey systematically registering the number of households in each locality of the rural districts in the autumn of 1352 are extant, and this survey can likewise be compared with the census of 1339 according to the standard assumptions established above for this type of estimate. With one exception, all villages and hamlets show either a sharp fall in the numbers of households between 1339 and 1352 or, in a few cases, stability in numbers. The exception is Sorniana, which is entered in the records with six hearths in 1339 and 17 in 1352, a sharp deviation from the general pattern that must be considered due to some sort of scribe's error, and is therefore here reduced from 17 to 7, which introduces Sorniana into the tiny category of localities with a stable number of households.

According to the census of 1339, the rural districts of the commune of Prato contained 1,796 hearths containing, on average, 4.3 persons, 7,723 persons in all. In 1352, the registrars recorded 1,032 hearths in the countryside which, when corrected for an underregistration of 6 per cent, indicates a more realistic figure of 1,098 hearths ≈ 1,100 hearths. In the three years elapsing from the Black Death to the redaction of the tax lists, the number of households would have grown by 2.25 per cent according to the standard assumption, but it would also have lost a comparable number of persons by emigration to the city. This means that the number of households recorded in the tax lists is reasonably similar to the number of households on the morrow of the Black Death; thus, these two factors cancel each other out and can be disregarded. These households contained on average 3.8 persons, corresponding to a total rural population of 4,180 persons. This means that the population decline in the period 1339–49 was 46 per cent. In order to take into account some possible population decline between 1339 and the arrival of the Black Death, it appears reasonable to conclude that the rural population of the commune of Prato probably suffered a mortality rate of around 45 per cent. The mortality rates in the ward of Porta Fuia in the city and in the 'contado' are conspicuously similar and could suggest that, in this

---

[20] According to Fiumi, another 10 hearths were 'non allibrati', entered in the records but not as taxable, presumably because they were uninhabited.

case, the mortality in the Black Death was about the same in the city and the country-side.

Thirteen hamlets (containing on average 11 hearths) of the 58 villages or hamlets in the rural districts of the commune of Prato in 1339 are not mentioned in 1352. They must be considered desolated by the combined effects of the Black Death and rapid desertion by the survivors when they suddenly had the opportunity to move to better tenements in larger settlements with a more comprehensive and intensive social life. Two of these deserted settlements are mentioned in the tax lists of 1372 as settled,[21] i.e., probably resettled.

On the other hand, five settlements have about the same number of households as in 1339 or, in one case, there is a small but significant increase. These settlements were probably passed over by the plague, although immigration may have veiled the fact that these settlements were also visited. These figures indicate that no more than five settlements or 8.6 per cent of the total number of settlements were passed over by the Black Death. Interestingly, this figure is quite similar to the figure for 215 villages in two merindads in the Kingdom of Navarre (in Spain), namely 6.8 per cent (see above).

In the census of 1339, the rural districts were divided into three sectors comprising mountain settlements, and two sectors comprising settlements in the plain. Compared to the tax records of 1352, it can be seen that the number of registered households had declined by 38 per cent in the plain and by 47.5 per cent in the mountains. This difference does not necessarily reflect any disparate impact of the Black Death. Instead, it could reflect that surviving families of the numerous rural proletarian classes of smallholders, cotters and sub-tenants in the mountain villages moved into the good vacant tenancies in the larger villages of the plain. In addition, it could reflect a stream of migrants in the aftermath of the Black Death from poor agricultural areas and marginal settlements colonized under the impact of extreme population pressure to better tenements associated with the larger villages in the more fertile old-settled areas in order to improve their economic situation and to seek a more gratifying social life. This may explain why nine of the deserted hamlets are found in the plain. Migration from the mountain settlements to the plain would take somewhat more time to filter through the difficulties inherent in moving and reset-tling at a distance. In such desperate times, it must also have been more difficult for the city government to organize material support for the distant parts of the 'contado' than for the city itself and its surrounding districts, which also could explain some of the difference.

According to these estimates, the commune of Prato suffered a mortality rate of about 45 per cent in the rural districts. The mortality rate in the urban centre remains more uncertain, because it has only been possible to perform an estimate for one of its eight wards containing about 10 per cent of the total number of households in 1339. The estimated mortality rate of 45 per cent (42.5–45 per cent) is conspicuously similar.

It appears possible to conclude that the Black Death caused a mortality rate of 45 per cent in the commune of Prato, and that possibly, also in this case, there was no or

[21] Fiumi 1968: 89–90.

insignificant difference in mortality between the small city and the rural districts of its 'contado'.

Within the region of Tuscany, there was at the time of the Black Death also another large independent city state besides Florence, namely Siena, which comprised both the city of Siena with over 50,000 inhabitants and a large 'contado'. Siena lies about 50 km south of Florence. At the time, the Italian towns and cities made great efforts to defend themselves, all men between 16/18 years and 60/70 years fit to bear arms were enrolled in military units according to wards or other administrative divisions. In Siena, the number of military companies was reduced from 43 on the eve of the Black Death to 21 in the immediate aftermath, i.e., by 51 per cent.

In this case, it is not necessary to consider the problems of underregistration, because two series of the same source in close proximity in time are compared. However, the representativeness of the mortality in the social classes that were recruited into these military units is a relevant issue. All men fit for military service were supposed to be registered, but they would see their individual interests served in evading registration both for economic and military reasons. The lowest classes of poor and destitute inhabitants consisted to a large extent of day labourers or industrial workers who often endeavoured to keep body and soul together by casual work. They constituted a fleeting social class that would move around between the wards of the poor or between the city and the countryside and could not be accurately registered whatever the ambitions and capabilities of the city's political leadership or the registrars. Members of these social classes could neither afford to acquire military equipment nor to pay taxes for procurement of arms, so the cost effectiveness of arming and training men of these social classes would be doubtful, as would the meaningfulness of continuous and meticulous registration. In this society, disease and disablement were rampant; many would not be registered because they would not be physically fit to bear arms, and the introduction of substantial numbers of unfit men into the registers would reduce their usefulness in times of military need.

As can be seen, problems of underregistration relate mostly to social classes and categories of people who would tend to suffer particularly high rates of mortality because they lived in overcrowded areas in overcrowded rooms in bad housing, and in unsavoury and filthy environments that would be ideal for rats, and which included relatively many persons handicapped by disablement or poor health. They were particularly vulnerable to secondary catastrophe effects, because they would have no or very sparse means by which they could acquire necessities of life when economic life broke down and the trickle of petty income they relied on for their livelihood dried up, and because elementary services for the diseased in the form of nursing care and feeding would tend to break down. In the words of the Florentine chronicler Marchionne di Coppo Stefani: 'many died by themselves and many died of hunger'. As underlined above, children were particularly vulnerable to neglect when their parents fell ill, and would for this reason suffer substantial supermortality, especially when they contracted the disease, but also if they did not.

Also, as pointed out above, children and adolescents have a particularly fulminant course of plague disease and accordingly suffer high case fatality rates. Women have an especially high risk of exposure because they spend more time than men in the houses where black rats with their consorts of fleas like to stay. Pregnant women invariably die from plague infection, and in those times a substantial proportion of women of fertile ages were pregnant at any time.

Consequently, the reduction in the number of military companies may cautiously be taken to suggest a proportional loss of men in the social classes from which they were recruited in the plague epidemic. The fact that the ruling political and bureaucratic groups suffered losses around 50 per cent may be said to provide some support for a mortality rate of around 50 per cent also for these social classes.[22] However, when we also take into account the arguments presented in the preceding paragraphs, it should be clear that the general population mortality must have been substantially higher, at least 55–60 per cent, and quite likely around 60 per cent.

There is an additional piece of interesting independent evidence relating to the city of Siena, in that the interments in the cemetery of the monastery of San Dominico are known by name in lists running from 1336. In the period up to the arrival of the Black Death, the average annual number of burials was 20, but one should note that this figure is affected by an increased rate of registration owing to the dearth of 1346–7. In the plague year, the registration suddenly breaks off in June when the epidemic is near its height of intensity, obviously because the person or persons in charge of keeping the registers died, and registration was not taken up again in a regular way until the end of August. Extrapolating the mortality curve for the period with no or only incidental registration, the total number of interments in 1348 can be estimated at 400–420.[23] This means that the mortality level in 1348 was 20–21 times higher than the average of the preceding twelve years.

Professor Massimo Livi Bacchi and Professor Lorenzo Del Panta, the two leading Italian historical demographers, who discuss these lists of interments, interpret them as reflecting the normal death rate in a representative sample of the general population. Del Panta assumes on unspecified grounds that normal mortality in the general population was 3–4 per cent, which means that he arrives at a mortality rate in the Black Death of 60–80 per cent. However, because medieval mortality rates were higher than early modern rates, the estimate according to this approach will be in the higher reaches of that range. Importantly, the average annual number of burials in the years following the Black Death was reduced by 60 per cent, which Del Panta considers as a significant corroboration of the estimate. It is not problematic that the implied mortality rate is significantly and even substantially higher in the recruitment area to this cemetery than in Siena as a whole, for considerable variation between wards and other subdivisions of the city is to be expected.

One could also raise the question of a possible deficit of infants and children in these lists, which is such a pervasive feature of medieval population records. However, the composition of the cohorts according to age is not given by the scholars, and one must believe that they have considered this problem without finding problematic aspects of this kind in the lists. If significant immigration supplemented the population in the post-plague years, these immigrants would also be recruited into the cemetery by the Grim Reaper and become registered in the post-plague lists. These social processes would tend to veil the real impact of the Black Death. In view

[22] Bowsky 1964: 18.
[23] Livi Bacchi 1978: 13; Del Panta 1980: 115.

of this likely development, a mortality rate of 60 per cent tends to take on the character of a minimum estimate. The tentative character of these comments must be stressed.

Before summing up this discussion of the demographic effects of the Black Death in the region of Tuscany, it is practical and useful to include valuable data from an adjacent area, namely the city of Bologna (province of Emilia Romagna), situated about 80 km north of Florence and containing at the time at least 35,000–50,000 inhabitants. As in the case of Siena, it is the military registers of men fit to bear arms that provide statistically usable demographic information on the impact of the Black Death. In Bologna, all men in the ages 18–69 were obliged to do military service. In addition to the general registers of armed men, a parallel series of military registers was produced in which each year the armed men were entered into lists quarter by quarter according to parish. Exceptionally, 46 of these lists are preserved for the year 1348 and 44 for the following year, and in twenty cases they relate to the same parishes and can be compared to identify the mortality rate in the Black Death. In 1348, they contained the names of 1,207 armed men, corresponding to about 12 per cent of the total number of armed men in the city on the eve of the Black Death. In 1349, the number of armed men had been reduced to 783, a decline of 35 per cent.[24]

However, as shown above in connection with Siena, it is easy to marshal arguments that indicate higher mortality rates in the general population than among men in ages 18 and older. For the same reasons, a decline in the number of registered armed men between 1348 and 1349 of 35 per cent indicates arguably a mortality rate of at least 40–45 per cent, and quite likely around 45 per cent, especially when the importance of secondary catastrophe effects on the lower classes is taken into account. In addition, in 1349, the survivors in the cohort of those young men who were 17 years and unregistered in 1348, would now be registered, and this cohort would be the largest of them all and far larger than the average of the 52 cohorts. Probably, they constituted an addition of at least 3 per cent to the lists of armed men.

The mortality estimates include cities, towns and rural districts and comprise a substantial proportion of Tuscany's population, although it is a weakness that there is a relative overrepresentation of urban populations. Estimates of rural populations are limited to those of San Gimignano and Prato. Perhaps, the rural mortality data can be supported somewhat by more flimsy and impressionistic evidence in the form of general contemporary assertions that acquire some credibility because they are consistent. They are consistent to the effect that the mortality in the Black Death was as high in the countryside as in the urban centres.

Matteo Villani, who finished his brother's chronicle, asserts in the second chapter that the Black Death made no difference between any sort of people within the confines of the city state: 'There died in the city, contado and rural districts of Florence of each gender and every age three out of [all] five [persons], or more.' Matteo Villani's view on mortality, that at least 60 per cent of the population of the city state of Florence died in the Black Death, is in accordance with the estimate of the mortality rate in the city of Florence. This accordance with the result of modern

---

[24] Pini and Greci 1976: 380.

demography and social science lends some credibility too to his assertion that the countryside was as badly ravaged. Boccaccio makes a similar assertion in the Introduction to Decameron. Herlihy summarizes this impressionistic evidence relating to the effects of the Black Death in Tuscany thus:

> There is, at least at present, no certain evidence that either of these two areas, town or countryside, offered consistently greater protection against the ravenous plagues of the late Middle Ages. Death, the great equalizer, seems to have taxed rural communities and urban communities with equal severity.[25]

There is some interesting variation in mortality rates at the consistently very high levels revealed by these estimates. The lowest mortality estimates pertain to Prato, where around 45 per cent of the population in the countryside and in the ward of Porta Fuia in the commune's small city perished in the plague year. This level is conspicuously lower than in San Gimignano, especially in the case of the town, and than in the industrial centres of Florence and Siena where mortality rates appear to have been around 60 per cent. It is difficult to explain this difference. An explanatory idea could be to consider differences in secondary catastrophe effects. One could take a keen interest in the fact that the governing elite of Prato initiated a complete registration of the population in 1339 in order to acquire vital knowledge of the need for supplementary grain and flour for the population in the face of increasing dearth. This commune may appear to have been particularly well and responsibly run, and it is interesting to note that the governing elite took immediate action to be prepared for a crisis that they could not know would take on a more serious character in the following year.

In these endeavours, the governing elite may have been helped by the fact that there was quite a good balance between the size of the city population and the rural population. In Florence, with its huge industrial proletariat, the task of securing the provisioning of the population in times of dearth and crisis would be much more difficult, not to say impossible, to realize in any efficient way. In other words, the industrial urban centres in Tuscany would suffer particularly high mortality rates in times of great crises or disasters because they had grown out of their medieval societal basis and taken on an early modern, capitalistic and industrial structure that the city governments were not mentally, administratively or technologically equipped to handle.

One should also keep in mind that the Black Death ravaged Tuscany in the crucial months of the agricultural year. Almost inevitably much of the normal agricultural production must have broken down when large proportions of the agricultural population fell seriously ill in an important period of agricultural work. In his study of the Black Death in Siena, Bowsky cites a contemporary chronicler on the situation in the 'contado': 'Almost all work ceased during the summer of 1348. Fields were neglected and animals left untended, as men were scarcely able to care for their own ill.'[26] This is another dimension of the secondary catastrophe effects: generally, serious plague epidemics reached the height of intensity in the summer and autumn and were followed by dearth and famine because agricultural work had broken down. The

[25] Herlihy 1970: 88.
[26] Bowsky 1964: 23, cf. passim.

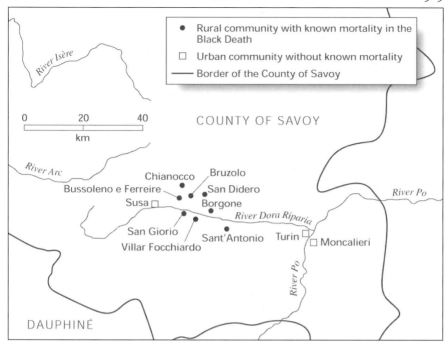

Map 4. Villages with known mortality in the Black death in the Piedmont

other dimension of secondary catastrophe mortality is also hinted at, that people had great difficulties in providing nursing care for the diseased.

Summing up the evidence on the mortality in the Black Death in Tuscany and Bologna (see Table 16 below), it becomes difficult to explain and defend the usual notion that the Black Death caused a mortality rate of a quarter or one-third of Tuscany's population, while it has become easy to argue for a mortality rate about twice as high. Actually, the orthodox low estimates appear to be without foundation in demographic studies, for all studies on statistically valid source material exhibit at least substantially and usually much higher mortality rates. Taken together, the present data suggest that 50–60 per cent of the Tuscan population died in the Black Death.

A few other mortality data reflecting the carnage wrought by the Black Death in Italy have been established for the north-western region of the Piedmont. Piedmont means 'mountain-foot', which in this case refers to the valleys and plain stretching south-wards from the foot of the western Alpine mountain range on France and Switzerland almost to the Mediterranean Sea. Most of the northern and central parts of the Piedmont belonged at the time to the County of Savoy. This is also the case with the localities for which useful mortality data are known, but the pertinent mortality data will be discussed here in the context of the territory of the modern province of the Piedmont within the modern national borders of Italy, while the other mortality of Savoyan localities will be discussed in the next chapter, on France.

These data pertain to eight villages situated on or close to the old road along the

Table 15. Number of hearths (households) in villages near Susa,
Piedmont 1335–67

Village	Hearths 1335	Hearths 1356	Hearths 1367
Sant'Antonino	50	40	24
Villar Focchiardo	116	61	56
San Giorio	129	70	50
Chianocco	71	45	38
Bussoleno e Ferreire	217	159	79
Total	583	375	247
Borgone	66	31	
San Didero	20	9	
Bruzolo	71	44	
Total	740	459	

Sources: Rotelli 1973: 87; Comba 1977: 75–7.

R. Dora Riparia between the city of Turin and the town of Susa, 52 km to the
north-west. They were situated considerably closer to Susa than to Turin, at a distance
of about 10–25 km, but not so far away from Turin than that at least some of them
could have substantial economic contact with this city (see Map 4). It is also clear that
communities with locations on or close to such an important route of trade and travel
would be particularly vulnerable to contamination of epidemic disease.

The data for these eight villages are based on registrations of households in 1335
and 1356 (Table 15). Such few and isolated data taken from sources at a significant
distance in time from the Black Death are difficult to mould into reliable generalized
information, but in view of the general scarcity of data they should not be passed
over. These villages were quite large, containing on average 92.5 households in 1335
compared with, for instance, an average of 32 households for the 56 villages and
hamlets in Prato's countryside. This reflects their attractive qualities: they were situated on or near the fertile bottom of the valley, and the advantageous proximity to
the quite large town of Susa ensured easy sale of surplus production at good prices,
which could be exchanged for the goods, services and social attractions of the town;
not far away was also the city of Turin, which offered more of the same attractions for
a somewhat higher input of effort. These factors must be taken into account in the discussion of the settlement developments in the decades around the Black Death.

Not much is known about average household size in the Piedmont at the time. In
1374, the commune of Moncalieri near the city of Turin produced a census aimed at
ascertaining the need for supplementary acquisitions of grain and flour for distribution in times of dearth. The purpose of the registration ensures that it will be quite
complete. The census registered 834 households that contained, on average, 4.32
members,[27] which is astonishingly similar to the Tuscan data on household size (cf.
Table 13 above).

[27] Rotelli 1973: 33.

Data on the number of households in six villages near Susa are available for the year 1331, which, when compared with the data of 1335, show insignificant change in this period. Thus, average household size should be expected to reflect the modest size associated with a stationary population, and a household size of 4.32 persons is easily compatible with this general picture. This was probably also the situation on the eve of the Black Death. The years of dearth in 1339 and 1347 did not have serious consequences in this sub-Alpine area where animal husbandry constituted a large part of the economy, a part that was not so vulnerable to the vicissitudes of weather as arable husbandry.

After the Black Death, in the years 1361–2,[28] the Piedmont was ravaged by the second wave of plague epidemics that spread across Europe. The strong decline in the number of households between 1356 and 1367 is a very conspicuous feature of Table 15, the proportional decline being almost as large as in the period 1335–56, which included the Black Death. The probable explanation for this feature is that a high proportion of the households had so few adult members on the eve of the next plague epidemic that they had little tolerance of further reduction and were liable to collapse. Such households could have various origins: many surviving households could have been decimated in the Black Death according to a pattern demonstrated by Gelting in the mountain hamlet of Grenis in Maurienne on the French side of the mountain range (County of Savoy), where every peasant household lost one or more members; others consisted of newly married young people who had moved out of their families of origin in order to settle on good vacant tenements (strong population pressures before the Black Death meant that there were few vacant tenements so that many marriageable young persons were forced to stay in the hearth); new cohorts of young persons of marriageable age grew up in the years after the Black Death up to 1356; others could have been formed by newly married living-in servants and maids who had moved out of their employers' households and settled on vacant good tenements; others could have been settled by young people from the mountain settlements who seized the opportunity to take up good vacant tenements in large villages with a more intensive social life, on or near the fertile valley bottom and in the proximity of the town with its attractions. Many reasons can be discerned for there to be many small and vulnerable households with a low proportion of adults in these villages when the next plague arrived.

However, these arguments do not really explain why this feature should have been especially marked in this area, and there is no means of distinguishing between the various factors that could make it possible to establish the real cause or the nexus of causes of household breakdowns in these communities. This line of argument makes it clear that the Black Death itself triggered a number of social responses that would tend to veil the real demographic impact of the epidemic as expressed in the number

---

[28] Comba 1977: 88. According to Comba's list of epidemics, there were plague epidemics in the large town of Alessandria in south-eastern Piedmont both in 1357 and 1360, and one outbreak in the small town of Cavallermaggiore in 1363. However, at the time the terms 'peste' and 'pestilenze' were generic for epidemic disease, and these singular dispersed outbreaks in quite distant areas of the Piedmont cannot be associated with general demographic developments in other parts of the region. The small town of Cavallermaggiore is situated only 40 km from Moncalieri, which today functions as a suburban area to the great city of Turin. When there is no hint in the sources about plague in Turin, it is not likely that there was plague in Moncalieri; the outbreak of an epidemic in Cavallermaggiore could be any noteworthy epidemic outbreak.

of households recorded in 1356. Undoubtedly, the demographic impact of the Black Death was substantially stronger than measured by changes in the number of households alone, and the unusual frequency of household breakdown after the second plague epidemic must reflect a high degree of vulnerability associated with a small average household size and relatively few adults after the ravages of the Black Death.

However, there is also a line of argument with a substantial explanatory potential that relates specifically to areas with this type of mixed agriculture. It could also be that widows had a better opportunity to establish themselves as householders by focusing on animal husbandry, which did not require the same high input of muscular strength as, for instance, ploughing.

In this region too, the population pressure characteristic of the last part of the High Middle Ages and the decades preceding the Black Death had occasioned the growth of a large proletarian class of sub-tenants, cottars and day labourers who were poorly registered because they did not bear any tax assessment. In the wake of the ravages of the Black Death, such humble people moved into vacant tenements and entered the taxpaying and rentpaying social classes. This is a social process that, for instance, is very much in evidence in a study of the Black Death in the castellany of Montmélian in the County of Savoy on the other side of this western Alpine mountain range (see below). This burst of upwards social mobility will veil some of the real impact of plague as measured in the number of registered households. This depletion of the proletarian classes also means that the percentage of unregistered households must have been significantly lower after the Black Death than before, because there were fewer households to be missed and fewer households that were of no real interest to the registrars and their employers.

The following assumptions constitute the basis for conservative population and mortality estimates: an average household size before the Black Death of 4.32 persons, which in the aftermath of the Black Death had declined to 3.82 persons according to the established standard assumption; a growth of 10 per cent in the number of households in the seven years from the Black Death to 1356, owing to the combined effects of the formation of numerous new families of diverse social and demographic origins and upwards social mobility of rural proletarians into the class of tenants. Converting the number of peasant households into the size of the peasant population according to these premises, the villages contained 3,197 ≈ 3,200 persons in 1335 and 1,598 ≈ 1,600 persons in 1349, a diminution of 50 per cent. A possible small decline in the populations of these villages caused by the dearths of 1339 and 1347 and not recuperated may be taken into account. However, when we also take into account a probable higher incidence of underregistration of households in 1335 than in 1356, these two factors will tend to cancel each other out. Supermortality of the poor and destitute social classes should also be taken into count according to the established standard assumption that it would usually raise the level of general mortality by 2.5 percentage points above the mortality level of the peasant classes. This indicates a central estimate of the general population mortality in these villages from the ravages of the Black Death of about 52.5 per cent.

The question of the representativeness of the demographic changes in these large villages in the proximity of a largish town in the sub-Alpine valley of Susa for the demographic developments in the Piedmontese region as a whole presents insoluble problems. The best that can be said for the estimate is that it is based on realistic assumptions and that the outcome accords with the other estimates of population decline caused by the Black Death. Consistency of independent estimates normally represents a strength for scholarly studies.

Summing up the Italian evidence on the Black Death's demographic effects, a population decline in the Black Death of the order of magnitude of 55 per cent is indicated as the central value, and most of the margins of uncertainty will be covered by a broader estimate of 50–60 per cent. Most of the margins of uncertainty are owing to the marked overrepresentation of urban data and the limited number of studies. The rather narrow territorial basis of these studies limits their evidential strength mostly to Tuscany and the adjacent regions (Table 16). However, the Piedmontese data expand the territorial horizon to include this region, because they fit so well into the general picture. Because the Piedmontese data relate to rural districts, they also serve to strengthen the impression that the countryside was ravaged in much the same way as the urban centres.

Table 16. Estimated population mortality rates (%) in the Black Death in Tuscany and two other Italian localities

Localities	Urban centres	Contado
Florence	60	
San Gimignano	66	52.5
Prato	(42.5–)45	45
Siena	60	
Bologna	45	
Valle Susa		52.5
'Italia'	50–60	

The available data do not really allow inferences for Italy as a whole. It has been speculated that other parts of Italy, for instance the southern half, may have suffered markedly lower mortality rates. However, the Black Death spread as powerfully in the countryside as in the towns and cities, and Italian mortality data are not different from mortality rates elsewhere in Southern Europe, in Spain (see above) or in Provence, south-central France or the County of Savoy (see below). The assumption that southern Italy suffered lower mortality rates than northern Italy has no factual basis.

30

France and the County of Savoy (including South-Western Valais in Present-day Switzerland)

The French studies of the demographic effects of the Black Death have the same strongly lopsided territorial character as the Italian. With one exception they relate to southern or south-eastern France, the exception being a town on the south-central plateau of Forez that can be considered adjacent to the areas of the other data. Provence and the County of Savoy are covered by a surprising number of good or at least fairly good data. This means that we have at best good data for roughly 6–7 per cent of France's territory of today, and, in addition, three sources of data for largish urban centres west and north of Languedoc, comprising in all something like 10 per cent of France, and probably a roughly corresponding proportion of France's population. Consequently, the available data do not really permit inference to the whole country. Nonetheless, they provide valuable information on the ravages of the Black Death in three regions containing large populations, vital urban centres and a productive agriculture.

Baratier's admirable study on the historical demography of Provence is still the centrepiece of information on the demographic impact of the Black Death and later plague epidemics in this region. The sources that can be used to estimate mortality rates in the Black Death are a type of fiscal registers called 'feu d'albergue' in which the whole population was supposed to be recorded according to hearths/households, along with the poor and destitute. Only the generally tax-exempted clerical and noble classes were left out as a matter of principle, social elites that constituted around 8 per cent of the Provençal population.[1] A significantly lower mortality among these privileged classes than among the non-privileged 92 per cent of the population is likely and would affect total mortality estimates only marginally. Pre-plague and post-plague records of this type are so comprehensive that they are well suited for comparison in order to identify general population changes in the intervening period.

No French fiscal records provide information on household size and composition. Baratier concluded that he would refrain from producing population estimates on the

---

1   Baratier 1961: 32–5.

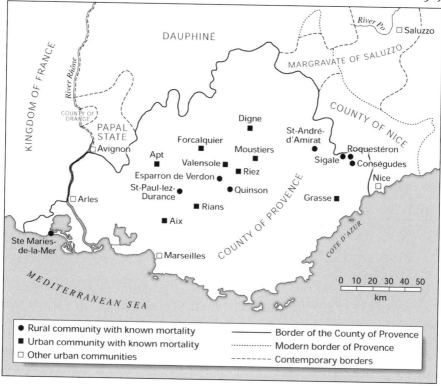

Map 5. Localities with known mortality in the Black Death in the County of Provence

basis of conjectures on average household size and would identify population developments only by comparing changes in the numbers of households over time.[2] This approach leads to underestimations of the real decline in populations caused by the Black Death, because households would tend to be significantly smaller on the morrow of the onslaught than before it. However, he also states that in Provence, with its strong Italian ethnic and cultural influences, a practical solution would be to introduce Italian data on average household size. In the years following the publication of Baratier's book, interesting Italian data on household size were produced, which have been presented and commented on above in connection with the discussion of the mortality rate(s) caused by the Black Death in Italy. These data show lower average household sizes than he imagined, namely of the order of magnitude of 4 and 4.5 persons in towns and countryside, respectively, before the Black Death and 3.5 and 4 persons, respectively, on the morrow of the epidemic (Table 13 above).

In the first half of the fourteenth century, the size of Provence's population appears to have been quite stationary, although this overall stability conceals some variation in different parts of the region.[3] According to Baratier, between one-fourth and one-third of the population lived in urban centres; today the lower proportion

---

[2] Baratier 1961: 58–61.
[3] Baratier 1961: 80.

appears the more likely. Although Provence was far more urbanized than most of Europe, at about the same level as Tuscany, it is still true that rural data showing mortality among the peasantry are more valuable and telling than urban data, especially for the development of notions on general population mortality rates.

Table 17 shows numbers of hearths/households in various localities in Provence before and after the Black Death, organized according to size of community and year of registration. The dividing line between rural communities and urban communities, which is assumed to lie around 1,000 inhabitants, corresponds to 220–250 pre-plague households. The table contains estimates for nine towns and seven rural communities. Except for Aix and Grasse, which were medium-sized towns with around 6,000 and 5,400 inhabitants, respectively, the others were more or less small; the largest rural community was Sigale with around 650 inhabitants, and several of the rural communities had probably below 200 inhabitants. The towns in the table contain over 7,000 of the 18,000 registered pre-plague urban households in Provence, i.e., 39 per cent. As they are distributed all over the region, there can be no doubt about the urban material's representativeness.

The rural households in the table have a useful territorial distribution, but represent only 1.3 per cent of all registered pre-plague rural households (45,000).[4] Because rural households constitute three-quarters of the Provençal population, this fact could jeopardize endeavours to approach the question of the regional mortality rate in the Black Death. However, the data in the table, reflecting registrations at various points in the 1340s and 1350s, show remarkable consistency: the decline in the number of urban households amounts to 52 per cent, while the decline in the number of rural households to 52.5 per cent. This consistency lends the figures considerable credibility, as does the conspicuous similarity to the Italian and Spanish estimates. This reflects the fact that there are no obvious biases in the material that has survived to posterity. Much material has been lost through the centuries, but the reasons for the losses have not had a selectively biased character with respect to the problem discussed in this chapter. In this situation, quite small samples will do – a fact modern opinion pollsters build on.

However, there can be no doubt that the real decline in the numbers of households caused by the Black Death was significantly larger. The data for six of nine towns relate to the years 1354–7, and four of the seven rural data relate to the years 1352–5. This means that the number of households constituting the populations of these communities had been affected by the surge in new marriages after the plague for a number of years before the tax lists were produced (as in Givry), especially in the towns that had, on average, an extra two years to recuperate compared to the rural areas, according to the dating of the various tax lists. It also means that we must assume a significant migration of people from the countryside into the towns in these years. A quite moderate assumption would be that these processes had caused an annual increase in the number of registered urban households of about 1 per cent, constituted by an internal growth rate of 0.5 per cent and an immigration corresponding to a growth rate of another 0.5 per cent; in both cases, rates would be higher in the first couple of years and, then, tend to taper off to more normal rates. The fact that 75 per cent of the Provençal population lived in the country-

---

4   The total figures of registered households are found in Baratier 1961: 67.

Table 17. Changes in the number of households before and after the Black Death according to hearths *d'albergue* in towns and villages of Provence[a] (cf. Map 5)

Locality	1340	1345	1349	1350	1352	1354	1355	1356	%
Aix		1486						810	45.5
Grasse	1360			738					45.5
Apt		926					444		52.0
Riez	680					213			69.0
Valensole	660					226			66.0
Moustiers	622					204			67.0
Forcalquier	600			281					53.0
Digne[b]	444						260		41.5
Rians	300		213						29.0
Sigale		144			75				48.0
Conségudes		40	12						70.0
Roquestéron		110			49				55.5
Saint-André		40	11						72.5
Saint-Paul		92	40						72.5
Quinson		122				66			46.0
Esparron	29					22			24.0
Totals		7655				3664			52.0

[a] Baratier 1961: 82, 128–9, 165, 179. This tax was collected from Michaelmas to Michaelmas. Except for 1349, all indications of year include most of the next year and should be read as 1340–1, and so on. Saint-Paul-le-Fougassier appears to be identical with Saint-Paul-lez-Durance north-east of Aix; as for Saint-André-d'Amirat, I have assumed that it is identical with the small village called Amirat in the district (canton) of Saint Auban, north of Grasse.
[b] The demographic developments in Digne with its 'bourg', its suburb, may appear somewhat unusual. In 1263–4, 440 households were registered in the town itself and 154 in its 'bourg', 594 in all; in 1315–16 the figures were 500 + 131, 631 in all; in 1323–4 the figures were 480 + 104, 594 in all; in 1332 the figures were 475 households in the town and 82 in the 'bourg', a significant increase in the town but an overall decline to 557 households, or by 6 per cent. This is the last fiscal registration that also includes the 'bourg'. In 1340–1 the town's 'feu d'albergue' contained, as given in the table, 444 households; in 1355–6 the number was 260. Seen in this perspective, it may appear that a decline in the urban centre's population commenced in the period 1315–24, and that this triggered a concomitant process of migration from the 'bourg' to the town. When we only have the figures for the town for the nearest pre-plague register and for the post-plague register, the result is that the migration from the 'bourg' into the town in the seven years following the Black Death will distort substantially the reflection of the carnage in the town. One must also take into account that the population could have continued to sag in the years from the last preserved pre-plague registration in 1340–1 to the arrival of the Black Death. Taken together, these considerations indicate that Digne should be taken out of the table and the synthetic estimates, because the real meanings of the figures are too unclear and problematic.

side means that an immigration rate corresponding to an annual increase in the towns' numbers of households of c. 0.5 per cent had so little impact on the development of the size of the population in the countryside that it can be ignored in this case. The population of the countryside will be assumed to have increased as measured in the number of households at an annual rate of 0.75 per cent, affected also by a great surge in marriage rates, as recorded in the marriage registers of Givry, for instance. This means that, on the morrow of the Black Death, at the end of 1348, the towns in Table 17 contained only 3,200 households and the villages 265 households (when the data of July 1349 are taken into account), 3,465 households in all. When these factors are taken into account, the diminution in the number of households in the Black Death was 54 per cent in the countryside and 55 per cent in the towns.

Next, the question of the decline in the corresponding population must be considered. This means that the households must be multiplicatively related to notions of household size, notions that must also take into account the reduction in the average household size caused by the Black Death. According to the standard assumption on this subject, average household size was reduced from 4.5 persons to 4 persons in the countryside and from 4 persons to 3.5 persons in the towns. Use of these household multipliers produces the following results: the total population contained in the registered households in Table 17 declined from 30,950 persons on the eve of the Black Death to 12,260 on the morrow of the epidemic onslaught, i.e., by c. 60.5 per cent; the towns' populations declined by 60.5 per cent, the villages' populations by 59 per cent. The difference between the urban and rural mortality rates is so small that it is well within the margins of uncertainty, and does not signal any need for further adjustment of the mortality estimate.

However, a third factor must also be taken into account, in that surviving members of the proletarian classes must be assumed to have moved into good vacant tenements and jobs in the aftermath of the plague and had joined the better-recorded taxpaying classes. Although these tax lists ('feu d'albergue') were also supposed to record the poor and destitute social classes, there can be no doubt that a significant proportion of them used to be passed over by the registrars, but would now be recorded in their new social positions. This development would tend to veil some of the impact of the Black Death. For the same reason, it must also be assumed that the post-plague registrations of the populations were more complete than the pre-plague registrations, because there now were not only fewer households, but also in relative terms substantially fewer proletarian households that could be insouciantly passed over. These considerations point in the direction that the estimate of population mortality in the Black Death should be rounded slightly upwards. However, the urban mortality rate based on a high proportion of urban households in Provence is slightly higher than the rural mortality rate based on a quite small sample of the rural households in the region, which means that a proportional representation of rural households would possibly or quite likely have tended to reduce slightly the estimate back to around 60 per cent.

The final question relates to population developments in the 1340s. According to Baratier, in most of Lower Provence the population continued to grow up to 1345 (when our pre-plague data are discontinued), and while the first symptoms of regression are noticeable in Upper Provence, the general impression is of overall stand still.[5] More than

5   1961: 80.

half of the pre-plague data in Table 17 are from registers produced in 1340–1, in other words produced during and in the immediate aftermath of the serious crisis of 1340. In the following years the population must be assumed to have recuperated gradually from possible supermortality, and, thus, to have become larger, i.e., comprising more hearths than indicated in the population data in the table. To a smaller extent this could also be the case with the data of 1345–6. On the other hand, it cannot be ruled out that this population was negatively affected by a smaller crisis caused by a poor harvest in 1347, from which it would not have had time to recuperate before the onslaught of the Black Death. These considerations tend to suggest that the pre-plague registrations of households most likely were not significantly different from the household populations in these communities on the eve of the Black Death.

Thus it appears reasonable to conclude that 60 per cent of Provence's population died in the Black Death, mainly by having contracted the infection, to some extent also by its secondary catastrophe effects.

Baratier concluded on the basis of the developments with respect to the numbers of hearths alone that all data showed a reduction of at least 50 per cent. Table 17 shows a general diminution of the number of hearths of 52 per cent. In addition, adjustments were made for the post-plague population developments in the years up to the redaction of the tax registers. These adjustments took the diminution up to 55 per cent, which must be considered a central estimate that accords well with Baratier's minimum estimate. The main reason that the estimate here is slightly larger than Baratier's is that a reduction in the average household size has been taken into account based on data that were not available to him.

There is also one other piece of evidence of the mortality in the Black Death in Provence, which, however, is based on entirely different type of records. In the south-westernmost corner of Provence, on the coast of the Camargue, the delta of the R. Rhône, lies the fishing village of Sainte-Maries-de-la-Mer. According to the customs of this village, males of age 15 and older were supposed to participate in the general assemblies of the community. In 1338, 258 male inhabitants were recorded as being present; in 1352 only 83 of them were recorded again in a similar register.[6] In order to be able to produce an estimate of the mortality in the Black Death, we need a realistic notion of the normal rate of attrition by death in this cohort of males over age 14. In the Middle Ages, life expectancy at birth in France was slightly below 25 years; actually it was 25 years still in 1700 (see above). Quite likely, life expectancy at birth for the general population in this local society before the Black Death was not higher, but could, of course, in this fishing village have been lower because of losses of men at sea.[7]

With this reservation, model life tables will be a useful tool for the analysis of these data according to the general presentation and discussion of model life tables made in Chapter 26 above. A general level of life expectancy at birth of 25 years corresponds to a mortality rate of about 4 per cent, but men's life expectancy may have

---

[6] Stouff 1962a: 290.
[7] There is, of course, always much variation between the individual communities that constitute societies, and the use of generalized assumptions in relation to the individual community implies considerable margins of uncertainty. However, the range of variation will be limited within the specific demographic system of the time and, again, also in the individual case it is far more likely to meet with the usual or ordinary than the unusual or extreme, which will occur only rarely.

been negatively affected by death at sea for fishermen. Nonetheless, the normal annual mortality rate for males over age 14 was much smaller than for the general population because the mortality among infants and young children was so great: according to model life tables 32 per cent of all infants will die, 20 per cent of young children in the age cohort 1–4. However, only 5 per cent of youngsters in the age cohort 15–19 would die, corresponding to an average annual mortality rate of 1 per cent, while adult males in ages 25–29 years would die at an average annual rate of 1.6 per cent. In other words, the fifteen youngest and by far largest cohorts (ages 15–29) would have a normal annual mortality rate of around 1.2 per cent, while all males in ages 15–39, comprising the great majority of adult males in the community, would die at an annual rate of 1.4 per cent.[8]

On the condition that all males in the cohorts over age 14 actually took part in the assembly and were recorded, and taking into account that people moved more around in old-time society than usually assumed, and that males in this population may have suffered significant supermortality at sea, it could be tentatively assumed that this male population was each year depleted by 2–2.5 per cent by death, including death at sea, and migration each year. This means that out of the original group of 258 males recorded at the assembly in Sainte-Maries-de-la-Mer in 1338, 215–205 were still present in the fishing village on the eve of the Black Death. In 1352, only 83 were still present. However, in the four years 1349–52, the survivors would be depleted at the same rate as before the plague, which means that 90–92 members of the original group of males would have still been alive on the morrow of the epidemic. This implies a mortality rate in the year of the Black Death of 55–58 per cent. Because there undoubtedly was significant and even substantial supermortality among children and women, this level of mortality among adolescent and adult men indicates that the general mortality rate in the community was 60 per cent or even somewhat higher. The tentative nature of this estimate must be underscored, but it fits quite well into the general picture of mortality in the Black Death. This outcome of the discussion of these data conforms conspicuously to the conclusion of the much larger material on the mortality in the Black Death in Provence provided by the hearths 'd'albergue'. As such it also provides independent confirmation not only of the credibility and validity of the mortality level but also of the tenability of the demographic techniques applied.

Baratier points out correctly that there is no real difference between the urban and rural mortality data, which also is supported by the outcome of the study of the ravages of the Black Death in Sainte-Maries-de-la-Mer, a fishing village.[9] This outcome conforms to the Italian pattern and underscores again that there is no basis for any assumption to the effect that mortality rates in the Black Death should have been lower in the countryside than in the urban centres. However, neither do these data conform to the assumption presented above on the basis of studies of Italian plague epidemics in the 1630s and data from the large plague epidemic in southern France in 1720–2 that morbidity and mortality rates were higher in the countryside than in the

[8]   Coale and Demeny 1983: 43.
[9]   1961: 82.

urban centres, although this view appeared to be corroborated by the Spanish mortality data.

Immediately to the north of Provence lies the region of the Savoy, at the time the County of Savoy,[10] which was not formally a part of France but of the loosely organized constellation of principalities and countries pompously called the Holy Roman Empire of the German Nation. As such the county functioned as an independent Savoyard state[11] with its own administration. This was quite efficient according to medieval standards: it produced some of the best medieval fiscal registrations of populations. However, it is important to note that the area of the contemporary County of Savoy was considerably larger than the two modern French départments of Upper and Lower Savoy: at the time the Savoy also included also the western part of the Swiss French-speaking canton of Valais and the northern and central parts of the modern Italian province of the Piedmont and Valle d'Aosta in present-day north-western Italy. This is a mountainous region.

This feudal territorial construction of the countyship of Savoy in the first half of the fourteenth century presents the author with several more or less unsatisfactory options with respect to the discussion of mortality data from this area. After much dithering I decided to discuss the mortality data of the areas of the Savoy covered by the two modern French départments and the adjacent Swiss border areas of the French-speaking canton of Valais in this chapter, where French data are discussed, while the Piedmontese mortality data are discussed in connection with the other Italian mortality data.

The available data on mortality rates in the Black Death are territorially distributed according to a pattern of localities associated with the road that runs southwards out of Chambéry; other march routes further into the countyship are likely but await discovery. The spread of the Black Death can be followed southwards to Montmélian, where it turned eastwards along the road that at a distance of about 15 km first branched off southwards towards the large valley of Maurienne, and at another crossroads about 20 km further to the east, at the town of Albertville, turned northwards into Upper Savoy.

At the time of the Black Death, the castellany[12] of Ugine lay about 60 km north-east of Chambéry, between the southern end of the Lake of Annecy in the Upper Savoy and Albertville. The mortality in the Black Death can be roughly estimated on the basis of the registers of subsidy accounts of 1331 and 1353.[13] These accounts record the taxpaying householders in their capacity as heads of their households. The urban element is so tiny that all hearths for all practical purposes can be considered peasant households. The numbers of householders in five of the seven parishes for which there are preserved registers are rendered in Table 18. It reveals that the number of such households had declined by 51 per cent.

The first question to be addressed is the probable development of the population

---

[10] The continental title of count corresponds more to the English title of earl, and a continental county corresponds, thus, more to the English earldom than to the English county.
[11] See Brondy, Demotz and Leguay 1984.
[12] The term castellany refers to the lordship of a castle and its district.
[13] Demotz 1975: 93–5.

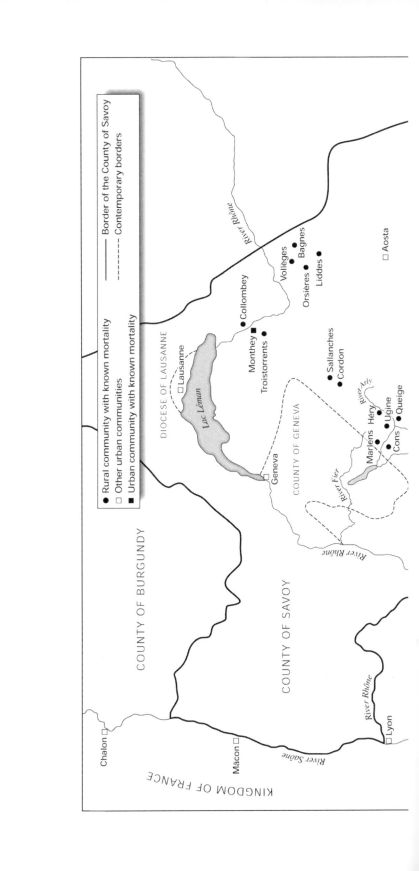

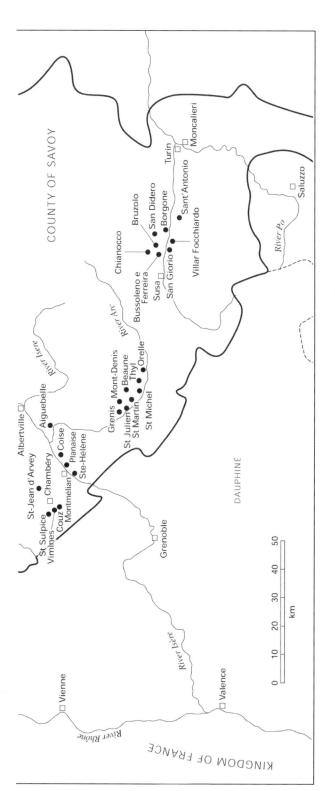

Map 6. Localities with known mortality in the Black Death in the County of Savoy and the County of Provence

between 1331 and the arrival of the Black Death. The author writing the medieval history of the castellany does not discuss this question, but other historians studying various areas and localities in the County of Savoy consider it. They are unanimous in their opinion that the population either continued to grow, or that growth tapered off into a stationary situation in the 1340s (see below). Consequently, an assumption to the effect that the number of households on the eve of the Black Death was identical to the number in 1331 will be cautious or conservative and will likely be the basis of a low mortality estimate.

Table 18. Decline in the number of subsidy-paying households in five of seven parishes in the castellany of Ugine between 1331 and 1353

Parish	Households 1331	Households 1353	Decline (%)
Ugine	333	156	53
Cons	31	17	45
Marlens	120	32	73
Queige	174	111	36
Héry	163	84	48
In all	821	400	51

On the other hand, it must be assumed that the population grew briskly after the plague for various reasons that have been presented and discussed above. Assuming post-plague population growth according to the standard assumption of 0.75 per cent, implies that the number of households was about 385 on the morrow of the Black Death, and that the real reduction in the number of households caused by the Black Death was at least 53 per cent.

However, because also the surviving households had lost members, the diminution of the population constituted by these subsidy-paying households must have been larger than for the householders alone. The standard assumption in this case is that average rural household size was reduced from a pre-plague level of 4.5 persons to 4 persons on the morrow of the Black Death, which implies that the better-off part of population constituted by the subsidy-paying households diminished by 58.3 per cent.

Taking into account supermortality among the poor and destitute classes of the population, which, according to the established standard assumption amounts to an addition of 2.5 percentage points, a loss of around 60 per cent of the general population becomes a likely estimate.

Although this level of mortality is awe-inspiring, the real mortality was undoubtedly significantly higher, because the adjustment for population growth between the Black Death and 1353 is in all likelihood much too small. This can be seen from Table 19, which renders the registrations of households in the subsidy accounts of 1353 and 1356. The comparison of the registrations of households in these two subsidy accounts show that, in the intervening three years, the number of households had grown by 16.5 per cent.

Table 19. Increase in number of households in the castellany of Ugine between 1353 and 1356

Parish	Households 1353	Households 1356	Increase (%)
Ugine	156	192	23
Cons	17	21	23.5
Marlens	32	39	22
Queige	111	118	6
Héry	84	96	14
In all	400	466	16.5

Such a high rate of increase must be owing to social mobility by local landless households of smallholders, cottars, sub-tenants and seasonal workers who moved into good vacant tenements, or by immigration by other proletarian households of diverse local origins, or rather a combination of these factors. Although migration at a distance by poor or destitute households was a demanding task that could take some time to realize, there can be no doubt that the first type of developments started immediately after the Black Death, the second shortly afterwards, and that they have contributed to increase the number of households significantly above the number of households that survived the Black Death as estimated above. For this reason, it cannot be inferred from the fact that the parish with the smallest loss of subsidy-paying households in the Black Death, namely Queige, with the lowest increase in the period 1353–6, was less attractive for resettlers than the other parishes. On the contrary, the reason could be that it was so attractive that most of the good vacant tenements had been resettled before the subsidy account of 1353 was taken.

About 30 km along the road that runs north-eastwards from Ugine lies the parish of Sallanches, which at the time also included the township of Cordon. In the years 1339–56, the number of peasant households in this parish declined by 43 per cent.

The 1340s was a hard time for the Savoyards facing increasing poverty, although there are no clear indications of a really serious demographic crisis caused by a combination of overpopulation and bad seasonal weather for agriculture. In the words of Brondy and his colleagues:

> Certainly, the Savoy was not subjected to the great famines that reappeared in the north of Europe at the beginning of the fourteenth century, but there was, no doubt, a certain scarcity in the supply of food.[14]

When the sources permit concrete glimpses of the demographic developments in the first half of the fourteenth century, they tend to show significant growth of peasant households at least up to 1339, when the last pre-plague subsidy account provides important information.[15] This means that at least in some areas, at least up to this

[14] Brondy, Demotz and Leguay 1984: 184. My translation from French.
[15] See., e.g., Dubuis 1990: 1/43–4; 1990: 2/67. See also below under the discussion of the mortality in the castellany of Entremont.

time, there must have been appreciable amounts of unused and underused agricultural resources that allowed the formation of quite a number of new peasant households, and not only growth in the impoverished landless classes. Another important reason was undoubtedly the emphasis on animal husbandry in the Savoyard areas, because this type of production was not so sensitive to seasonal weather as arable husbandry. Better balance between these two types of production provided greater stability and predictability of yields. Nonetheless, mortality may have increased, and it appears realistic or at least reasonably cautious to assume that the population was stationary in the decade preceding the Black Death.

On the other hand, the post-plague surge in the marriage rate must be assumed to have caused a significant increase in the number of households in the seven years elapsing from the time of the Black Death until the register of hearths was recorded in 1356. According to the standard assumption this was probably at an annual rate of about 0.75 per cent, constituting roughly 5 per cent in the course of those seven years between the Black Death and the time the subsidy account was recorded. This indicates that the diminution of the number of peasant hearths was in the order of magnitude of 48 per cent.

If we also take into account that surviving households of the landless classes had entered good vacant tenements in significant or even considerable numbers in these years and had thus swelled the numbers of the peasant classes, it is hard to imagine that the decline in the number of peasant households on the eve of the Black Death was not appreciably higher. Also the surviving peasant households had suffered losses, according to the standard assumption at a rate corresponding to a decline in average size from 4.5 to 4 persons, which in this case constitutes an additional diminution corresponding to 5.5 percentage points.

The question of general population mortality (which includes the mortality of the poor and destitute classes that went unrecorded because they did not bear any tax assessment) remains to be addressed. If the usual significantly higher mortality among the poor and destitute classes is taken into account, representing according to the standard assumption an addition of 2.5 percentage points to the estimates on the mortality among the peasant population, a level of general population mortality around 60 per cent is indicated (or at least of 55–60 per cent).

Data on mortality caused by the Black Death are available for three parishes near Chambéry, based on records registering small money payments by the households for permission to collect firewood.[16] The particularly valuable feature of these lists of rural householders is that new lists were produced each year and thus reflect directly the impact of the Black Death; they also appear to comprise the landless classes who likewise had a need for firewood for cooking and heating. Some households may not be registered, sub-tenants for instance, who could probably base their consumption of firewood on the permission acquired by the peasant householder.

16 Brondy 1988: 88.

Table 20. Decline in number of households and population size in parishes near Chambéry 1348–9

Parish	Households 1348	Households 1349	Decline (%)
Couz et Vimines	129	64	50
Saint-Sulpice	127	72	43
Saint-Jean d'Arvey	147	48	67
Households	403	184	54
Population	1814	736	59

As can be seen from Table 20, in these three parishes 54 per cent of the recorded households disappeared in the period of the Black Death. There was considerable variation of mortality between the three parishes, but consistently at very high levels ranging from the disastrous (43 per cent) to the truly catastrophic (67 per cent). Taking into account also that average household size had been reduced by the plague, applying here as elsewhere the standard assumption of 0.5 person, a diminution of the population of almost 60 per cent is indicated. In view of a probable small deficit of poor and destitute households that could avoid paying this feudal due (sub-tenants) or could not find the means to pay, it appears reasonable to round up the estimate of the population decline caused by the Black Death slightly to 60 per cent.

Immigration to Chambéry has not affected this estimate significantly for three reasons: first, because the second registration of households came so close after the Black Death; second, because Chambéry was a small town containing 495 taxpaying households in 1339,[17] which means that would-be immigrants from the three parishes would have to compete with other would-be immigrants from the quite densely populated surrounding region for a quite small number of vacant positions whatever the ravages of the Black Death; and third, because Chambéry was not an ordinary commercial town, but mainly an administrative centre, much of the havoc wrought by the Black Death would have been on persons and households associated with the count's administration who could not be substituted by peasants or rural labourers. Instead, the peasant households in the three parishes enjoyed the important advantage of having a good market for their produce in the nearby town.

Some 13 km south-east of Chambéry on the road to Maurienne lies the town of Montmélian on the R. Isère, which was the administrative centre of the castellany. A bridge toll provides very interesting data: peasant households on the left side of the R. Isère paid for permission to cross the bridge with their produce for sale in Montmélian or in Chambéry. Extant toll lists for eight parishes show a decline from 411 households in 1347 to 197 in 1349, i.e., a decline of 52 per cent.[18] Unfortunately, the specific data for these parishes are only given for three of them, which means that the full variation in mortality rates cannot be ascertained, and this is also the reason

[17] Brondy 1988: 88.
[18] Duparc 1965: 253, 271, 275. New tax lists were also produced during the epidemic, which show that at that point 328 households were still in operation, i.e., a reduction of 20 per cent.

for the form of Table 21. The standard assumption as to the normal reduction of average household size caused by the plague implies that the peasant population of these communities was reduced by 57 per cent.

Table 21. Decline in number of peasant households in eight parishes near Montmélian 1347–9

Parish	Households 1347	Households 1349	Decline (%)
St-Pierre	108	55	49
Ste-Hélène	108	61	44
Coise	195	81	59
Seven parishes[a]	303	142	53
Eight parishes[b]	411	197	52

[a]   Sainte-Hélène-du-Lac, La Chavanne, Planaise, Villard d'Héry, Coise, Pied-Gauthier, Hauteville et Châteauneuf. The seven parishes include also Sainte-Hélène and Coise, but not Saint-Pierre de Soucy.
[b]   Namely the seven and Saint-Pierre de Soucy.

In order to approach a realistic notion of general population mortality, we must make an addition reflecting the supermortality of the landless classes, which according to the standard assumption amounts to 2.5 percentage points. This means that general population mortality appears to have been of the order of magnitude of 60 per cent.

The existence of a large rural proletariat that gladly entered into the vacant good tenements is vigorously confirmed by the developments in the ensuing years. Already in 1352, the decline in the number of households had been reduced to 346 households or 16 per cent. The scholar undertaking the study explains this development with reference to serious overpopulation in pre-plague society, which created a large class of (all-but-)landless people, and which made it difficult for young adults to attain the economic basis for marriage. Also, one must take into account the possibility of migration by survivors in more marginal settlements and smallholders elsewhere who would readily enter the good tenements near the towns of Montmélian and Chambéry registered in the bridge-toll lists. An indication of the possible importance of medium-range and long-range post-plague migration can be seen in the fact that most of the new households were not established immediately after the Black Death but in 1351 and 1352, as movement and resettlement at a distance would take some time to organize for common people in those times.

Another 25 km down the road lay the castellany of Aiguebelle. A study of lists recording taxpaying households in four parishes in 1347 and in 1356 shows a diminution of 34 per cent. The scholar compiling the study points out that many new households had entered tenements vacated by the Black Death, and assumes tentatively that actual mortality among taxpaying householders in the epidemic was over 50 per cent.[19]

---

[19]   Commanay 1963. This is an unpublished thesis, the main results of which are briefly rendered by Gelting 1991: 9.

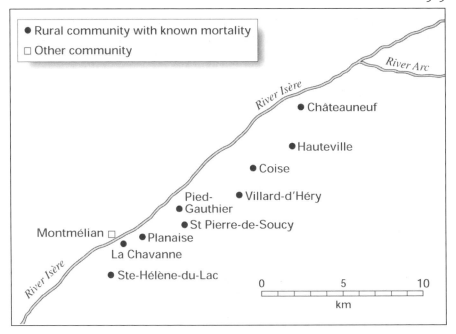

Map 7. The Black Death in the district of Montmélian

In the present context, the new households that moved into the tenements deso-lated by the plague must be deducted in order to reach a realistic notion of the proportions of households on the eve of the Black Death that survived the ordeal or succumbed to it. These new households could have three social origins, especially surviving landless households and newly married couples, but also poor immigrants. The importance of social advancement receives strong support from the preceding study of parishes near Montmélian where a decline in the number of households of 52 per cent in 1349 had been reduced to 16 per cent by 1352. For the sake of consis-tency and comparability we must stick to the standard assumptions that indicate a growth in households of around 10 percentage points, implying a real decline in the number of households of 44 per cent. Applying the standard household multipliers, this gives a mortality rate among the peasant population of 50 per cent. In order to approach a realistic notion of general population mortality it is necessary to include the supermortality among the poor and destitute social classes. According to the stan-dard assumption on this point, this supermortality will normally be covered by an addition of 2.5 percentage points to the mortality among the peasant population, which implies that the general population mortality was around 52.5 per cent.

Lastly, the Danish scholar M. Gelting has made a fine study of a number of parishes in the castellany of Maurienne on the basis of tax lists contained in the subsidy accounts of 1346–7 and 1359, and running data from death duty lists redacted annually.[20] The 1340s was a difficult decade for the common population, as can be

<hr />

[20] Gelting 1991: 7–45.

seen from the fact that 17 per cent of the count's tenants and over one-half of the local gentry's tenants were exempted because of poverty, and many of these impoverished peasant householders had obviously been among the taxpayers in the previous subsidy of 1331–2. In addition, peasant society contained a high proportion of proletarian households, cottars, day labourers and sub-tenants, who were not registered because they did not hold land, and could not pay any taxes or subsidies whatsoever.

The tax lists of 1346–7 contain the names of 1,352 peasant householders holding tenements of the count, distributed according to 'métralies', the main administrative divisions of the castellany, and within the 'métralies' according to parishes. The scholar selects for study 281 male householders in six parishes in the 'métralie' of Saint-Michel. This area comprises topographic and economic diversity that permits comparison between a privileged market borough, namely Saint-Michel, the wine-growing river–valley parish of Saint-Martin-la-Porte and typical mountain parishes like Orelle, Beaune, le Thyl and Montdenis. One should note that according to the number of households in the privileged market borough, it really was a smallish village and should be considered a rural community with relatively lively commercial contacts and functions in the area. In 1346, the 281 households of the six parishes contained 317 male taxpayers who constitute the cohort that will be followed through the epidemic in order to identify the mortality.

The Black Death also killed persons who would have died anyway for other reasons in that year, not least children. Nonetheless, they died from the Black Death's mortal microbiological agents or from its secondary catastrophe effects and must be considered part of plague mortality. This also means that in localities ravaged by the Black Death and losing, for instance, 50 per cent of the population, mortality for other reasons would be sharply reduced. The difference between net plague mortality and general population mortality in the plague year of a community will, therefore, be only about one-half of normal annual mortality.

Ten of the 317 male householders can be shown to have died in 1346–7, representing an annual mortality rate of 1.6 per cent, an estimate that is compatible with the mortality data Herlihy and Klapisch-Zuber estimated for 'non-poor' adult Florentine men in 1425–7, namely 1.5–1.9 per cent.[21] In England, Zvi Razi has shown that of about 210 male tenants on the manor of Halesowen about 3.5–4.5 would die in normal years in the first half of the fourteenth century, corresponding to a normal death rate of 1.66–2.15 per cent. This English population of male peasant householders contains a substantial portion of cottars and smallholders, which makes its social composition somewhat different from that of the peasant householders of Maurienne.[22] This suggests that the normal mortality rate in the English case should be expected to be somewhat higher than in the Savoyan case. Thus, this discussion ends up with an outcome that seems consistent and indicative of this aspect of the medieval demographic regime.

However, the normal annual mortality rate estimated on the basis of the material relating to these six parishes in the 'métralie' of Saint-Michel is disregarded by the scholar, ostensibly because it is too low. Instead, he analyses the material for the privi-

[21] 1978: 459–60.
[22] Razi 1980: 35–41. See also the valuable comments on related questions by Postan and Titow 1958–9: 400.

leged borough of Saint-Julien, which in reality was a middle-sized village, a material so poor that the outcome must be expressed as between 1.2 per cent and 2.4 per cent. Within this range of possibilities the scholar opts for the highest rate. Applied on the material of the six parishes, this view implies that 15 and not 10 householders had died in the two years 1346–7, which implies that the scholar has missed one-third of the pre-plague deaths in this cohort. In relation to the material of Saint-Julien it means that the initial cohort of 111 peasant householders in 1332 had been reduced to 77 men by 1348, i.e., by 34 persons, while he has been able to identify only 18 of them in the sources as having died in the period, or just above one-half of the estimated number of deaths. This introduces a major element of uncertainty with respect to the quality of his data that endangers the usability of his source material for demographically valid estimates.

However, according to Model West life tables[23] showing the rate of diminution by age of a population with life expectancy at birth of 25 years both for men and women, corresponding to a mortality rate for the general population of 4 per cent, the cohort of male persons aged 20–24 will die at a rate of c. 1.6 per cent, the cohort of persons at age c. 39 will die at a rate of about 2 per cent, while the rate of 2.4 per cent preferred by the scholar is the mortality rate of males at c. age 40 – elderly men according to the medieval mind as well as to medieval demography. The most important reason for this shape of male adult mortality rates is the very high mortality rates among infants and young children in ages 1–4, 30–32 per cent and around 20 per cent, respectively. In view of the basic form of the age pyramid, in this case shaped according to a pattern of dying (and surviving) in ages 20 and older in which one-half of those reaching age 20 would be interred by their early fifties, and according to the fact that the largest cohorts have the lowest mortality rates, the normal average death rate for adult men in this population will quite likely be around 2 per cent. If we take into account that we are relating to middling and upper-class males both in the case of Florence and in the case of the peasant householders in Maurienne, these categories of persons should be expected to have lower mortality rates and better life expectancy at birth than the general population.

This discussion has, thus, confirmed the good quality of Gelting's source material and that the number of identified deaths in these cohorts of men in 1346–7 is trustworthy. Consequently, it is technically and factually justified to retain the view that, in the borough of Saint-Michel, the male population of householders at risk on the eve of the Black Death consisted of 307 persons after having experienced a normal average annual mortality rate for this social category in the preceding two years of 1.6 per cent. Similarly, the population of male peasant householders in Saint-Julien would have been reduced to 87 persons, which means that the scholar has missed only six deaths in the cohort of the years 1333–47, confirming, thus, the good quality of his source material and its suitability as a base for valid demographic estimates.

Of the 307 male householders in Saint-Michel who presumably were alive and kicking on the eve of the Black Death, 132 householders can be positively identified as survivors in the following years, which means that 57 per cent of the peasant

---

[23] On model life tables, see above p. 249.

householders in the cohort had died in the year of the Black Death. It cannot be entirely ruled out, of course, that a few surviving householders died in the immediately following years before proof of their existence was entered into records. However, one should expect that the count's keen interest in rents and fines from his tenements and from death duties, which were meticulously taken care of by his effective and dedicated administration, would have resulted in registration in connection with the official transfer of the deceased householders' tenements to new holders, be it to their children, relatives or others.

The mortality rate among the population constituted by the middling and upper-class peasant households in these parishes must have been significantly higher than among their householders. Gelting has found material that enables him to study the fate of most of the constituent members of the eleven peasant households contained in the mountain hamlet of Grenis in the Maurienne during the Black Death and has presented them in the form of 'mini-biographies' (above, Table 11). These biographies show that not a single household escaped unscathed from the Black Death. It attests to the caution of the standard assumption used in this book to the effect that surviving households had lost, on average, 0.5 person; in fact, it indicates not caution but quite certain underestimation. Nonetheless, applying a standard deduction of 0.5 persons from 4.5 persons to 4 persons in average household size gives a mortality rate for the middling and upper-class peasant population in these parishes of 62 per cent.

In order to approach a realistic notion of general population mortality, we must also include the landless households and take into account the usual supermortality of the poor and destitute that in medieval society of the time appears normally to have constituted close to or around one-half of the population. According to the cautious standard assumption on this point the normal supermortality among the proletarian classes has been estimated at about 5–6 percentage points, which, in view of the usual proportion of this population segment in the population, will largely be taken into account by adding 2.5 percentage points to the mortality rate of the peasant population. This implies that the general population mortality rate was about 65 per cent.

The scholar has also attempted to estimate plague mortality in the privileged borough of Saint-Julien, which, as mentioned, really was a medium-sized village with relatively lively commercial contacts. However, in this case no subsidy account of 1346–7 is available, and instead the subsidy account of 1332 must be mobilized (see above). In this connection, the question of the normal mortality rate of the adult males of this middling and upper-class cohort could become devastating. However, as shown above, an annual pre-plague mortality rate among adult male peasant householders of 1.6 per cent in this village has a solid basis in the local source material, confirms the credibility of the sources' quality and produces an outcome that fits readily into the established pattern for Maurienne and southern France.

The number of taxpaying peasant householders in 1332 was actually 125, but for various reasons this number must be reduced to the 111 adult peasant householders that constitute the cohort. At the end of 1347, an annual mortality rate of 1.6 per cent would have reduced this cohort to 87 persons at risk on the eve of the Black Death. Thirty-five of these men are known to have survived, which gives a mortality rate in the year of the Black Death of 60 per cent. (If we alternatively assume a pre-plague death rate of 2 per cent, 82 householders would be alive on the eve of the Black Death and 57 per cent of them would have perished in the plague year.)

The mortality rate of the peasant population constituted by these households can be estimated by multiplying the standard pre-plague and post-plague household sizes with the numbers of pre-plague and post-plague householders. This gives a mortality rate for this middling and upper-class population of 64 per cent (or 62 per cent in the case of an annual pre-plague mortality rate among the householders of 2 per cent). If we also take into account that the mortality rate must be assumed to have been significantly and even considerably higher among the numerous rural proletariat of (all-but-)landless households, the standard assumption on the supermortality of the poor indicates a general population mortality in this medium-sized village of Saint-Julien of the order of magnitude of around 67 (65) per cent, or rather, perhaps, of 65–70 per cent. In reality, the mortality in Grenis was, of course, even higher, because the average intra-household mortality was higher than the 0.5 person presumed by the standard assumption.

Lastly, there is in this connection the study of the small mountain hamlet of Grenis in the parish of Montdenis (today in Saint-Julien) that has been referred to several times. In 1346, Grenis contained 11 taxpaying households constituting the peasant population. After elimination of one female householder, we are left with a tiny cohort of 10 male householders that is comparable to the other studies. All of these householders appear to have been alive on the eve of the Black Death. Of these men six appear to have died in the plague year, giving a mortality rate for the peasant householders of 60 per cent, about the same rate as in the other communities. When the standard pre-plague and post-plague household averages are multiplied with the corresponding numbers of peasant householders, the outcome indicates that the peasant population of Grenis consisted of 45 persons on the eve of the Black Death and of 16 persons on the morrow of the plague, corresponding to a mortality rate among the peasant population of 64.5 per cent. Again we must assume that also this mountain hamlet contained households of the landless classes that suffered significant supermortality, which indicates a general population mortality rate of 67 per cent, or again rather, perhaps, of 65–70 per cent.

Thus, summing up the data on the mortality in the Black Death in the castellany of Maurienne, the central results for the six parishes in the 'métralie' of Saint-Michel, in Saint-Julien and in Grenis, respectively, amount to mortality rates of 57–60 per cent of the peasant householders, 62–64 per cent of the peasant household population, and 65–70 per cent of the localities' general population.

Summing up the mortality data on the Black Death's ravages in the Savoy, a very consistent and frightening picture again emerges: 50–60 per cent of the peasant households disappeared in the epidemic, 55–65 per cent of the peasant populations died, and 60–70 per cent of the general population of the various localities were swept away by the merciless epidemic killer.

All localities are rural communities, a fact that underscores the validity of the observation that the Black Death made such a tremendous impact because it spread at least as effectively in the countryside as in urban centres. There is a tendency in the territorial configuration of the mortality estimates that mortality rates were somewhat higher in the mountain communities of the castellany of Maurienne than in the more central rural communities of the lowlands. The proportional diminution of the number of households in the Savoy's lowlands appears to be the same as in Provence. However, the general picture is of a surprising consistency in mortality rates.

Across the eastern mountain range of Upper Savoy lies what is today the large French-speaking Swiss canton of Valais, although at the time of the Black Death western Valais was part of the County of Savoy. There are available some interesting data on the ravages of the Black Death in this area that should be discussed in relation to the other data of the Savoy.

About 15 km east of the present-day Savoyard border as the crow flies lay the Alpine castellany of Entremont, comprising six parishes containing 1,025 peasant households in 1313. There are extant subsidy accounts for the years 1339 and 1356 that record the number of taxpaying peasant households at these two points in time for four of the parishes, containing over 91 per cent of the castellany's peasant households in 1313. These data are given in Table 22.[24]

Table 22. Numbers of taxpaying hearths in four parishes in the castellany of Entremont 1313, 1339 and 1356

Parish	Hearths 1313	Hearths 1339	Hearths 1356	Decline (%) 1339–56
Vollèges	115	150	76	49.5
Bagnes	355	411	236	42.5
Orsières	304	402	259	35.5
Liddes	161	160	90	44.0
Total	935	1123	661	41.0

The data in Table 22 are taken from the same subsidy accounts as the data for Sallanches (see above), and the same approaches and standard assumptions should be used to develop the data on peasant households into mortality rates for the general population in the Black Death. Also the mortality rates among the peasant classes were about the same: 43 per cent in Sallanches, 41 per cent in Entremont. In this case, it can be shown that the peasant population had been growing significantly from 1313 to 1339, by 20 per cent.

This indicates, as mentioned above, that there were available significant amounts of unused or underused agricultural resources, which allowed population growth to find an outlet in the lively formation of additional new peasant households and not only in an increasing pauperization in the form of a rapid growth of the landless classes. Again, Alpine agriculture, with its strong emphasis on animal husbandry, was not as vulnerable to bad seasonal weather as arable husbandry, and this gave the communities greater stability of production. Presumably, therefore, the population in this area did not become significantly more exposed to demographic crises by its continued growth, and, as mentioned above, there is no evidence of serious economic or demographic crises in the

[24] Dubuis 1990: 1/38, 47–8; 1990: 2/66, 68.

sources.[25] It seems reasonable on the conservative side to assume that the number of peasant households and the number of persons they contained were not smaller on the eve of the Black Death than in 1339.

It must also be reasonable to assume that the population grew quite briskly after the plague, increasing in the eight years to 1356 by 4–6 percentage points, which must be subtracted. However, we must also assume that surviving poor households that did not bear any tax assessment before the plague had entered good vacant holdings and swelled the ranks of the peasant classes that were taxed in 1356; these households must also be deducted in order to identify the cohort of surviving peasant households on the morrow of the Black Death. Relatively arbitrarily but cautiously, this point could be approached by assuming that this upwards social mobility by poor households constituted also about 5 per cent of the households in 1356. Such a premise will take the number of surviving households down to 600 and indicates that the real decline in the number of peasant households caused by the Black Death was 46.5 per cent. In addition, it must be assumed that average size of the surviving peasant households declined, according to the established standard assumption from an average of 4.5 persons to 4 persons, which implies that the peasant households suffered a mortality rate of 52.5 per cent.

However, we must again assume that the landless classes were significantly and even substantially more harshly ravaged than the peasant classes. The general mortality rate of the population in these four parishes must, therefore, have been significantly higher, according to the standard assumption, in this case about 2.5 percentage points higher, which indicates a general population mortality of around 55 per cent. In 1313, the population density of this castellany was 1.6 household per sq. km, showing that great dispersion of the population and low population density did not dampen the Black Death's disseminative powers.

Some 35 km north of the castellany of Entremont lay the Alpine castellany of Monthey. The small town of Monthey that was the administrative centre of the castellany in the fourteenth century and the parish of Troistorrents and the community of Collombey-Muraz contained together in 1329 685 taxpaying peasant households. In 1352 the number had declined to 404 households, i.e., by 41 per cent (Table 23).[26]

The question of the population development in the period 1329–48 becomes important for an assessment of the plague-specific mortality in Monthey in the Black Death. In the case of Provence, Baratier concluded that the population grew through most of the first half of the fourteenth century and then stagnated into an overall stationary size in the 1330s and 1340s, an overall standstill that, however, veiled some local variation of

[25] It seems to this author that Dubuis holds exaggerated notions as to the average size of households, being, as it seems, quite sympathetic to an average of 6 persons. Dubuis 1990: 1/43–4; 1990: 2/67. This is a much higher household multiplier than registered for pre-plague areas anywhere else or assumed by other scholars for France or Italy. Of course, an average of 6 persons is not impossible, but requires that the average size of tenements was higher than usually assumed, making it possible that either the incidence of living-in servants was high, the incidences of joint or multiple families were high, or that the incidence of sub-tenements was high, or some combination of these factors. In that case, the average number of persons living within the territories of the tenements could be high, but be registered only under the name of the peasant householders. If this cannot be shown to be the case, and Dubuis does not produce any evidence to this effect, average household size should be assumed to be 4–5 persons; 5 persons will indicate rapid population growth, 4–4.25 probable standstill and 4.5 slight population growth.
[26] Dubuis 1979: 148–52.

Table 23. Decline in the numbers of registered taxpaying peasant households in the castellany of Monthey from 1329 to 1352

Locality	Households 1329	Households 1352	Decline (%)
Town of Monthey	264	152	42.5
Parish of Troistorrents	270	142	47.5
Community of Collombey	151	110	27.0
Total	685	404	41.0

continued small growth or a slight tendency towards diminution. Above, Brondy has been cited to much the same effect with regard to the County of Savoy, and Dubuis uncovered an increment of 20 per cent in the number of taxpaying peasant households in the castellany of Entremont in the period 1313–39. It cannot be taken for granted that some of this growth had not taken place also in the 1330s, but the size of the increase makes it seem likely. This means that an assumption to the effect that the population size was stationary between 1330 and the arrival of the Black Death must be considered cautious and tend to produce a mortality rate on the low side.

Nonetheless, the diminution was certainly larger than shown by Table 23: the records of 1352 comprised not only the remaining peasant householders of the cohort of householders at risk on the eve of the Black Death, but also a significant element of formerly poor and destitute households that had used the opportunity to take up good vacant tenements in the aftermath of the Black Death. These 'newcomers' to the peasant class must be deducted in order to reach a more realistic notion of the mortality caused by the Black Death. Much of this socio-demographic movement would have taken place in the 3–3.5 years since the Black Death (from c. mid-1349 to mid-1352). Above, evidence has been adduced of an intensive influx of households from the landless classes within the same time frame in parishes near Montmélian. However, the use of standard assumption requires a cautious approach, and a much smaller addition of households of this social background corresponding roughly to 1 per cent per year in this early phase. The population as measured in the number of households must also be assumed to have grown through the formation of new households by marriage in the same years: according to the standard assumption on post-plague growth, it can be cautiously estimated at about 2.5 per cent. This means that around 5 per cent of the peasant householders recorded in 1352 must be deducted in order to approach a more realistic notion of the number of surviving peasant householders on the morrow of the Black Death. This implies that the number of surviving peasant householders was 384, and had declined by about 44 per cent. If we take into account the usual standard assumption to the effect that average household size had diminished from 4.5 persons in the pre-plague population to 4 persons in the immediate aftermath of the Black Death, the peasant population appears to have declined by 50 per cent. In addition, the normal supermortality among the poor and destitute social classes must be taken into account, which, according to the standard assumption, indicates a general population mortality of 52.5 per cent.

The parish register that Dubuis discovered in the parish church of Saint-Maurice situ-

Table 24. Mortality rates in the Black Death in the County of Savoy, in Upper Savoy (nos 1–2), near Chambéry (nos 3–5), castellany of Maurienne (nos 6–8) and the Savoyard area of Valais (nos 9–10)

	Localities	Peasant householders	Peasant population	General population
1	Castellany of Ugine	53	58	60
2	Parish of Sallanches (and Cordon)	52.5	57.5	60
3	3 parishes near Chambéry[a]	54	59	60
4	8 parishes near Montmélian	52	57	60
5	4 parishes near Aiguebelle	44	50	52.5
6	6 parishes, métralie of Saint-Michel	57	62	65
7	Village/borough of Saint-Julien	60	64	65–70
8	Hamlet of Grenis	60	64	65–70
9	4 parishes in Entremont	46.5	52.5	55
10	3 communities in Monthey	44	50	52.5

[a] The sources for these parishes also comprise most of the landless classes.

ated at a short distance south of Monthey covers only a part of the Black Death (see above), and cannot be used for estimating mortality.[27]

The estimates of population losses in the Black Death in various localities within the borders of the Savoyard state, including the communities in the present-day canton of Valais in south-western Switzerland, are presented in Table 24, and can now be summarized. Mortality rates were at consistently very high levels, varying between 50 and 70 per cent. In four out of ten localities, the mortality rates were around 60 per cent, in three of ten localities of the order of magnitude of 65–70 per cent, in the remaining four localities of the order of magnitude of 52.5–57.5 per cent. This indicates that the total loss of population was probably of the order of magnitude of 60 per cent. Such mortality rates are almost incredible, but in this case, as in the case of Provence, they are based on good source material. They are supported by the usual set of epidemiological, demographic and sociological analytical techniques and considerations, which indicate that the level of general population mortality was about 7.5 percentage points higher than for male peasant householders.

The mortality rates are highest in the castellany of Maurienne, a feature that may be taken as support for the hypothesis that plague spreads most effectively in dispersed types of settlement.

Unfortunately, only three additional sources of data on mortality in the Black Death are available from French areas, two of them also from south-central France, and one from Auvergne, a hilly region situated to the north of south-central France; they all relate to largish urban communities.

The small city of Millau on the R. Tarn lies in the modern département of Aveyron, about 130 km west of R. Rhone and 200 km west of Provence's south-western contempo-

[27] Dubuis 1980b: 1/20; 1979: 149–53.

rary border. The municipal archives contain tax records, the so-called 'cadastral penny', for quite a number of years from 1280 and onwards, organized according to hearths and the name of the householders. In the two decades preceding the Black Death, the number of registered taxpaying households declined slightly, from 1,598 in 1326 to 1,541 in 1346, i.e., by 3.5 per cent. Almost the whole diminution occurred between 1336 and 1344 and was very likely caused by the bad harvest of 1340. This means that this city and area appears to have had considerable resilience in the face of dearth, which probably was mainly owing to the good fertility of the countryside and the fine balance between arable and animal husbandry. This also means that it is justified to assume that the number of households was quite stationary between the redaction of the tax records of 1346 and the arrival of plague only a year and a half later.

In 1353, the number of hearths/householders had suddenly diminished to 918, i.e., by c. 40.5 per cent. Interestingly, the number of households sagged in the following years, by 2 per cent to 899 in 1358. This could suggest that the Black Death had caused significantly higher mortality in the countryside than in the city. Higher mortality rates in the country-side than in the town would undermine the livelihood of more of the artisans and shop-keepers by reducing the number of their customers and their productive basis proportionally more than their own losses. Thus, a scenario can be discerned in which a few years after the disaster, when the boom in new marriages and immigration of opti-mistic and enterprising persons from the countryside had petered out, a relatively larger decrease in the rural population than in the urban population began to depress the commercial activities as a lasting situation. Consequently, the urban population began to decrease slowly by emigration to other towns or to the countryside. According to this scenario, it can be assumed that the population had not grown in the five post-plague years, 1349–53.

Professor Philippe Wolff, the distinguished historian supervising the study that had been undertaken by one of his students,[28] assumes, as does the author of this book, that the average size of the pre-plague households was 4 persons, and that the average had been reduced to 3.5 persons on the morrow of the plague. This means that the population contained in these middling and upper-class taxpaying households was reduced from 6,164 persons to 3,213 persons, or by 48 per cent. However, registra-tions were presumably better after than before the Black Death, according to the stan-dard assumption corresponding to 1.5 percentage points. This point suggests that the mortality rate among these social classes should be rounded off upwards to around 50 per cent.

The municipal archives also contain a number of lists of communicants, which indicates a much larger population, and, thus, by implication the existence of large classes of poor and destitute people in the city, which quite likely may have consti-tuted roughly half of the population. If we also take into account probable substantial supermortality among the poor and destitute social classes, according to the standard assumption corresponding to 5 percentage points, the mortality in the plague year was quite likely around 52.5 per cent.

Another of Professor Wolff's students made an equally interesting and useful study of the small city of Albi, situated on the R. Tarn about 80 km west of Millau,

[28] Wolff 1957: 501–5.

and which gave the modern département its name.[29] In the archives of Albi are still extant two so-called 'compoix', from 1343 and 1357, respectively, in which the population is registered according to households and their assets are surveyed in order to assess their taxability. Unfortunately, the 32 opening pages of the records of 1357 have been lost, containing most of the assessments of the householders in the quarter of Verdussa, where some of the richest persons in the city lived in 1343, and five or six pages at the end of the records have been lost as well. In principle, all Albi's households should be recorded, including the poor and destitute, which would not bear any tax assessment but are present in the form of names of householders without valuations of assets or tax contribution. In fact, this is the case with 42 per cent of the householders in 1343, and 28 per cent of the householders in 1357. Nonetheless, a significant number of poor households have undoubtedly been passed over because the futility of registration was too obvious and not really worth any effort. As in Millau, the proportion of the poor and destitute quite likely exceeded half the pre-plague population. And, then, there were the exempt classes of clergy and noblemen. The much lower proportion of poor and destitute households in the post-plague population than in the pre-plague population confirms the general assumption in this book with respect to post-plague social-class developments, and also implies that the post-plague populations will be more accurately recorded because the registrars will pass over fewer households that will obviously not bear any tax assessment. However, in this case, where most of the poor and destitute households in the pre-plague population must be assumed to have been registered, any adjustment for this factor will be too small to really be worth paying regard to.

The tax-assessment records of 1343 contain 2,669 names of householders, while the extant tax-assessment records of 1357 contain only 952 such names. In this case about 250 names must be added in order to compensate for the lost pages, which brings the total up to c. 1,200 householders. It seems reasonable to assume that Albi and its surrounding hinterland had been ravaged by the Black Death in much the same way as Millau and its hinterland, and apply the same explanatory scenario. Consequently, the pre-plague figures can be used as they are for the purpose of estimating the mortality in the Black Death, while the post-plague figures should be adjusted a couple of percentage points upwards to about 1,225 in order to compensate for an assumed slight diminution in the years 1353–7.

This means that the number of recorded households fell by 54 per cent from 1343 to 1349. However, a standard reduction in the average household size from 4 persons to 3.5 persons must be taken into account. This indicates that the recorded population had diminished by 60 per cent on the morrow of the Black Death. When it is also taken into account that there still remained a significant population element of unregistered poor and destitute households that must be assumed to have suffered even more severely, and that the registration of the post-plague population presumably was more accurate than the pre-plague registration, it appears reasonable to conclude that the central estimate for Albi's population loss in the year of the Black Death is at about 62.5 per cent.

---

[29] Prat 1952: 15–18. Cf. Wolff 1957: 495–8.

Table 25. Mortality in the Black Death in south-central France (%)

Locality	Tax-assessed households	Tax-assessed population	General population
Millau	40.5	50	52.5
Albi	54	60	62.5
Mortality			57.5

Unfortunately, the summing up of data on the mortality caused by the Black Death elsewhere in southern France is easy, because they represent only two localities, as set out in Table 25. However, the consistency of the mortality rates is conspicuous: in Albi about 62.5 per cent and in Millau about 52.5 per cent. The study of the onslaught in Perpignan in the south-westernmost part of present-day Languedoc has been discussed under Spain (Chapter 28), because it was under the Crown of Aragon at the time. Although this study focuses on certain social elites and, therefore, does not allow inference to general mortality on its own, the results certainly fit well into the general picture obtained for southern France.

The level of mortality in the Black Death indicated by these two urban data from south-central France is quite similar to the mortality found in Tuscany, and could be slightly lower than the level of mortality indicated for Provence and the County of Savoy on the basis of more numerous data. The internal consistency of these data and their consistency with the much broader-based findings for south-eastern France combine to give the few data of south-central France a certain level of credibility. This corresponds to a general rule of the thumb to the effect that one should expect to find data that reflect ordinary or normal courses of events exactly because they are usual, while extreme events are by nature rare and will rarely be met with.

On the basis of the data on mortality in the year of the Black Death obtained and discussed for Provence, the County of Savoy and south-central France, large regions that include a large part of Mediterranean France and the south-eastern mountain region, it appears possible and justified to conclude that around 60 per cent, or at least close to 60 per cent, of the population in this part of France died in a cataclysmic catastrophe. Taking into account the likely margins of uncertainty, this central estimate can also be expressed as 60 ± 5 per cent.

The last piece of information on the mortality in the Black Death in France comes from the hilly and mountainous region of Auvergne. In the largish town of Saint-Flour, lying about 100 km north of Millau in the modern département of Cantal, 1,540 households paying the familiar tax called the 'taïlle' were registered in 1345, 843 within the walls and 697 in the suburbs; in 1356 the corresponding numbers of taxpaying households had diminished to 805, 548 within the walls and 257 in the suburbs, a decline of 48 per cent in the town as a whole (Table 26).[30] If some post-plague growth of a couple of per cent is cautiously assumed to have occurred since the Black Death, and the standard adjustment for improved post-plague registration is also taken into account, the esti-

---

[30] Audisio 1968: 260–1.

mated decline in the number of taxable households in the epidemic can be rounded off upwards to c. 51.5 per cent.

Table 26. Decline in number of fiscal hearths in Saint-Flour 1345–6

Part of the town	Hearths 1345	Hearths 1356	Decline (%)
Within the walls	843	548	35
Suburbs	697	257	63
Total	1540	805	48

These data that show a strongly differentiated decline in the proportions of fiscal hearths within the walls of the town and in the suburbs provide another important confirmation of two of the central assumptions of this part of the book: (1) the Black Death caused considerably higher mortality among the poor and destitute, which constituted the large majority of those living in the suburbs outside the walls, than the better-off social classes who mostly lived within the walls; (2) the Black Death caused lively social mobility. The mortality among the taxpaying households in the suburbs was quite likely higher than among their social equals within the walls, because the suburbs contained a much larger proportion of poor and destitute people that would increase the general exposure to infection. However, this cannot explain why the diminution of fiscal hearths in the suburbs was almost twice as high as within the walls.

Assuming the standard decline in average household size, the population contained in the fiscal households declined from 6,160 persons to 2,818, or by 54 per cent. In this phase of the discussion, the case of Albi, 150 km to the south of Saint-Flour, should be kept in mind: 42 per cent of the recorded householders in 1343, and 28 per cent of the householders in 1357, bore no tax assessment; and the fiscal hearths comprised less than 60 per cent of the registered households before the plague and less than three-quarters afterwards. This highlights one of the main themes of this part of the book: the existence of a large proletariat in the first half of the fourteenth century that often remained unrecorded in contemporary society, because they could not bear any tax assessment and, consequently, were ignored by registrars, and, for the same reason often have been passed over by historians as well. The same point is underscored by historians of Auvergne.[31] It is a general observation that for several reasons, underlined above, proletarian classes suffer supermortality in epidemic crises. Consequently, the mortality among the whole population must have been higher than 54 per cent, and according to the standard assumption quite likely around 57 per cent. One should note that contemporary sources contain a number of references to catastrophic mortality in the Black Death in the region of Auvergne.

One could have hoped that the extant French parish registers would furnish usable data on mortality in the Black Death. However, the parish register of Lyons, about 180 km north-east of Saint-Flour, is not usable because it breaks off too early in the

---

[31] Boudet and Grand 1902: 138.

epidemic, obviously because its keeper(s) died. Neither are the almost complete parish registers of Givry, about 120 km north of Lyons, usable because the size and social composition of the population at risk and the social-class representativeness of those entered in the registers are not known. According to Biraben, the average number of marriages recorded in the marriage registers in the pre-plague years probably reflects a population of around 2,000 persons, while the average number of burials in the pre-plague years could reflect a population of around 1,000 persons.[32] Until these registers are published and the various types of information provided in the entries can be scrutinized in detail, the population represented in the marriage registers remains uncertain. Was, for instance, the population of couples that got married in the parish church of Givry recruited only from the town's own population, or was it swelled by couples from the countryside who wished to get married in the more beautiful church in Givry? Again the historian must give in, so far.

The account books of the churchwarden of the parish of Saint-Germain-l'Auxerrois in Paris contain entries on donations to the church made by persons who had subsequently died. A study of these wills has uncovered an abrupt increase at the end of August 1348.[33] While the average annual number of wills in the period April 1341 to June 1348 represented five dead persons, 361 deaths were reflected in this way in the 1.5 years from 11 June 1348 to December 1349, corresponding to an average annual rate of 235 persons or a monthly rate of 19.5 persons, forty-six times higher than the pre-plague average. This is clear evidence that the making of such wills was strongly affected by mass psychosis in the face of terrifying mortality, and of course many of those who made such wills would be survivors at the end of the epidemic. Again, the historian has to give in.

A related type of source is known from the city of Caen in Normandy. The archives of five parish churches contain cartularies where donations to the church for the purpose of acquiring prestigious burial places (usually in the church itself) were entered. In the fourteenth century as a whole, including the time of the Black Death, there were made 84 such donations, i.e., 0.84 donation per year. Seventeen of these donations were made in 1348, twenty times more than the annual average in this century, and fifteen of these donations were made in the last three months of this year.[34] If the plague year is deducted from the total with the exception of one donation (which will roughly represent the normal annual incidence of donations), the number of donations increased by almost twenty-four times in the plague year compared to the remaining ninety-nine years of the century. Unfortunately, the significance of this estimate is not at all clear, partly because there was a much smaller population in Caen in the second half of the century that would make donations, and partly because the frequency of donations in the plague year was affected by mass psychosis in the face of the triumph of death, which means that there is no clear mathematical correlation between the number of donations and the level of mortality.

*

[32] Biraben 1975: 160.
[33] Mollat 1963: 510–11, 515, 518–26.
[34] Jouet 1972: 270–2.

As mentioned above, the data for Mediterranean France and the County of Savoy show a surprising consistency and can be legitimately synthesized into a general expression of the level of mortality in the Black Death. The usable mortality data based on sources suitable for demographic estimates end in Saint-Flour in Auvergne. As can be seen from Table 27, for these large regions the mortality rates in the Black Death are consistently in the order of magnitude of 60 per cent, which must also be the synthetic mortality rate of all data taken together.

Table 27. Mortality in the Black Death in France (%)

Region/country	Taxpaying householders	Taxpaying population	General population
Provence[a]	54.5	60	60
Albi, Millau, St Flour	50–55	55–60	60
County of Savoy	50–55	55–60	60
'France'	50–55	55–60	60

[a] The progression of the figures rightwards is somewhat different for Provence compared to the other regions because the registers of 'feu d'albergue' also comprise (most of) the poor classes.

The few more impressionistic data available from more northerly parts of France are not at variance with the data from southern France. No demographically valid data are available that can support a view that is sometimes presented to the effect that mortality rates in the Black Death were lower in central and northern France than in the south.

In French historiography, it has been quite usual to emphasize the importance of the Hundred Years War for the national calamities and catastrophes that visited France in the Late Middle Ages and to play down the causal role of the Black Death and ensuing plague epidemics for the decline in population and its duration. Indeed, the regions invaded and ravaged by the English troops were seriously affected, price materials and other economic indicators show sharp fluctuations and gyrations, albeit only in the short term. However, the data on the mortality in the Black Death generally come from French regions that were little affected by war. They confirm the good sense in Postan's dictum that one should not explain by the Hundred Years War what can be explained by a hundred years, and, certainly, one should not explain by the Hundred Years War what can only be explained by the Black Death and ensuing plague epidemics.

31

Belgium

There are a few pieces of information on the mortality of the Black Death in Belgium, more specifically in the County of Hainault (for terrritorial and administrative terms, see above, Chapter 13). Manorial account books registering traditional death duties payable by tenants in the form of the holding's best beast, so-called 'heriots', reveal sharply increased death rates among the peasants in the countryside of the southern and central parts of the County of Hainault from the summer of 1349.[1] Unfortunately, there are no earlier registers that can serve as a base for comparison and estimates of the relative increase in mortality. If the numbers of deaths in the corresponding period of 1358–9 are used as a comparative basis constituting the index of 100, the level of mortality in the district of Ath (35 km north of Valencienne) in the period 24 June 1349–11 April 1350 was more than five times higher, namely 533;[2] in the district of Maubeuge (about the same distance east of Valencienne) the level of mortality was 480; and in the district of Soignies (15 km north of Mons) 253. There can be no doubt that these figures underestimate substantially the real increases in mortality, because the population in 1358 must be assumed to have been much smaller than on the eve of the Black Death in the summer of 1349. In addition, the mortality figures relating to the time of the Black Death are minimum figures, because the registers are in such a bad state that parts of the folios are missing or the writing has become illegible.

The death of heads of households/tenants would often, of course, create human and social problems that easily could cause delayed payment of heriots. Nonetheless, at least a considerable part of the quite high numbers of payments of heriots in the ensuing years reflects, undoubtedly, that the Black Death was still spreading in this very densely populated countryside of Belgium: the district of Maubege, for instance, which had suffered 231 deaths as reflected in payments of heriots in 1349–50, suffered an additional 98 deaths in the period 25 April 1351–1 May 1352.

Two villages situated centrally in the district of Ath in western Hainault, namely Hyon and Hon, are registered with 14 and 7 payments of animal heriots, respectively,

1   Sivéry 1965: 431–47. Cf. Sivéry 1966: 56–7.
2   More accurately, within this district the small town of Ath itself and surrounding areas were only lightly hit, while the small town of Chièvres and surrounding areas were severely ravaged and made most of the contribution to the level of mortality. Sivéry 1965: 435, 437.

in 1349–50, and with only 1 and 0, respectively, in 1353–4. Although nothing is said in the tax registers about the cause of death of so many tenants in 1349–50, no doubt, the Black Death was to blame.[3]

Table 28. Decline in number of households in two hamlets in Artois 1347–86

Year	Izel	Esquerchin
1347	61	28
1351	45	23
1377	31	20
1385	23	11
1386	29	10

There are also two possible glimpses of the mortality in the Black Death in the two small villages of Izel and Esquerchin, east of Arras in eastern Artois, an area that today belongs to Belgium but at the time was under the French Crown. A tax payable in kind by these villages makes it possible to estimate the number of taxed households, with the usual reservations concerning tax evasion and special arrangements.

As can be seen from Table 28, in these villages, the reconstructed number of taxpaying households declined by 26 and 18 per cent, respectively, between 1347 and 1351. Applying the standard assumption with respect to the reduction in the average size of households between the pre-plague populations and the surviving populations from an average of 4.5 persons to 4 persons in the countryside, these figures indicate that the populations contained in the taxpaying households in the two villages were reduced by 34.5 per cent and 27 per cent, respectively. This may be correct in relation to the facts on the ground, but, then, it could also be quite far off the mark. As in Montmélian in the County of Savoy, surviving households from the large landless classes (of cotters, day labourers and sub-tenants) could have moved rapidly into the good vacant tenements after the ravages of the Black Death. In Montmélian, the number of peasant households declined by 52 per cent from 1347 to 1349, but already in 1352 the decline had been reduced to 16 per cent. This is not to say that this is what happened in Izet and Esquerchin, only that it is fully possible.

It is a conspicuous feature of Table 28 that the number of fiscal households continued to fall so sharply that by 1385/1386 their numbers had diminished to 37.5/47.5 per cent and 39.5/35.5 per cent of the pre-plague level. The sharp fall in the number of households in the two villages between 1377 and 1385 could reflect a thinning out of the households that eventually triggered numerous breakdowns. This could be taken to indicate that there was a relatively larger diminution in the size of the households than envisaged by the standard assumption, as also seems to have been the case elsewhere, and that, in this area, the households tried harder than in most places to scrape through as long as possible for economic, social, cultural or religious reasons.

---

[3] Sivéry 1965: 436–8.

However, the sudden leap in the number of fiscal households in Izel between 1385 and 1386 gives occasion to some doubt as to the social, economic and demographic realities reflected in the table. The representativeness of these two isolated data remain in doubt, and they could be compared to the mortality in Esparron-de-Verdon in Provence.

Also interesting is a so-called *obituary*, a register in which a religious institution entered notices on the death of brothers, sisters, other spiritual staff or dignitaries, and of donors. *The Obituary of the Hospital of Our Lady of the Potterie* in Bruges records 60 deaths in the hundred years 1301–1400. In fifty-eight of these years there was no death at all; in thirty-four of the years there was only one death; in five of the years there were two deaths; in one of these years, in 1400, three names were entered. And then there are two years that stand even more clearly out as special cases: in 1349 there were nine deaths and in 1351 four deaths. It should be added that a serious plague epidemic ravaged Flanders in 1400, so that plague must be considered the cause also of the three deaths registered in this source that year. This means that plague was the cause of 26.5 per cent of all mortality among the spiritual staff at the hospital and its donors. If we subtract the deaths due to plague around 1350, there was, on average, 0.5 deaths each year in the remaining ninety-eight years of the four-teenth century; thus, plague mortality in 1349 was eighteen times higher than the average for these years. Furthermore, this dramatic increase took place in the course of four months. Also the deaths in 1351, representing the second highest annual level recorded in hundred years, must be assumed to have been caused by the Black Death, and the real mortality could, therefore, quite likely have been appreciably higher.

Why was no mortality recorded in 1350? There are mainly two possible explana-tions: (1) there could have been a reintroduction of contagion in Bruges in 1351 from surrounding areas – it has been shown above that the Black Death lingered on unusu-ally long in the Low Countries, and plague mortality was obviously quite widespread also in 1351; (2) it may have been a temporary breakdown in some of the hospital's administrative functions in 1350 as a consequence of the extreme loss of members of the staff, with some names of persons who died this year possibly being entered in the obituary only in 1351. The relevance of the second line of argument is strengthened by the fact that in the city of Ghent, for instance, no accounts for any institution are preserved for the years of the Black Death.[4] One should note that these two adequate explanations are not contradictory alternatives, and both could be true at the same time. Also this line of argument on the basis of information provided by the obituary indicates that the real mortality rate caused by the Black Death in this upper-class demographic segment was considerably higher than suggested by the figures of 1349.

These few pieces of evidence on mortality can only be considered suggestive of the level of mortality caused by the Black Death in Belgium, but they are obviously comparable and compatible with the levels of mortality obtained for Spain, Italy and French-speaking Europe.

Blockmans also concludes that the Black Death appears to have caused lower mortality in the Low Countries than in most other countries or regions of Europe.[5] This is in accordance with the current epidemiological theory of plague as presented

---

4   Blockmans 1980: 839.
5   Blockmans 1980: 843.

above. The main reason for this important feature of the Black Death's history in this part of Europe is the extreme population density. Large parts of the population lived in town-like environments with particularly low mortality rates in plague epidemics, or in cities with higher mortality rates than in towns but still with considerably lower mortality rates than in more sparsely settled rural areas.[6] A country with Belgium's demographic characteristics, high population density and high intensity of inter-local and inter-regional interaction should be expected to be blanketed by the Black Death but suffering, nonetheless, lower mortality rates than regions characterized by rural socio-economic structures.

Because late-medieval Belgium was particularly intensively involved in international trade, plague would be more often imported in the following centuries than in most other regions of Europe. The net demographic effect of Belgium's plague history in the Late Middle Ages was quite likely a diminution of the population of much the same size as in other countries, although the mortality effect of the individual epidemic was less severe. Blockmans presents a related view when he states that 'the demographic effects of plague in the Low Countries in the course of the 14th and the 15th centuries are probably more due to a regular recurrence of the epidemic than to the phenomenon of the Black Death itself'.[7] That is certainly true for all Europe, but even more so for the Low Countries.

[6] See above, pp. 30–34.
[7] Blockmans 1980: 850.

32

England[1]

Data on the mortality of the Black Death in the British Isles are only available for England. In England, as in other countries, the vast majority of the population lived in the countryside, gaining their livelihood from agriculture. Only a disease with exceptional powers of spread in the medieval countryside could cause such extreme mortality as to lead to a tremendous diminution of the population of momentous historical significance. This was indeed the case, as stated by Ziegler: 'the story of the Black Death in England is above all the story of its impact on the village community'.[2]

In contrast to the plague mortality data from south-western Europe, English mortality data relate almost entirely to the countryside, to mortality among manorial populations and the rural clergy.

In his pioneering book of 1948 on English medieval demography Professor J.C. Russell made an estimate of the mortality in the Black Death among the tenants-in-chief, the class of noblemen that held land directly from the king, using documents reflecting transfer of such feudal land following the death of the possessor in the epidemic.[3] However, this material is too unrepresentative both with respect to social class and age structure to be of any use in this context. Russell's claim that the mortality of the noble class was representative of general population mortality must be dismissed out of hand. This has been done emphatically by a number of scholars.[4]

A number of studies on the mortality among the beneficed parish clergy are of great interest, because they include thousands of persons living all over England in relatively well-known circumstances and, thus, constitute a social category suitable for meaningful statistical analysis and discussion of mortality. Their territorial distribution would by and large correspond to the distribution of England's population and must be considered satisfactorily representative in this important respect. Nonetheless, there are, unfortunately, many problems associated both with this source material and with the studies.

---

1 British historiography on the Black Death is commented on above in the introduction to the chapter on the Black Death's epidemiology.
2 Ziegler 1970: 122.
3 Russell 1948: 216.
4 See. e.g., Titow 1969: 68; Razi 1980: 100.

First, the beneficed parish clergy are a special social category with a specific behavioural pattern, living in social and economic circumstances that generally were much better than those of the general population. Studies on this social category, whatever their qualities, primarily yield information on mortality among the beneficed parish clergy. The desire to use studies of these beneficed clerics to approach the question of the mortality among their parishioners, the ordinary rural populations, in order to obtain notions of mortality at the national level of analysis meets with serious problems of comparative sociological and epidemiological translation: it must be possible to identify and estimate the significance of various economic, social and behavioural similarities and dissimilarities characteristic of the beneficed parish clerics and the ordinary population that would affect their relative risk of exposure to the disease and their chances of survival if infected.

The serious problem inherent in the question of the representativeness of special social categories can be illustrated by comparing the mortality rates of bishops and parish priests in the Black Death: whereas English bishops suffered a mortality rate of 18 per cent, at least 45 per cent of the parish priests died,[5] as we shall see. When the death rate of bishops can be shown to be entirely unrepresentative for what happened to their parish clergy, claims to the effect that the mortality of parish clergy should be representative of the mortality among their parishioners can easily be thrown in doubt, and the need for intensive comparative analysis and independent evidence becomes very much emphasized.

When a beneficed parish priest died, his bishop would institute a successor to the cure. The use of institutions of parish priests as sources for the demographic study of mortality among the beneficed parish clergy in the Black Death involves a number of source-critical problems. Some of these problems have been discussed above in connection with the use of the same material for epidemiological analysis of the pace and the spatio-temporal pattern of spread of the Black Death in England. However, when mortality is brought into focus, other aspects of the source-critical problems become central, but they all relate to two basic questions: (1) the identification of the population of beneficed parish priests at risk on the arrival of the Black Death; (2) the proportion of them who died in the epidemic (or, alternatively, the proportion still alive on the morrow of the epidemic).

Surprisingly, so far no attempt has been made to make a comprehensive and in-depth discussion of the source-critical problems pertinent upon the use of this material. Opinions on the interpretation of these mortality data and their suitability for inference to general mortality may appear to be based on rather incomplete premises. However, in the context of this book, this task cannot be avoided. Six principal categories of *source-critical problems* can be identified.

(1) The population of beneficed parish clergy at risk was not identical with the holders of benefices at the time of the Black Death.[6] In a significant number of cases,

---

[5] Coulton 1947: 496. In France, the mortality among the bishops was much the same. The annual mortality rate in the decade 1330–39 was 6.08 per cent, in the plague years 1348–9, 24 of 97 bishops, or 24.74 per cent, died. Cazelles 1962: 295–6. It is erroneous to deduct the normal mortality rate for two years in order to estimate net plague mortality, because many of the bishops who would have died anyway actually died of plague and must be included in the plague mortality rate.

[6] The proportion of parish benefices that were normally vacant and waiting to be filled is also a question that could be legitimately asked. As shown both above and below, the normal mortality rate of upper-class

the benefices fell vacant more than once because not only did the incumbent priest at the outset of the epidemic die, but also his successor(s). Deaths among subsequent holders of benefices during the epidemic must be deleted because there is no way of comparing the incidence of their deaths with the number of persons constituting the pool of non-beneficed clergy from which they were recruited.[7]

(2) In a significant and even considerable number of cases, benefices became void by resignation during the time of the epidemic, which means that the cause of the institution of a new priest to the benefice was not the death of his predecessor from plague, but could have been the incumbent's wish to avoid the dangers inherent in the administration of the last rites among his parishioners, and to acquire a legal opportunity to flee from the epidemic disaster. In all fairness, it must be said that many resignations arose from an exchange of livings: incumbents could also resign in order to enter a better living that had been vacated by the Black Death in another parish.[8] In the ecclesiastical year running from Lady Day (25 March) 1349 to Lady Day 1350, 1,025 institutions were performed in the diocese of Lincoln; of these 201, or 20 per cent, were owing to resignation.[9] In the case of the diocese of Bath and Wells (= the medieval county of Somerset), for instance, it appears that as much as a quarter of the new institutions were the result of the resignation of the previous incumbent, rather than his death.[10] The cases of resignation must for obvious reasons be identified and deleted from the material in order to avoid significant and even substantial overestimation of mortality rates.

(3) Next, there are the problems represented by pluralism and absenteeism. It was quite usual that clerics in the service of the king or a noble patron held more than one living and, by implication, some clerics were absent from their livings for this reason. They would be represented in the parishes by non-beneficed clergymen who acted as their vicars. Ordinary rectors who held only one benefice were quite often also, for varied reasons, allowed to be non-resident, on condition that they arranged with a non-beneficed clergyman to perform their functions for pay or a share in the living's income, in other words to be his vicar. Whatever the mortality among these non-beneficed vicars who functioned as parish priests, their death would not lead to institutions. The significance of this problem in the present context is enhanced by the fact that the mortality among the pluralists was much smaller than among the ordinary parish priests. Hamilton Thompson underscores this point in his pioneering studies of the mortality among the parish clergy in the dioceses of York and Lincoln. He notes that even in the chapters [of the cathedrals] of York and Lincoln 'those who died were comparatively insignificant persons' and that the number of pluralists who died in these two large dioceses 'is hardly worth regarding'.[11] The effect of pluralism

---

males with the age distribution of parish priests is about 3–3.5 per cent. Above p. 278. The administrative delay between the death of an incumbent and the institution of his successor is 4–6 weeks. Therefore, the proportion of benefices that were normally vacant and, in this case would be vacant on the eve of the Black Death, is too small to merit consideration in this context.

[7]   I cannot agree with Hollingsworth, who would like to include every death by clerics holding benefices in the parishes, 1969: 235.

[8]   Coulton provides many data on the incidence of resignations taken from Dr Lunn's now-lost Ph.D thesis, 1947: 498–9.

[9]   Thompson 1911: 316.

[10]   Ziegler 1970: 130.

[11]   Thompson 1914: 99–100.

and absenteeism was to shrink the initial clerical population of benefice holders attached to the parish churches, and it was only their deaths that were recorded, because they led to institutions of new priests. If unrecognized, the effect on an estimate of mortality will be to produce an underestimation because the clerical population at risk was actually considerably smaller in relation to the number of livings than assumed. Because the 'number of non-resident clergy was very considerable',[12] this represents a considerable problem.

(4) Another problem that presents a serious problem for the study of this matter in many dioceses is the fact that the bishops did not have the right of institution to all parish benefices. This right could with varying frequency have been transferred to other prelates: archdeacons could possess this right in their archdeaconries, for instance, although they formally were subordinated to their bishop in the hierarchy of the Church. In the diocese of York, for instance, the number of parishes was somewhat below 1,000, but the bishop had the right of institution to only 536 benefices. In contrast, the bishop of Lincoln had almost the exclusive right of institution in his diocese.[13] Thus, it is of crucial importance that scholars studying clerical mortality rates in the parishes recognize the problem and take it into account in the material forming the basis of their estimates. The number of institutions made in the period of the Black Death must be related to the number of benefices for which the bishop had the right of institution. Otherwise, if the number of institutions entered in the bishop's register as owing to the incumbents' death is compared to the total number of parochial benefices in the diocese, the estimate could be seriously flawed and take on the character of a substantial underestimation of the mortality.

(5) Another problem affecting this material is that some institutions were not entered in the bishops' registers, presumably because the number of new institutions were episodically so extreme that the officials in charge of arranging for them and keeping the records did not manage to cope with their tasks. Another cause of deficient registration of institutions was that they were continuously made while the bishop was circularizing in his diocese; his officials took preliminary notes of these events in order to enter them in the bishop's register later. Such notes could easily be lost when they died from the epidemic. Although this problem is of noteworthy significance, it does not appear to be a serious one, but it will tend to affect estimates in the direction of being on the low side.[14]

(6) The last significant source-critical point has been made by Jessopp:

> In a period of dreadful mortality, if the parsons died off in large numbers, it would be inevitable that the impoverished livings would 'go begging'. It might be difficult to get the most valuable pieces of preferment filled – it would be impossible to fill such as could not offer a bare maintenance. Hence the Institution Books can only be accepted as giving a part of the evidence with regard to the clerical mortality. However startling the number of deaths of clergy within a certain area during a given period may appear to be, they certainly will not represent the whole number – only the number of such incumbents as were forthwith replaced by their successors [. . .] within any

---

[12] Thompson 1914: 98.
[13] Thompson 1914: 100–2.
[14] Thompson 1914: 99.

diocese the *larger the number of institutions* recorded in a given time, the *more incomplete* will be the record of the deaths among the clergy during that time.[15]

This demographically relevant point was made also by contemporaries, although in a more implicit way because the focus was entirely on the religious side of the matter. William Dene, a monk of Rochester (in Kent), renders parts of a mandate issued 27 June 1349 by the bishop of Rochester at a time when the plague was still raging but in a subsiding mode,[16] containing, among other things, the following statements:

> And some priests and clerics refuse livings, now vacant in law and fact, because they are slenderly provided for; and some, having poor livings, which they had long ago obtained, are now unwilling to keep them, because their stipend, on account of the death of their parishioners, is so notoriously diminished that they cannot get a living and bear the burden of their cure. It has accordingly happened that parishes have remained unserved for a long time, and the cure attached to them has been abandoned, to the great danger of souls.[17]

Thus, estimates of mortality among the beneficed parish clergy will tend to be underestimations, additionally for the reason that not all deaths among them will be reflected in the institution of a successor in the living, which for this reason will remain vacant.

This comprehensive presentation and discussion of the source-critical problems relating to the use of the bishops' registers of institutions is not entirely exhaustive, but it includes all significant factors. Conspicuously, only the two first problems could cause overestimation of mortality rates, and four of the six source-critical problems will tend to cause underestimation. Because several of these four source-critical points could affect estimates substantially, estimates of the mortality among the beneficed parish clergy in the Black Death will undoubtedly tend to be too low. This point has only been recognized by Richard Gyug.[18]

However, *epidemiological factors* relating to the relative chances of dying or surviving in the Black Death of the beneficed parish clergy and their parishioners must also be discussed. There are three main epidemiological or physiological problems relating to the normal mortality rate of this special social category: their level of exposure to infection, the significance of the parish priests' advantageous social and economic situation, and the significance of their relatively high average age.

(7) Undoubtedly, to the extent the parish priests personally discharged their spiritual obligations of administering the last rites to their parishioners when the Black Death broke loose in their local communities, they would have a particularly high

---

[15] Jessopp 1922: 194. Jessopp's italics.
[16] Shrewsbury 1971: 93.
[17] Gasquet 1908: 121–2.
[18] 1983: 387–8.

degree of exposure to infection. However, both the extent of exposure and its epidemiological significance are not obvious and should be discussed.

Population pressures were as much a part of the life of clerics as of the manorial populations. This point is vividly illustrated in the course of the epidemic: although a large part of the English parish priesthood was swept away by the Black Death, it appears not to have been a serious problem to find successors to the cures. Thus, in pre-plague society, there was a large pool of clerically qualified men competing for clerical livings and promotion. Preliminary research indicates that, in pre-plague society, the number of the non-beneficed clergy in the parishes was about equal to that of the beneficed clergy, although this numerical or proportional relationship varied considerably between the dioceses and between their main divisions into archdeaconries or deaneries.[19] Quite likely this is a conservative estimate, because, according to the poll tax of 1377, when surviving unbeneficed priests in great numbers had entered the livings vacated by the Black Death and three subsequent (smaller) plague epidemics, the number of unbeneficed priests was only slightly smaller than the number of the beneficed parish priests.[20]

It was usual that beneficed parish priests were assisted by auxiliary priests and hopeful successors. Hollingsworth maintained that auxiliary priests may have performed many of the dangerous spiritual services that the parish priests were supposed to perform.[21] This affects the appraisal of the parish priests' exposure to dangerous rat fleas relative to the ordinary population, which is dependent upon the extent to which they actually visited the houses of the peasants and the working classes in order to administer the last rites. The answer to that problem is only partly known: the great mortality among the parish priests proves that the majority of them must have personally and heroically discharged their obligations to their parishioners in a time of tremendous spiritual need and in the face of terrible personal risk. An important reason for this could be that they did not really have much choice, because the non-beneficed clerics in the parishes were not obliged to offer their services and expose themselves to great personal danger. This point was bluntly made by a contemporary observer, namely William Dene, a monk of Rochester (in Kent):

> In this pestilence, many chaplains and paid clerics refused to serve, except at excessive salaries. The bishop of Rochester, by a mandate addressed to the archdeacon of Rochester, on the 27th of June, 1349, orders all these, on pain of suspension, to serve such cures.[22]

Although many auxiliary priests may have refused to enter houses with dying parishioners, many of them, or at least a substantial proportion of them, fearful of their own salvation, have undoubtedly fulfilled their religious duties to prevent the loss of the parishioners' souls for want of the last rites. By doing so, they have also contributed to a significant reduction in the mortality of the beneficed parish clergy that will tend to veil some of the demographic realities to the prying eyes of modern scholars. They may have mostly performed spiritual services that the parish priests

---

[19] Hollingsworth 1969; 233.
[20] Russell 1948: 134–7.
[21] For some interesting points, see Hollingsworth 1969: 232–5.
[22] Gasquet 1908: 121.

did not find time or strength or courage to carry out personally. This does not mean that it could not have been quite usual for parish priests to leave a disproportionate part of this dangerous work to their devoted auxiliary priests; nor does it rule out that a significant proportion of parish priests was so concerned with their personal safety that they left most or all the dangerous work to their non-beneficed auxiliary priests. The fact that the number of resignations in some counties was exceptionally high supports a notion to the effect that it is realistic to take into account that the beneficed parish clergy, in the face of disastrous epidemic mortality, in general terms tended to modify their behaviour in ways that significantly reduced their risk of exposure. According to Coulton, the testimony of contemporary chroniclers 'is overwhelmingly against any distinctive clerical self-sacrifice: a unanimity all the more remarkable because they themselves were nearly all clerics, often monks or friars, and sometimes their criticism touches not a rival order, but their own'.[23]

(8) In relation to an epidemic of plague, the question of housing becomes important for the discussion of the relative risk of exposure of various social classes or social segments, because of the crucial part played by the house rats and their fleas. Social-class differences in the quality of housing with relevance to its suitability for rats must therefore also be considered. This question has attracted considerable interest in relation to early modern plague epidemics. In Italy, Cipolla and Zanetti have collected assertions by contemporaries to the effect that the poor suffered serious supermortality because they lived in small, overcrowded and unsanitary housing.[24] Professor Paul Slack has studied the plague epidemics in Bristol in the period 1540–1650, and underscores the much higher mortality among the poor than among the better-off social classes, presenting the following explanation: 'The vital determinants behind this association were of course variations in standards of housing and hygiene which might attract or repel the rats and fleas which carried plague.'[25]

Actually, the habitation of the peasantry contributes to explain why the Black Death could wreak such havoc in the countryside. The hovels of the peasants were built in wattle and daub, i.e., with interlaced rods and twigs or branches in walls and roofs that were plastered with clay or mud, materials that offered no real resistance to the movement and settling of rats. Inside, there were grossly unsanitary conditions: pigs and chickens and even cows and sheep would live in the same rooms as the peasant household who would sleep on hay directly on the earthen floor. Higher temperatures and much filth and dirt were living conditions very much to the liking of house rats. In the humorous but apt words of Ziegler: 'The medieval house might have been built to specifications approved by a rodent council as eminently suitable for the rat's enjoyment of a healthy and care-free life.'[26] Much the same can be said about the urban housing of the poor and destitute classes. In fact, much the same can be said about the housing of common people all over Europe and not only in England.

[23] Coulton 1947: 500.
[24] Cipolla and Zanetti 1972: 198–202; Cipolla 1974: 280–3.
[25] Slack 1977: 49–62. Cf. Wilson 1963: 172.
[26] Ziegler 1970: 157; Dyer 1986: 19–45; Hurst 1988: 898–915.

The significance of the fact that the beneficed parish clergy were much better housed than the ordinary population has important epidemiological aspects that are generally overlooked: to the extent that they lived in houses of stone, and to a significant degree also if they lived in half-timbered houses,[27] their habitations would contain smaller or fewer rat colonies than peasant houses. Thus, they would be exposed to fewer rat fleas in the time of plague for the time they stayed indoors, at night, at meals, at times of leisure and rest. This point accords also with John of Fordun's statement in his chronicle to the effect that the Black Death in Scotland 'everywhere attacked the meaner sort and common people [. . .] seldom the magnates'.[28]

Summing up, although the parish clergy exposed themselves to infection when visiting their dying parishioners, the extent of overexposure relative to the risk of exposure of the ordinary population may have been overrated.

(9) It is generally assumed that the normal mortality rate of the medieval beneficed parish clergy was higher than for the general population because their average age was much higher. This assumption is taken to support an inference to the effect that the mortality rate among the general or national population in the Black Death was probably significantly lower than for the beneficed parish clergy, or that it would contribute to such a tendency within the framework of various factors affecting mortality.[29] The implied causal explanation is that the immunological and physiological competence of resistance to serious disease was much weaker in the beneficed parish clergy than in the normal population because of their high average age.

This important assumption, because it has been so influential on the interpretation of the clerical mortality data, is not based on any specific medieval material. It appears that no information is available on the average age of priests at the time of institution in their benefices. Recently, it has been shown that the average age of heads of religious houses at the time of promotion was forty-three years and that they lived, on average, for another sixteen years.[30] This corresponds to the pattern predicted by Model West life table level 3, life expectancy at birth of 22.8 years,[31] and is, thus, in accordance with the other English medieval mortality and survival data.[32] Presumably, parish priests were somewhat younger at the time of institution than abbots and priors and died at about the same age, being ordained at 35–40 years and dying at about age 60. If one takes into account that those who were ordained parish priests had usually served as auxiliary priests for quite a number of years and were survivors in very unhealthy environments, one should rather assume that their basic immunological competence was above average and had not deteriorated much below any hypothetical average for the national adult population for much of their time as incumbents. Their living standards were usually much above that of the ordinary population, which should also contribute to a noticeably higher life expectancy. This is suggested also by the age-specific mortality rates contained in Table 29.

---

[27] Hurst 1988: 915–20.
[28] Dodgshon 1981: 13.
[29] Russell 1948: 230; Ziegler 1970: 131; Hatcher 1977: 23.
[30] V. Davis 1998: 115–16.
[31] See discussion of life tables in Ch. 26 above.
[32] The use of life tables and the English medieval demographic data are discussed above in Ch. 26.

Table 29. Average mortality rate at ages 0–70
according to Model West, life table, level 4
(compare Table 10)

Ages	Mortality
0	32.2
1–4	4.9
5–9	1.0
10–14	0.7
15–19	1.0
20–24	1.4
25–29	1.6
30–34	1.8
35–39	2.1
40–44	2.6
45–49	2.9
50–54	3.7
55–59	4.4
60–64	5.8
65–69	7.4

Russell made estimates of age-specific death rates on the basis of Inquisitions Post Mortem pertaining to the transfer of land subsequent to the deaths of tenants-in-chief, the noblemen and barons holding land directly from the king. His conclusion that the plague fell more heavily on older men than on the young was challenged by Goran Ohlin, who demonstrated that Russell's source-critical and statistical approaches were flawed and that age, according to this source material, made no difference to this particular risk of death.[33] Ohlin's finding agrees with other studies of the age structure of plague mortality. Plague mortality is mainly decided by exposure, by the risk of exposure to plague infection and the risk of exposure to secondary catastrophe effects. Children have a particularly high level of exposure in both cases, children's play-related behaviour increases their exposure to infection, they are especially susceptible to the debilitating effects of lack of nursing care, and they also suffer from a specific biological susceptibility insofar as plague disease tends to take a particularly fulminant course reflected in a particularly high case fatality rate (see above). Predictably, Zvi Razi found indirect evidence in the court rolls of Halesowen in northern Worcestershire that 'child mortality in the Black Death was very heavy'; in fact, 'child mortality in the plague must have been catastrophic'.[34]

In view of the fact that the normal case fatality rate in bubonic plague is c. 80 per cent, and that women and children have supermortality for physiological reasons (see above), it appears almost impossible that a hypothetical marginally higher case fatality rate for parish priests can explain much.

[33] Russell 1948: 216–17; Ohlin 1966: 78–80.
[34] Razi 1980: 104.

Several scholars have pointed out that the beneficed parish clergy, as a social category, were much better housed, fed and clad than ordinary people in their parishes, but they have been very reluctant to assign significance to these factors for the relative levels of morbidity, case fatality and mortality. However, several of the points mentioned are variables of considerable importance for the demographic effects of the Black Death, particularly with respect to risk of exposure and secondary catastrophe effects: mortality caused by the breakdown of economic production and social relations.

(10) Dearth and famine were a usual consequences of the Black Death (and later plague epidemics), because normal work both in agriculture and urban industries tended to grind to a halt under the impact of the epidemic onslaught, with severe consequences for production and income. That could be very serious indeed for the great masses of poor and destitute people, and could cause substantial secondary supermortality from the debilitating effects on the immune apparatus of serious undernutrition and starvation. The beneficed parish clergy were economically cushioned from any serious effects of agricultural failure.

(11) Strangely, the significance of nursing care for physiological competence and survival has been overlooked. In the great wave of plague epidemics that spread from China to many countries in Asia, Africa and America from the mid-1890s and raged with great severity in the first decades of the twentieth century, medical scholars engaged in combating the epidemic noted that the case fatality rates of Europeans were much lower than among the native populations, about 40–50 percent, instead of around 80 per cent. Because no medication was available the reasons for this difference were exactly the same that shaped the mortality of the beneficed parish clergy: they were better housed, fed and clad, and of particular importance is the fact that they were much better nursed and cared for in time of illness.[35] The relatively low level of mortality in cases of untreated bubonic plague that are well-nourished and enjoy the benefits of a good level of nursing care is confirmed by recent American experience.[36]

Because plague is transmitted to human beings by rat fleas released from a strongly decimated colony of house rats, there is a strong tendency for members of the same household to contract plague much at the same time, which will occasion a breakdown in normal functions of nursing care. It is an important point that the beneficed parish priests would normally enjoy the services of one or more servants, and their parochial staff also lodged with them, 'which could amount to four or five persons'.[37] Furthermore, parishioners would have very strong motives for doing their very best to take care of their parson when he fell seriously ill under circumstances in which they all looked death in the eyes and the need for final rites as a necessary precondition for evading perdition must have seemed all too likely. No doubt, the parsons would be well nursed if they contracted the Black Death.

---

[35] Simpson 1905: 173; Hirst 1938: 690; Hirst 1953: 145; Pollitzer 1954: 418, 509; Benedictow 1993/1996a: 146–56.
[36] Reed, Palmer, Williams et al., 1970: 483.
[37] Hurst 1988: 916.

It cannot be assumed that the case fatality rate of the parish clergy was reduced to the twentieth-century level for non-medicated persons in or from western countries. They may have enjoyed an ample diet, but it may not have been a healthy diet according to modern standards. Did they really consume a varied diet of vegetables and fruits? It is quite possible that many were gourmands or gluttons, with diets containing too many calories and animal fat and too few vitamins and other valuable nutritional elements, diets that would cause unhealthy obesity and concomitant physiological malnutrition. It will never be possible to calculate the real case fatality rate of the beneficed parish clergy, but some simple arithmetic will illustrate the potential of the line of argument. If the case fatality rate of the beneficed parish clergy was reduced from the average of 80 per cent to 60 per cent, this implies that a mortality rate of 40 per cent reflects that two-thirds of them contracted the disease. A mortality rate of 45 per cent corresponds to a morbidity rate of 75 per cent, and a mortality rate of 50 per cent corresponds to a morbidity rate of 84 per cent, morbidity rates that accord with our assumption above that parish priests would tend to become physically involved in the epidemiological process in the early epidemic phase in their parishes.

In short, although the beneficed parish clergy may have had a significant overexposure to infection with a correspondingly higher morbidity rate, it must be considered probable that their case fatality rate was substantially lower.

Additionally, supermortality from secondary catastrophe effects must have been much lower among the clergy than among the ordinary population, especially among the poor and destitute, and among children. When whole families fell ill more or less at the same time as a mass phenomenon, often no healthy person would be left that could take properly care of the ill, provide them with food and drink, maintain elementary standards of sanitation and hygiene, and so on.

(12) The epidemiological line of arguments includes some other points that have also been discussed in the general introduction to plague mortality. The course of plague disease is particularly fulminant in children and to some extent in adolescents. Women are more susceptible to contracting the disease than men, because they spend more time inside the houses where the infective rat fleas lurk. Pregnant women invariably die, and married women were often pregnant in those days when they were exposed to natural fertility (see above). As pointed out several times, adult men must be assumed to have had lower morbidity and case fatality rates in plague epidemics than the ordinary social categories of women and children with which they constituted general populations.

Taken together, the epidemiological arguments underpin an inference to the effect that the mortality among the beneficed parish clergy was not higher than in the ordinary population. On the contrary, they indicate that mortality may have been significantly and even considerably lower. Among English historians, Thomas Hollingsworth and A. Hamilton Thompson have doubted the conventional wisdom of considerable supermortality among the beneficed parish clergy as compared to the general population, assuming, instead, that the mortality rates for these two social categories were about equal;[38] Maud Sellers, J.Z. Titow and R. Lomas appear to be the

---

[38] Hollingsworth 1969: 234; Thompson 1911: 321–2.

only historians who have envisaged that the mortality among the rural populations was even higher,[39] Sellers stating bravely as long ago as 1913:

> It is probably owing to the preponderance of information from ecclesiastical sources that the belief has become so general that the clergy suffered more than any other class of the community [from 'the Great Pestilence'], but a careful study of the limited material other than ecclesiastical does not bear out this assumption.

The two lines of arguments that have been pursued in order to establish a general basis for assessing the mortality of the beneficed parish clergy compared to that of the ordinary population, namely the source-critical arguments and the epidemiological arguments, can now be summed up and generalized. First, four (nos 3–6) of six important source-critical factors will tend to contribute to underestimation of the beneficed parish clergy's mortality rate. Several of these factors will tend to affect the data in ways that will lead to significant underestimation; thus, the total level of underestimation on these grounds may be quite considerable.

Summing up the epidemiological line of arguments, taking into consideration all factors of importance that would affect the risk that resident beneficed parish priests would contract plague and would die from it, it is not at all likely that they, as a social category, would suffer a higher mortality rate than the ordinary population. Five (nos 8–12) of the six epidemiological factors, excluding specific exposure to infection, will tend to produce higher morbidity and mortality rates among the ordinary population than among the beneficed parish clergy. They have quite likely had a significantly higher risk of exposure with consequent higher morbidity rate, but their case fatality rate was probably substantially lower. Furthermore, the beneficed parish clergy did not suffer significant supermortality caused by breakdown in nursing care when they fell ill. It must also be taken into account that the beneficed parish clergy were quite safe from the economic secondary effects of the plague that were such a dire menace to the health and survival of the large classes of poor and destitute people in those days, especially in those rural parts of England that were ravaged in the high seasons of agricultural work.

Summing up both the source-critical and epidemiological lines of argument, it appears clear that the mortality among the beneficed parish clergy must be assumed to be significantly underrepresented in the bishops' registers of institutions, and that the epidemiological factors affecting their chances of surviving the carnage would give significantly lower mortality rates (or higher survival rates) than among the ordinary population.

We now have at our disposal a solid basis for discussing the estimates of the beneficed parish clergy's mortality rates according to dioceses given in Table 30 below. The registers of institutions for the dioceses of Durham and Carlisle in northern England are lost or only partially extant, so no contributions to the present subject can come from these areas. The majority of the estimates are marked with an asterisk. They are taken from Dr Lunn's thesis, which is now lost; hence it cannot be ascertained to what extent his estimates have been produced with due consideration to the various

---

[39] Sellers 1913: 442; Titow 1969: 6; R. Lomas 1989: 130. Cf. Gyug 1983.

source-critical and epidemiological problems discussed above. Professor Coulton, who had access to the thesis and renders most of these figures, does not comment on the source-critical problems, which may give cause to scepticism. Shrewsbury, who also used this thesis, refers to two important points made by Dr Lunn: the importance of resignations, and that some other prelate than the bishop or the king could have the right of institution.[40] Thus, we may infer that Dr Lunn has taken into account some of the source-critical factors, while he seems to have ignored the epidemiological factors, possibly except the probable higher risk of exposure inherent in the administration of the last rites during the epidemic.

Another danger signal can be seen in the fact that in the case of the three dioceses for which we have independent and competent studies of the mortality rates among the beneficed parish clergy, namely for the dioceses of Exeter, Lincoln and York, Dr Lunn's figures are markedly lower in two of them, and in the case of the diocese of Coventry and Lichfield his estimate is slightly miscalculated on the low side. Dr Lunn has estimated a mortality rate of 39 per cent for the beneficed parish clergy in the diocese of York, while Hamilton Thompson, in a study that can be scrutinized and confirmed to be of a fine standard, has estimated a mortality rate of 44.2 per cent; Dr Lunn's estimate for the diocese of Exeter is 48.8 per cent, while Ransom Pickard has estimated it at 51.5 per cent (331 first institutions owing to death in 642 parishes).[41] Thompson's and Pickard's estimates are preferred over Dr Lunn's in Table 30, because they can be examined and found to be the outcome of competent studies. The estimated death rate for the diocese of Coventry and Lichfield, based on 459 benefices to which the bishop instituted, in which there were 184 first institutions owing to the death of the incumbent, should be 40.1 per cent and not 39.6 per cent as calculated by Dr Lunn.[42]

Two other scholars in addition to Dr Lunn have studied the clerical mortality in the Black Death in the diocese of Ely, comprising Cambridgeshire and the Isle of Ely. K.L. Wood-Legh found 90 institutions in 1349, whilst J. Aberth in a recent study found only 83.[43] It is unfortunate that Aberth does not argue why his figure should be more accurate than Wood-Legh's; consequently both figures must be taken into account.

One reason for some of the difference could be that Wood-Legh found only one resignation, while Aberth found three. On the condition that Wood-Legh has overlooked that two of the institutions she registered were resignations, the real difference is five institutions (88 and 83).[44]

Unfortunately, Aberth's and Wood-Legh's approach is incomplete and unsatisfactory: they do not actually consider the question of the total clerical mortality in the parishes caused by the Black Death, but refer to the more limited question of the extent of clerical mortality in the year 1349 and the institutions that these deaths occasioned. In the pre-plague years, there were two institutions in 1345 and in 1346, and five institutions in 1347 and in 1348. Consequently, the average annual death rate

40   Shrewsbury 1971: 94.
41   Pickard 1947: 22, 24–5.
42   Figures rendered by Shrewsbury 1971: 77.
43   Wood–Legh 1948: 158; Aberth 1995: 278–9.
44   It cannot, of course, be entirely ruled out that she just found more institutions, and that the figure of 90 should be maintained.

among the beneficed parish clergy in this diocese in these years was 3.5 clerics. According to Aberth's figures for institutions in 1350 and 1351, there were 13 and 11 institutions, respectively, 3.7 times and 3.1 higher than the pre-plague average, while the figures for the ensuing years show that the situation was normalized, with a sudden drop to four and three institutions in 1352 and 1353, respectively, and none in the following two years. This pattern reflects presumably to some extent that the Black Death was still active at the beginning of 1350, but, because the number of institutions was so high also in 1351, probably reflects mainly that there were more clerical deaths than there were at the time clerical recruits to the vacated benefices in the parishes. This could be owing to a variety of reasons: some stayed away for fear, other took the chance to succeed immediately to the good vacated benefices, which consequently were filled quite soon after the incumbents' death, while the poor cures had a hard time finding a new incumbent. It could also be owing to extraordinarily high mortality.

Because the great number of new beneficed clerics must have reduced the average age of the parish priests, clerical mortality must be assumed to have fallen noticeably in the following years. This consideration is corroborated by the fact that the average annual number of institutions in the four-year period 1352–5 was 1.75, exactly half of the pre-plague incidence of institutions. Consequently, about twenty of the twenty-four institutions in 1350–1 should on statistical grounds be assumed to have been caused by the Black Death, and this number of institutions should be added to the numbers of institutions identified for 1349. This means that the number of plague-death-related institutions in the diocese was probably 108 or 103. Second institutions in the same benefice, of which there were seven, should be subtracted from both these sets of figures, which gives a total of 101 or 96 institutions related to the subsequent deaths of beneficed clerics resident in the parishes on the eve of the Black Death. These must be considered minimum figures, because neither Wood-Legh nor Aberth considers the question whether there could have been plague-related institutions in the autumn of 1348. However, according to Frances Page, the Black Death's onslaught on the manors of Crowland Abbey, a few kilometres north of the town of Cambridge, began in October 1348 (see above).

The number of benefices in the parishes at the time of the Black Death is not known with certainty. One could have hoped that it would have been possible to reconstruct the number of parishes from the bishop's register. Instead, Aberth uses an ecclesiastical tax register of 1291 that records 176 parish benefices. From this figure seven cases of non-resident priests must be subtracted, which takes the total of resident parish priests in the diocese on the eve of the Black Death down to 169. This means that either 59.8 per cent or 56.8 per cent of the parish priests were carried away by the Black Death. This extraordinary figure can also explain why it took so long to fill up the vacancies. Remarkable mortality seems also to accord with the economic effects in Cambridgeshire outlined in a contemporary statement of Thomas de Chedworth:

> lands in very many and innumerable places lie uncultivated, not a few tenements are daily and unexpectedly destroyed and ruined, rents and services cannot be levied nor will it be possible just now for them to be collected therefrom in the usual manner, but by a great habitual necessity they are of lesser value than they were wont to be.

Table 30. Mortality rates of the beneficed parish clergy according to dioceses (see also Table 31 and Map 8)

Diocese	Medieval counties	Mortality (%)
Exeter	Cornwall, Devonshire	51.5
Bath and Wells*	Somerset to the R. Avon	47.6*
Winchester*	Hampshire, Surrey	48.8*
Ely	Cambridgeshire	57/60
Norwich*	Suffolk, Norfolk	48.8*
Worcester*	Worcestershire, Gloucestershire, Warwickshire	44.5*
Hereford*	Herefordshire, Shropshire to the R. Severn	43.2*
Lincoln	Oxfordshire, Buckinghamshire, Hertfordshire, Bedfordshire, Huntingdon, Rutland, Northamptonshire, Leicestershire, Lincolnshire	40.2
Coventry/Lichfield*	Shropshire, Staffordshire, Derbyshire, Cheshire, Lancashire to the R. Ribble	40.1*
York	Nottinghamshire, Yorkshire (to the R. Tees and R. Humber), Lancashire (from the R. Ribble)	44.2

* refers to information in Dr Lunn's thesis, now lost (see pp. 352–3).

For the same reason, the incomes of a chantry de Chedworth had founded in Anglesey Priory in Cambridgeshire in early 1349 and which he had endowed with lands and rents that should suffice to maintain two priests who would say masses for him, his family and his ancestors had fallen so strongly in the wake of the Black Death that they could maintain only one priest.[45] This means that the mortality among the customary tenantry was so high that the survivors among the very numerous (all-but) landless classes were too few to provide successors to all the vacancies although they apparently constituted more than half the pre-plague population (see above).

Because an annual average of 3.5 parish priests died in the pre-plague years, about half of this number could be assumed to be beneficed parish priests who died from other reasons than the Black Death, while the other half would have died anyway, but actually died from the plague and, therefore, should be included in the estimate of net mortality among the beneficed parish priests. This gives an adjusted estimate of 58.7 or 55.7 per cent, respectively, but because such adjustments have not been made in relation to the other estimates, the unadjusted figures will be used in Table 30 to ensure comparability.

The mortality rate among the diocese of Ely's parish priests found by Dr Lunn and passed on by Professor Coulton is 'only' 48.5 per cent. This could indicate that also Dr Lunn relates only to the institutions performed in 1349, and not to the totality of institutions that must be assumed to be plague-related. This gives further occasion to suspect that Dr Lunn's estimates tend to be on the low side. Alternatively, the discrepancy could be explained by assuming a scribal error on the part of Professor Coulton,

---

45 Cited by Aberth 1995: 285.

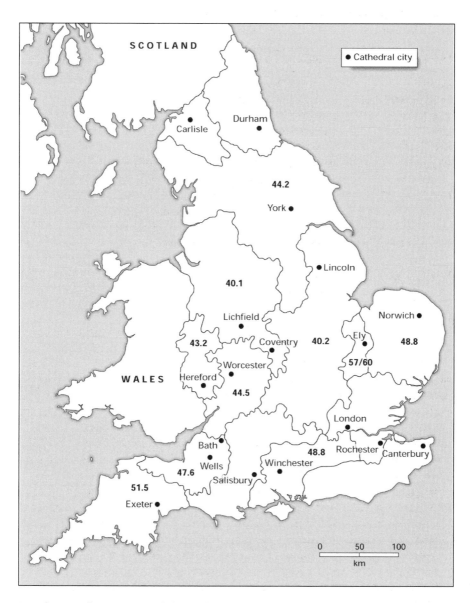

Map 8. Mortality among English parish priests in the Black Death

that Dr Lunn's figure was 58.5 per cent and not 48.5 per cent. In Table 30, the testable estimates based on the studies of Wood-Legh and Aberth are used instead of Dr Lunn's, because the evidential premises are known and apparently trustworthy within small margins of uncertainty, in the range of 60–57 per cent (on the somewhat unlikely condition that no parish priests in the diocese died from the Black Death in the autumn of 1348).

No scholar considering these figures has seriously taken into account all the six epidemiological and physiological factors discussed above. They have all focused one-sidedly on the increased risk of exposure for the parish priests consequent upon visiting of houses of dying parishioners, neglecting to take into account the five factors that will tend to produce underestimation. Neither have they taken into account all the source-critical factors bearing upon the estimates, or considered that four of six factors will tend to skew the estimates in the direction of underestimations. Taking into account all significant factors that would affect the mortality of the beneficed parish clergy and the quality of its reflections in the bishops' registers with respect to demographic studies, the figures in Table 30 should either be considered minima or more likely underestimations. Death from other causes than the Black Death must have been about halved in relation to normal death rates, and represents a counteracting deductive factor of around 1.5 per cent (which has not been deducted in Table 30).

There is a discernible geographical tendency in this material, indicating slightly higher mortality in the southern half of England than in the northern half. The reason for this is not clear. It could possibly be that while the Black Death was unleashed in spring and could spread undisturbed or little hampered by cool or cold seasonal weather in the southern half of England, the epidemiological processes could have become extinguished by cold winter weather in some places as it moved into the northern half of England. The tentative or hypothetical nature of this line of argument must be emphasized. It could also be that parish priests tended more to flee, resign or leave their duties to their auxiliary priests as the news of the disastrous mortality rates of the approaching epidemic had more time to sink in.

It has also been possible to glean a few urban data from various studies, which are rendered in Table 31. Because no study on good source material has so far been published on the mortality among any urban population,[46] mortality rates of the beneficed parish clergy in these urban centres are the only urban data available. The representativeness of this small sample of data can be challenged. As they stand, they

---

[46]   The small exception is Megson's study of 370 prosperous Londoners registered in a tax-assessment list of 1346. Of these 370 persons, 359 were alive on the eve of the Black Death; 29 per cent can be positively identified as having died in the Black Death, 38 per cent are known to have survived, but the heart of the demographic problem in this case is that 32 per cent of the names just disappear. This author would tend to believe that at least the great majority of these prosperous and active Londoners disappear from the sources because they were dead, which would take the mortality of this wealthy category of persons up to 50–60 per cent. If the source material relating to these persons is so poor that this is not the case, that a large proportion of these 116 persons should be expected to disappear from the records in the ensuing years, it should be assumed that there was also a great loss of members in the years 1346–8, much larger than the 11 persons who are identified as having died in this period and are subtracted from the original cohort in order to identify the cohort exposed to the Black Death. This destroys the usability of the material both in its pre-plague and post-plague versions. In short, if that is the case, the conclusion must be that the mortality was between 29 and 61 per cent, which is not of much use. Megson 1998.

suggest that the mortality among the beneficed parish clergy was markedly higher in urban centres than the general averages for their corresponding dioceses. Because the urban populations constituted such a modest proportion of the English population, this degree of supermortality among the urban parish clergy will have meant little for total mortality among this social category. It is interesting to note that these four cases of mortality rates among the beneficed parish clergy in English urban centres have an average that is quite similar to the mortality of their colleagues in Barcelona.

Table 31. Some urban mortality rates of English beneficed parish clergy according to first institutions compared to diocesan rates (%) (see also Table 30 and Map 8)

Diocese	Diocesan mortality	Town/city[a]	No. of benefices	No. of deaths	Urban mortality
Exeter	51.5	Exeter	19	11	58
Lincoln	40.2	Lincoln			60
Worcester	44.5*	Bristol	18	10	44.5
York	44.2	York	21	17	81

[a]   Pickard 1947: 25; Thompson 1911: 326; Boucher 1938: 36; Shrewsbury 1971: 110, referring to Sellers 1913. Boucher forgets to deduct two second institutions, so the mortality rate among the parish clergy holding benefices on the eve of the Black Death is therefore not 55 per cent, as estimated by him, but 44.5 per cent.
* refers to information in Dr Lunn's thesis, now lost.

It is unfortunate that the bases of these diocesan mortality estimates for the beneficed parish clergy, namely the numbers of parish benefices within the bishops' right of institution and the numbers of first vacancies caused by death, are not specified in most cases. This means that the two categories of figures cannot be summarized and the average be calculated. Considering this question on the basis of a more rough evaluation of the diocesan estimates and the spatial distribution of the English population[47] it appears reasonable to infer that they indicate an estimated general mortality rate of the beneficed parish clergy at around 45 per cent. Seen in relation to the source-critical and epidemiological discussion above, and the indications to the effect that Dr Lunn's estimates tend to be low, it appears reasonable to conclude that this must be an unrealistic minimum figure. Instead, in contrast to previous comments on this material, it appears more likely that the real mortality rate of the beneficed parish clergy in the Black Death was significantly higher, and 50 per cent may seem a quite moderate adjustment. Urban mortality among this social category appears to have been around 60 per cent, about the same as for the beneficed clergy of Barcelona.

A less interesting category of people is the monastic communities living in religious houses. However, the religious houses were widely distributed, and a large proportion was situated in the countryside. As a social category they must be considered to belong to the upper classes, enjoying the advantages of far better food, clothing, services and nursing care in time of illness than the ordinary population. Not least, they would often also enjoy the important advantage in relation to plague of living in houses of stone that were far less amenable to colonies of black rats than ordinary English housing at the time. J.C. Russell has collected information on twelve religious houses and found an average mortality rate of 44 per cent.[48] Presumably, the regular clergy, with its more secluded life than the secular clergy, would have been less exposed to the Black Death than the beneficed parish clergy. The mortality rate suggests that this was the case, but, perhaps, to a smaller degree than expected. It is an interesting aspect of these two types of clerical mortality in the Black Death that the epidemiological and sociological analyses of the respective social circumstances support a presumption to the effect that the mortality in the ordinary population was higher (and not lower, as some scholars have hypothesized).

A comparative test of the validity and representativeness of these conclusions on the mortality among the beneficed parish clergy can be obtained from studies of the mortality among rural classes of customary tenants, sub-tenants, cotters, demesne workers and day labourers. According to the basic assumptions with respect to the social distribution of mortality in the Black Death established above and used in the present Part 4 on mortality, it should be expected that the mortality rates were even higher among the ordinary population than among the beneficed parish clergy or the regular clergy in religious houses. This view is supported by the epidemiological discussion of factors affecting the mortality of the beneficed parish clergy. As underscored several times, the study of the mortality among the rural populations in the Black Death is much more important than of any other social category, because almost everywhere they constituted 85–95 per cent of the national populations.

In this part, the term tenants will refer to peasants holding land in significant amounts that would at least more or less suffice to maintain the household by subsistence farming. Those who held no land or insignificant amounts of land, namely cotters, sub-tentants and day labourers, will be referred to collectively as the landless classes; the class of smallholders will tend to straddle this divide in varying degrees.

The main categories of sources for the study of rural populations have been produced within a manorial context, namely rentals, cadasters, manorial court rolls and account rolls, and have been commented on above in the introduction to Chapter 15, on the epidemiology of the spread of the Black Death in England. This means that also in the case of England, the main type of information on mortality among rural populations in the Black Death will relate to tenant householders who represent the better-off social classes of manorial peasant society. In the technical language of English medieval agricultural history, the sources can mainly give information on the mortality among the customary tenantry.

The classes of the rural poor had grown vigorously in the thirteenth century and the first half of the fourteenth century, and had equalled or outnumbered the classes of fully-fledged customary tenants defined as holders of tenements of the size of half-virgates (roughly 15 acres) or larger that would about suffice for subsistence

---

[48] Russell 1948: 222–3.

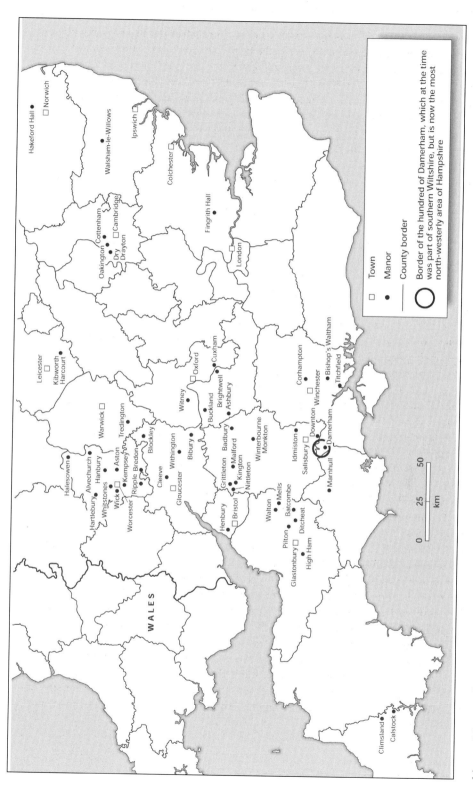

Map 9. Manors of southern and central England with known mortality in the Black Death

Table 32. Death rates in per cent on 15 manors belonging to the diocese of Worcester, as mentioned in Table 33. Locations are shown on Map 9

W = Warwickshire   G= Gloucestershire

Manor	Death rate (%)
Alvechurch	43
Aston	80
Bibury G	76
Blockley	54
Bredon	60
Cleeve G	35
Hanbury	64
Hartlebury	19
Henbury	19
Kempsey	50
Ripple	55
Tredington W	45
Whitstones	21
Wick	36
Withington G	60
Total	42

farming (18 acres).[49] For instance, on the six manors of Glastonbury Abbey in Somerset there were 260 fully fledged customary tenants and 350 holders of five acres and less, of whom at least 150 were cottars.[50] The surviving manorial extents for thirty of Glastonbury Abbey's manors show that the total number of landless men ('garciones') was of the same order as the number of tenants.[51] On the eve of the Black Death, the social scene in the English countryside was characterized by strong population pressure. There was strong competition for land, the lords of the manors could demand high rents and fines and exact heavy labour services from their tenants. Cottars, day labourers, smallholders and other poor people who were dependent on work for wages in order to scrape together a livelihood had to compete for work opportunities and work hard for little pay. In short, they were hard times for the poor and destitute who constituted large proportions of the rural populations.

This means that in pre-plague society there was a vast pool of people who could only dream of acquiring a good tenement. Great numbers of those who survived the Black Death saw their dreams come true. This process of sudden upward social mobility by a great many households of the landless classes caused by the Black Death was a general European feature that has been commented on many times above in relation to various countries, especially because it tends to blur or conceal the real mortality suffered by the tenantry in the Black Death.

[49] Kitsikopoulos 2000.
[50] Postan 1950: 242.
[51] Ecclestone 1999: 14.

In addition, English sources tend to make it difficult to follow a well-defined cohort of individually known tenants through the epidemic and ascertain their fate with respect to dying or surviving in the Black Death. When Christopher Dyer estimates that 15 manors belonging to the bishopric of Worcester had a total reduction in their number of tenants of 42 per cent (see Table 32 and Map 9), this figure cannot be taken to indicate the real mortality rate among the tenants. The estimate is based on post-plague registrations of tenants of 1351 and 1353, a time when an unknown, but certainly substantial number of cottars and sub-tenants and other landless people would have taken up good tenements escheated to the lord for lack of heirs, a point also emphasized by the author.[52] The point can also be illustrated with evidence relating to the manor of Titchfield, which contained about 150 tenants, but where 155 tenants were registered as dead in the period late October 1348 to early May 1349.[53]

On the other hand, the tenant population of age 20 and older can often be quite well reconstructed on the basis of rolls of the manor court, because it is unlikely that tenants would not appear in them: they would be mentioned making suit of court or fealty to the lord or for default of either, making transfers of land, payments of fines, for disposing of the tenement by surrender at death, and so on. The crucial point is that the court rolls provided customary tenants with evidence of title, so that it was in the interests of the heir or the new tenant to have the transfer of property following a death properly registered.[54] In addition, rentals often give good information on the size and composition of a manor's tenantry and their holdings. The main source-critical problem is that not all tenants died while holding land: the sick, disabled or aged might surrender their land and retire, and their deaths would not be mentioned. Strictly speaking, the number of deaths appearing in court rolls is the number of tenants who died while in possession of a holding.

Table 33 contains all good data on the mortality among the tenantry[55] and the very important data on the mortality among the landless men of age 12 and older on 17 manors of Glastonbury Abbey. It is a comprehensive material with strong evidential powers, comprising 51 manors and 28 townships, 79 rural communities in all. This manorial material has a wide spatial distribution in southern and central England, although it is also possible to discern a narrow band of counties stretching north-wards from Sussex without manorial mortality data. There is an obvious deficit of mortality data north of Worcestershire and southern Leicestershire, where a line can be drawn through Halesowen and Kibworth Harcourt, respectively. North of this line we have at our disposal mortality data only for the north-easternmost corner of England. With data for 26 townships County Durham is actually well covered, and studies of three manors in the south also comprise three of these townships. The two townships in Northumberland for which mortality data are available are situated on the border with County Durham and in close proximity to a number of the town-ships in County Durham and must be considered to reflect much the same social and economic context (see Table 34 and Map 10). On the other hand, the quite large parts

---

[52] Dyer 1980: 237–9. See also comments in note m, Table 33, below.
[53] Watts 1998: 24–5.
[54] Dyer 1980: 220.
[55] There are a few other studies of very small manors, which, taken together, show the same mortality pattern as on the larger manors in the table. See, e.g., James 1998: 13–15.

Table 33. Manorial death rates among tenants. Manors of the diocese of Worcester and their specific death rates are specified in Table 32, of the priory of Durham in Table 34, of the abbey of Glastonbury in Table 36. Locations of manors in southern and central England are shown on Map 9; locations of manors in northern England are shown on Map 10

Possessor of manor(s)	Manor	County	Mortality (%)
Duchy of Cornwall[a]	Calstock	Cornwall	62
Duchy of Cornwall	Climsland	Cornwall	42
Glastonbury Abbey[b]	17 manors	4 counties[c]	57
Diocese of Winchester[d]	Bishop's Waltham	Hampshire	65
Diocese of Winchester[e]	Witney	Oxfordshire	65
Abbey of Titchfield[f]	Corhampton	Hampshire	54.5
Diocese of Winchester[g]	Downton	Wiltshire	66
Diocese of Winchester[h]	Brightwell	Berkshire	29
Merton College, Oxford[i]	Cuxham	Oxfordshire	65
Crowland Abbey[j]	Cottenham	Cambridgeshire	57/49
Crowland Abbey	Oakington	Cambridgeshire	70
Crowland Abbey	Dry Drayton	Cambridgeshire	47
Earl of Oxford[k]	Fingrith	Essex	63
Earl of Suffolk[l]	Walsham-le-Willows	Suffolk	60
Lay lord[m]	Hakeford Hall	Norfolk	+50
Abbey of Halesowen	Halesowen	Worcestershire	40–46
Diocese of Worcester[n]	15 manors	Worcestershire	(+)50
Merton College, Oxford[o]	Kibworth Harcourt	Leicestershire	64/70
Durham Cathedral Priory[p]	Billingham	County Durham	55
Durham Cathedral Priory	Newton Bewley	County Durham	59
Durham Cathedral Priory	Wolviston (free tenants)	County Durham	41
Durham Cathedral Priory[q]	28 townships	County Durham	+50

[a]   Hatcher 1970: 105. For some problems relating to the use of heriots (death duties), see below.

[b]   Eccleston 1999: 25–6. All 17 manors and the relevant figures are presented in Table 36 below. Cf. Titow 1969: 71. This figure of 57 per cent is based on the study of head-tax lists of males of age 12 or older that held no land on the manors. Thus, this is a study of the rural proletariat and the estimate of the mortality in the Black Death relates to this social category. However, Eccleston points out that a number of males of this social category who died in the Black Death presumably were not registered, and that the real mortality was somewhat higher, presumably about 60 per cent. The mortality among this social class must be assumed to be significantly higher than among the customary tenantry, and a standard assumption of 5–6 per cent has been discussed in Chapter 27 and has been used throughout the book. In accordance with other findings on the proportional distribution of taxable–nontaxable or rentpaying–nonrentpaying social sections of the populations, Eccleston too finds that this landless section of the manorial population constitutes about half the population. These are the reasons that the figure of 57 per cent is used here as representative of the general manorial population.

[c]   Somerset 6, Wiltshire 8, Berkshire 2, Dorset 1. Damerham is today situated in the north-westernmost part of Hampshire, but in the Middle Ages was situated in Wiltshire, as indicated on Map 9.

[d]   Manor of Bishop's Waltham, 264 of 404 tenants died in the Black Death. Titow 1969: 69–70.

[e]   Ballard 1916: 195–6.

[f]   James 1999: 6.

[g]   Ballard 1916: 213. The basis of Ballard's estimate is not completely clear in this case. It is based on the payment of heriots, which are death duties paid on the death of the tenant for the right to transfer it to an heir. In 1349, the bishop received 106 farm animals as heriots from his tenants who, according to an extent of 1376–7 numbered 152, but this number is now said to comprise also the cottars. This is rather unusual, because

cottars would often not have at their disposal farm animals, and either transfer of the cottage to an heir did not require payment of a heriot or the heriot was payable by a small money payment. On the manor of Brightwell, which also belonged to the bishopric of Winchester, cottars did not pay heriots, as Ballard himself points out. 1916: 208. Whatever the case, the inclusion of cottars means that this estimate of mortality among tenants is not directly comparable to the others, because cottars must be assumed to suffer higher mortality than the customary tenants.

[h] Ballard 1916: 207–8.

[i] P.D.A. Harvey 1965: 135–6.

[j] Page 1934: 120–5. The basic figures for the three manors are 58, 50 and 42 tenants at Cottenham, Oakington and Dry Drayton, respectively, on the eve of the Black Death, of whom 33, 35 and 20 died. Taken together, this means that 88 of the 150 tenants on the three manors died in the Black Death, corresponding to a mortality rate of 58.67 per cent. Ravensdale has recalculated the mortality rate among the tenants on Cottenham, and has found a significantly lower mortality rate than Page did, namely 49 per cent. Ravensdale 1984: 198. It is somewhat disquieting that both scholars are very confident about their results.

[k] Fisher 1943: 13–20. I must admit that I have found Fisher's information somewhat bewildering. He states that the number of tenants was 60–65 in 1348. If this estimate of the number of tenants is related to the number of tenants that had died in the plague, namely 55, the mortality rate will be a mind-boggling 88 per cent. However, Fisher also asserts that the number of tenements on the manor was 88. If we relate the number of dead tenants to this figure, the mortality rate is 62.5 per cent. Cf. Hatcher 1977: 22.

[l] Lock 1992: 316–21. Of 176 tenants 71 survived.

[m] Campbell 1984: 96. Campbell states that over half of the 198 tenants named in the pre-plague listings of 1349 were dead by December 1350, but the number of deceased tenants given in his Table 2.2 is 98, i.e., 50 per cent.

[n] Dyer 1980: 236–9. See also Table 32 containing the names of all 15 manors and their respective death rates. As mentioned above, Dyer cannot follow a cohort of tenants through the Black Death, but bases his estimate on the pre-plague and post-plague numbers of tenants, in the latter case on tenants registered in 1351 and 1353 As it is, Dyer's material produces an estimate of tenant mortality of 42 per cent. However, Dyer points out himself that it would be unjustified to infer that this was the real mortality rate caused by the Black Death, because the figures for the various 15 manors reflect to a varying degree 'recovery in the aftermath of the epidemic'. Actually, the process of replacement by new tenants started during the epidemic. Dyer's figures show great variation in mortality between the manors: for Aston and Bibury the tenant mortality rates were 80 per cent and 76 per cent, respectively, while for Hartlebury and Henbury the rates were 19 per cent. Dyer points out that this variation is 'explicable in terms of the different rates at which tenants took up vacant holdings. Recovery may well have been rapid at Henbury, Hartlebury and Whitstones, and relatively slow at Bibury and Hanbury, because land was in greater demand on the first three manors.' Dyer 1980: 238. For these source-critical reasons, Dyer's estimate is obviously markedly too low. I have, therefore, taken the liberty of rounding off his total estimate upwards to 50 per cent in order to approach a more realistic mortality estimate, which still, however, must be considered a minimum estimate.

[o] C. Howell 1983: 16–17, 42. The manor was endowed by Bishop Merton of Rochester for the foundation of the Oxford College named after him. The data are somewhat unclear, but there appear to have been 69 tenements before the plague and that 44 of the tenants died in the Black Death. R. Lomas has estimated the mortality rate of tenants at Kibworth Harcourt at over 70 per cent. 1989: 131.

[p] T. Lomas 1984: 259–60. Billingham, Newton Bewley and Wolviston all lie in the south-eastern part of the county: see nos 24, 25 and 26 in Table 34 and Map 10. In a rental of 1347, 84 tenants are listed under Billingham, 22 under Newton Bewley and 66 under Wolviston of which 29 were free tenants. The records of Durham Cathedral Priory contain three surveys of tenants who died during the period of the Black Death. They show that 46 tenants in all died at Billingham, 13 at Newton Bewley and 12 of the free tenants at Wolviston. T. Lomas mentions that there were in addition 15 bondage tenants at Billingham, held exclusively for labour services, but because he does not mention how many of them died, this group must be deleted from the material. This means that the mortality rates on Billingham, Newton Bewley and Wolviston were 55 per cent, 59 per cent and 41 per cent, respectively; average mortality for the three manors was 53 per cent.

[q] R. Lomas 1989: 129. See also Table 34, note a, and Map 10.

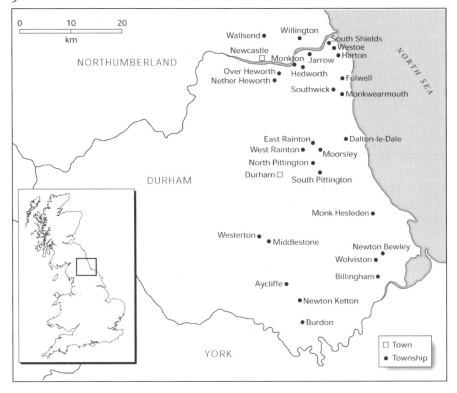

Map 10. Townships in Northumberland and County Durham with known mortality in the Black Death

of England that are covered by data contained a large proportion of England's population.

Even a quick glance at Table 34 will show that the assembled data confirm that the mortality rate of the customary tenantry, predominantly male householders, exceeded 50 per cent. Again, it is not possible to summarize all the basic data in order to produce an average estimate for them, but it is plausible to approach this question in a more approximate fashion. More than half the material is constituted by the 17 manors of the Glastonbury Abbey (see Table 37 and Map 9) and the 15 manors of the Worcester diocese (see Table 31 and Map 10), with average mortality rates of 57 per cent and around or probably rather somewhat above 50 per cent, respectively. The significance of the mortality data relating to Glastonbury Abbey's manors is enhanced by the fact that the manors have a quite wide geographical distribution over four counties. Taking into consideration the remaining twenty or so manors that tend to exhibit an even somewhat higher average death rate, it appears reasonable to conclude that the mortality rate of the English tenantry in Black Death was about or at least close to 55 per cent.

This finding is certainly supported by the study of the mortality in 28 townships in north-eastern England that show a collective mortality rate of over 50 per cent (see Table 34 and Map 10).

For various reasons discussed above, the mortality among the tenantry as a social

Table 34. Mortality (%) for the 28 townships of the priory of Durham mentioned in Table 33. Locations are shown on Map 10, each specified by the number in the first column. N = Northumberland.[a]

No.	Manor	Death rate (%)
1	Willington (N)	20
2	Wallsend (N)	43
3	South Shields	50
4	Westoe	56
5	Harton	45
6	Jarrow	78
7	Monkton	21
8	Hedworth	27
9	Over Heworth	36
10	Nether Heworth	72
11	Fulwell	56
12	Southwick	53
13	Monkwearmouth	67
14	Dalton-le-Dale	69
15	East Rainton	29
16	West Rainton	34
17	Moorsley	45
18	North Pittington	56
19	South Pittington	52
20	Monk Hesleden	44
21	Middlestone	70
22	Westerton	61
23	Aycliffe	61
24	Newton Bewley	48
25	Wolviston	47
26	Billingham	45
27	Newton Ketton	42
28	Burdon	64
Total		+50

[a] In his paper of 1989, R.A. Lomas specifies the death rates for only a few of the individual townships. I am sincerely grateful to Dr R.A. Lomas for providing me in a personal communication with the individual data for all 28 townships as rendered in Table 34. Because the size of the individual manorial populations and the number of deaths on each of them is not known, the total number of persons exposed to the Black Death cannot be summarized and related to the total number of deaths among them. Consequently it is not possible to indicate more accurately the death rate for these townships taken together than the figure of +50 per cent given by Dr Lomas.

category and as manorial demographic cohorts must be assumed to be lower than among their children and wives and, thus, among the general tenant population; it must also be assumed to be lower than among the poor and destitute classes of a manor: consequently, the mortality among manorial demographic cohorts of tenants must be assumed to be significantly lower than for the general manorial population. As mentioned above, no English evidence has been produced that provides information on the intra-household mortality and its effect on household size.[56] The specific mid-fourteenth century data that so far is available relate to Tuscany and a mountain village in the Savoy. In this case, we must rely on the pointers inherent in the general analysis of the workings of plague epidemiology in the social settings of households and neighbourhoods[57] and its accordance with the scant empirical material on the matter that is available. This material indicates that the net effect on the average size of surviving households in a general population as a result of losses among their own members and of admission of surviving relatives or children of other families, was a decline of 0.5 person, in Tuscany from 4.3 household members to 3.8.

Supermortality among the poor has been confirmed by Razi's study of the population on the manor of Halesowen, and by Ecclestone's study of the mortality among the landless males of age 12 or older on 17 manors of Glastonbury Abbey. Ecclestone's study indicates a supermortality among this social class in relation to the usual mortality rate among the tenantry of about 5 per cent.[58]

Applying the standard assumption with respect to the development of the household multiplier gives the result that the English tenant population was reduced by about 60 per cent. In addition, it must be assumed that the landless classes and other social categories that were particularly susceptible to secondary catastrophe effects suffered considerable supermortality for various reasons discussed above, so general population mortality must, therefore, have been noticeably higher. The standard assumption on this point implies that general population mortality, which also includes the supermortality of the lower manorial classes, was of the order of magnitude of 62.5 per cent.

In some cases, special types of sources have allowed scholars to construct pre-plague cohorts of men that are somewhat wider with respect to age and social class than the tenantry. Frankpledge was a basic element of local jurisdiction in medieval England.

---

[56] Professor Richard Smith praises M. McIntosh for applying a household multiplier of 4.5 in 1251 and one of 3.0–3.5 in 1352. Smith 1991: 42. This assumption does not appear to be based on any specific evidence, but the tendential direction of the line of reasoning is in general accordance with this book. At the mid-1200s the English population was still growing quite briskly, while in the pre-plague decades it appears to have been oscillating around a quite stationary size, which means that average household size would have been significantly smaller, quite likely in the order of magnitude of 4.25 persons, as in Tuscany. This reduces the difference somewhat. The post-plague reduction in household size envisaged by them has a poor evidential basis, and it is easier to argue for a stronger reduction in average household size in the intermediate aftermath of the plague than three years later, when many of the households that had lost a parent and one or more children had fused by marriage with other households with a similar fate, and therefore made for a significant incidence of quite large households. The cautious line pursued throughout this book in the construction of standard assumptions will also be maintained for the sake of the regularity of argument and the comparability of outcomes.

[57] An interesting case showing the strong tendency for plague to hit all members of a family or household because it is based on rat plague within the house is given by Gasquet 1908: 120.

[58] See Table 33, note b in relation to Glastonbury Abbey and Table 37 below.

A frankpledge jurisdiction was constituted by several tithings. Every member of a tithing was answerable for the good conduct of, or the damage done by, any one of the other members of the tithing. The tithings originally contained ten members, but at the time there were usually from eight to fifteen members.[59] All males aged 12 or older and resident within the frankpledge jurisdiction for at least a year were required to be sworn into tithing. Women, clerics, wealthy freemen, and the gentry were excepted. The tithings were liable to render a cash payment, and in many communities this 'tithingpenny' payment became a fixed sum paid annually by the community as a whole. However, in some communities it still represented a payment of a halfpenny or penny from each member of the tithing in the fourteenth century, and thus fluctuated from year to year in accordance with the tithing's membership, and, consequently, with the resident population of adolescent and adult males. The need to keep the frankpledge system updated, integrate new age-qualified cohorts and new members of the communities, and to fill up the tithings, ensured quite continuous records that, in theory, are suitable for demographic and statistical treatment.[60]

Series of annually fluctuating tithingpenny data pertaining to some Essex localities are still extant and have been studied by the two American scholars, Professor J.C. Russell and Professor L.R. Poos. They have used tithing lists to study the ravages of the Black Death in three and four communities, respectively, in southern and central parts of Essex (see Map 11); one of these communities is included in both studies, so there are data for six different communities in all. The data are rendered in Table 35, but need some further discussion and analysis: in the view of this author, the tithing data are fraught with source-critical problems of various kinds when used to estimate mortality in the Black Death.

The effects of social mobility and migration on the tithings' membership are problems with the potential to seriously undermine the usability of such records in order to gauge the demographic effects of the Black Death. The crucial source-critical problem in the case of the pre-plague and post-plague tithing lists is whether or not or to what extent they record the same cohort of persons so that the reductions in their membership numbers reflect their mortality rates in the Black Death. Unfortunately, the two scholars have not attempted to establish cohorts of individually known named males and follow the constituents through the Black Death. They have only counted the number of males on specific manors named in the tithing lists closest in time to the Black Death, measuring the decline in their numbers in the intervening years.

The earliest post-plague tithing lists are from 1351, 2.5 years after the plague. In the meantime much could have happened that could have affected the tithing lists' demographic usability or trustworthiness for two main reasons: because of the abrupt changes in the social composition of the manorial population that took place when many surviving landless families moved into vacant tenements that had escheated into the lord's hand for want of heirs, and because poor families could improve their lot by migration[61] now that there were good tenements to be taken up everywhere.

---

[59] Poos 1986: 6.
[60] Poos 1985: 519–21; Poos 1986: 5–17; Smith 1991: 37–8.
[61] Poos 1991: 108, 159–64.

The point can be illustrated by A.E. Levett's comments on some relevant developments on the diocese of Winchester's manors in the immediate post-plague years:

> Of 18 manors examined 5 had absolutely no vacant tenements in September 1349, 2 had none in September 1350, 4 had none in 1351, while in 1354 4 had none, and 2 had only one still vacant [. . .] a very large proportion of the tenements must have been occupied again by 1351.[62]

The fact that the earliest post-plague tithing lists are from 1351, and most of them are even later, implies that the tithings in the meantime had probably gone through radical change brought about by a substantial influx of new members of diverse origins, especially by upwards social mobility of poor people in local society, and by immigration. This is the reason that in order to carry out a realistic mortality estimate showing the diminution of the original cohort of tithing members in the plague, the lists must be studied at the individual level of analysis so that newcomers can be identified and deleted from the material. Actually, Poos has used tithing lists to show the high turnover rates of tithing membership and among local populations more generally in the first half of the fourteenth century.[63]

The longer time a manor had to adjust to the radically new situation after the ravages of the Black Death and find ways to attract new tenants from other townships, and the smaller it was, the easier it would be to replace annihilated tenant families, and the more the Black Death's demographic impact on the tithings would become veiled. The manor of Seaborough Hall, where the first extant post-plague tithing list is from 1355, almost seven years after the disaster, can serve as an instance illustrating this point. If this manor is deleted from Table 35, the average mortality rate indicated by the tithing lists of Russell's three manors increases from c. 43 per cent to over 47 per cent, and the total for all remaining manors will be c. 47 per cent.

In fact, source-critical problems abound. People did not only have motives for evading taxes, they would also draw significant benefits from evading frankpledge registration and enrolment in tithings, with the associated social and economic liabilities. Also the Israeli scholar Zvi Razi has made the point that the use of 'frankpledge dues as a measurement of plague mortality might underestimate the actual mortality if before the plague a number of villagers succeeded in evading these dues'.[64] It is also easy to imagine that the members of the tithings would be loath to take in persons that were not able to contribute economically or were liable to activate their economic responsibilities by amerciable behaviour, or both, implying a social undercurrent of non-admission and possibly ejection. Quite likely such problems would be rife in pre-plague society when such high proportions of the rural population lived in great poverty. Large fleeting classes of day labourers and seasonal workers could hardly be well organized within the tithing system, which at base was founded on stability and economic accountability.

In the aftermath of the Black Death, when a large proportion of the population had been swept away, and when surviving poor families of cottars, sub-tenants, day labourers and seasonal migrant workers in large numbers had moved into good

---

[62] Levett 1916: 82.
[63] Poos 1986.
[64] 1980: 101.

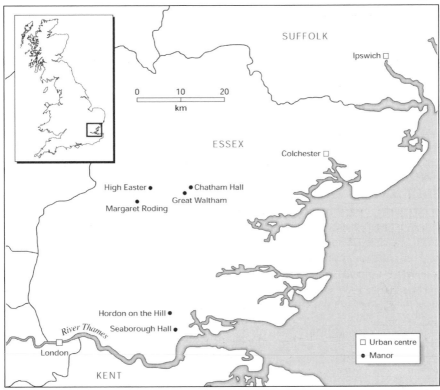

Map 11. Manors in Essex with known mortality in the Black Death

vacant tenements escheated to the lord and had joined the more stable and observ-able tenantry, the social scene in the countryside had become far more transparent, and most people were in a social and economic situation that would fit well into the tithing system. Consequently, one should expect that the enrolment of males of age 12 and older in tithings to be significantly more complete after the Black Death than before.[65] One should also note, that there is generally no sign of administrative break-down within the manorial society and economy. In the words of A.E. Levett: 'On some sixty manors in the south of England, of which exactly contemporary accounts

---

[65] For this reason, Poos's line of argument on this matter is not really convincing. He points out that studies of tithings in the light of the poll-tax lists of 1377 and even of Early Modern parish registers confirm that the tithing lists recorded quite accurately males of age 12 and older that had been resident on the manors for at least one year, and 'that in most places evasion was probably minimal on the part of those eligible for membership, even well into the sixteenth century'. However, at the same time he acknowledges that there were quite numerous 'short-term residents' that would not be sworn into tithings. Poos 1986: 16–17. The crucial point in this context is that these fleeting social classes of 'migratory agricultural or unskilled craft workers, and especially servants, who in the fourteenth century (as later) typically entered employment under annual hiring terms and might change place of employment yearly' were much larger before the Black Death than afterwards. Consequently, these social classes would affect the efficiency of recruitment to the tithings and the social representativeness of tithings differently in pre-plague and post-plague society. Unfor-tunately, this differential impact must be assumed to affect negatively the credibility of tithing lists as sources for estimates of mortality in the Black Death.

Table 35. Decline in number of tithing members in 4 + 3 Essex communities 1345–1356 (%)

Community	Year	Males	Year	Males	Decline (%)
Great Waltham	1346	187	1351	104	44.4
High Easter	1346	199	1351	92	53.8
Chatham Hall	1345	56	1356	31	44.6
Margaret Roding	1347	39	1352	29	25.6
Four communities		481		256	46.8
Chatham Hall	1345	56	1355	30	46.4
Hordon on the Hill	1349	16	1352	8	50.0
Seaborough Hall	1349	12	1355	10	16.7
Three communities		84		48	42.9
Seven communities		565		304	46.2

Source: Poos 1985: 524; Poos 1991: 106–7; Russell 1948: 226–7.

are preserved, there is no sign whatever of chaos [. . .] the Accounts were continued without a break and without change in form during the two plague years.'[66]

Professor Poos points out that, in 1355, great efforts were made on the two manors of Great Waltham and High Easter in order to force into tithing resident males who had escaped recruitment during the previous few years: especially vigorous demands were recorded that eligible males be sworn into tithing, and the juries of chief pledges were ordered to compile new lists of tithing members. As a consequence of these efforts 86 males were registered who should be sworn into tithings on the two manors. Only a minority of these 'newcomers' can be identified as having had previous recorded links to these communities, and some doubtless moved on again without ever being enrolled into the local tithings.[67]

This highlights the type of problems encountered when a social category of persons in some locality that is recorded systematically in registers at various points in time is not shaped into demographic cohorts that can be followed at the individual level, particularly when the intention is to use them for the purpose of analysing the demographic events that happen to these persons over a specified period. The well-established members of the tithings would no doubt stay registered throughout the period, but, in addition, other people of various origin, from inside and outside the manor, would to a varying degree have been sworn into tithing at the time the extant tithing lists were redacted. In short, while the tithing lists reflect truly the numbers of pre-plague and post-plague membership in tithings, and thus the decline in the registered membership, they do not any more reflect truly the decline in the original cohort of tithing members. Under this approach, all newcomers will reduce the real mortality rate among the members of the tithings on the eve of the Black Death as reflected in the sheer numbers of members. This introduces a substantial margin of error and uncertainty, and, in this case, it means that the entries of new members will

[66] Levett 1916: 72.
[67] Poos 1985: 524; Poos 1991: 107–8.

inflate the number of tithing members so that estimates of the reduction caused by plague will inevitably become underestimates, quite likely substantial underestimates. It has been shown that in every case when comparison is possible, township population data derived from poll-tax data of 1377 exceed that based on tithing membership.[68]

Summing up, as used by Russell and Poos, the tithing data will tend to underestimate the real mortality in the Black Death in Essex. It is for the time being impossible to determine by how much with any degree of accuracy, but the characteristic 'substantial' is probably justified. Arguably, the tithing material could imply much the same mortality level for tithing members as the manorial data for the tenantry, around 55 per cent, which could be a ground for increased suspicion that the landless classes were underrepresented in the tithing lists. This tentative conclusion regarding the level of mortality in the Black Death indicated by the tithing data can be seen in the same light as the manorial data for the tenantry, in which males in ages 12–19 comprise too small a proportion of the tithings to constitute a decisive difference. When we take into account that: (1) most of the tithing members were householders, (2) the standard reduction in average household size between pre-plague and post-plague society, and (3) the supermortality of children and women both from the epidemic itself and from secondary catastrophe effects, the crude data imply a general population mortality rate within the frankpledge jurisdictions of over 50 per cent, the adjusted mortality data suggest rather a general population mortality rate of close to or around 60 per cent.

Interestingly, a study has been made of the tithingpenny lists of the manor of Kibworth Harcourt in Leicestershire, which has also been studied independently by two scholars who have made two separate estimates of the mortality among the tenantry in the Black Death. This affords the opportunity to approach the promises and problems of tithingpenny data by comparing the results. In principle, the tithings should include the males of age 12 and older of the landless social classes on the manor, and the mortality rate estimated on the basis of tithing lists should be expected to be noticeably higher than the mortality rate among the tenantry if the registration was carried out in accordance with the principles of tithing registration.

Unfortunately, the scholar performing this tithingpenny study does not give the number of tithing members of the preserved lists for each year, but organizes his data in a sort of 'pin-code' figure where the height of each pin indicates the number of tithingmen when compared to his figure's vertical axis and the pin's place on the horizontal axis gives the specific year. Read in this way, it appears that there were 78 tithing members in 1348 and 38 in 1351, a reduction of 51 per cent.[69] This figure compares badly with the two estimates of the mortality among the manor's tenantry of 64 and 70 per cent, respectively. This disparity can be explained in two ways: by the source-critical problems discussed above that implied deficient registration, and by social developments in the couple of years after the Black Death until the first extant post-plague tithing lists were compiled; they can function as independent sufficient explanations, or they can also be combined.

The probable solution to the problem can be found in the same scholar's study of

---

[68] Poos 1991: 104–6.
[69] Postles 1992: 45.

Table 36. Tithingmen in Kibworth Beauchamp 1346–54

Year	Males
1346	96
1347	108
1348	122
1349	40
1350	72
1351	84
1354	96

the views of frankpledge of the adjacent manor of Kibworth Beauchamp in the years around the Black Death, which provides the data rendered in Table 36.[70] The decline in the number of tithing members between 1348 and 1349 from 122 to 40 corresponds to a mortality rate of 67 per cent, which agrees well with the estimates of the mortality among the tenantry at Kibworth Harcourt. The sudden rise in the number of tithing members in the following years contains a likely explanation for the much lower decline in the number of tithing members at Kibworth Harcourt in the years 1348–51 than the mortality among the tenantry caused by the Black Death: a similar surge in the number of tithing members there in the years following the Black Death would conceal the plague's real impact.

However, the sudden surge raises serious questions about the quality of tithing data. Although some of the rise can be explained by immigration, it indicates a substantial underregistration of males in the pre-plague tithing lists, particularly of the proletarian classes that in the wake of the plague entered good vacant tenements and were subsequently registered in the views of frankpledge. This may also explain the similarity of the mortality rate among tithing members at Kibworth Beauchamp, which can be estimated on the basis of continuous records, with the mortality among the tenantry at Kibworth Harcourt. However, the strong rise in the number of tithing members at Kibworth Beauchamp from 96 to 122 in the two years preceding the Black Death does not really fit into the picture: it could, of course, be explained as a sudden strong improvement in the registration of males in the views of the frankpledge, but, if that was the case, there should not still be a large pool of unregistered males containing so many survivors that the number of tithing members could reach the level of 1346 once more in 1354. Thus, source-critical problems continue to haunt the use of tithing data in order to obtain demographic data. Nonetheless, the tithing data do support a conclusion to the effect that the manorial populations were reduced by over 50 per cent. In view of the direction of the effects of the specific source-critical problems discussed, the real diminution of the number of tithing members caused by the Black Death may quite likely have been substantially higher.

Fortunately, in a couple of cases scholars have found material that provides insight into the mortality of the landless classes on the manors. On the manors of Glastonbury Abbey there lived a specific category of males called 'garciones',

[70] Postles 1992: 47.

comprising all males attached to the manor, aged 12 and older, who did not hold property and did not pay rent. For 17 of these manors records of an annual head-tax payable by these 'garciones' are preserved that permit calculation of their death rates in the Black Death. The outcome of a thorough discussion and analysis of this evidence, including the exempted categories of persons, is rendered in Table 37.[71]

Table 37. Plague mortality among landless men on 17 manors of Glastonbury Abbey (1348–50) in S = Somerset, W = Wiltshire, B = Berkshire, D = Dorset

Manor	Nos 1348	Recorded deaths	Mortality 1348 (%)	Nos 1350	Decline 1350 (%)
High Ham S	65	27	42	26	60
Ditcheat S	46	25	54	18	61
Pilton S	75	46	61	22	71
Batcombe S	39	21	54	9	77
Mells S	79	46	58	19	76
Walton S	31	19	61	12	61
Marnhull D	28	10	36	9	68
Damerham W[a]	156	100	64	57	64
Idmiston W	58	29	50	21	64
Winterbourne M.W	24	9	38	15	38
Kington W	57	32	56	9	84
Nettleton W	62	30	48	21	66
Grittleton W	43	27	63	13	70
Christian Malford W	79	52	66	15	81
Badbury W	45	34	76	7	84
Ashbury B	20	11	55	5	75
Buckland B	70	42	60	22	69
Totals	977	560	57	300	69

[a] Today situated in the north-westernmost corner of Hampshire.

According to Table 37, 57 per cent of the landless men liable to pay head-tax on these manors on the eve of the Black Death died in the epidemic. The scholar points out that 'it is possible indeed that some deaths went unrecorded so that the mortality may even be under-estimated'. This suggests that the mortality estimate should be rounded off upwards to around 60 per cent.

The figures in Table 33 on the mortality among the tenantry were taken to indicate an average of about 55 per cent. Again a supermortality of around 5 per cent among the poor sections of the population is indicated. The mortality among the landless classes as a whole must be assumed to have been significantly higher than 60 per cent: if we also take into account the usual supermortality among women and children as reflected in the reduction of average household size and according to the standard

---

[71] Ecclestone 1999: 25–6. There are also a couple of other studies of such lists of 'garciones' that I have not had the opportunity to read, both unpublished theses, see Ecclestone 1999: 28, n. 12.

assumption, a general mortality rate among the rural proletarian classes of close to or around 65 per cent is suggested.

The evidence also reflects the expected surge in social mobility, that many landless households took up many of the tenements left vacant by the Black Death: the decline in the numbers of landless males is substantially higher in 1350 than the decline caused by the Black Death in 1348, 69 per cent and 57 per cent, respectively. Ecclestone mentions also quite briefly that the number of 'garciones' on thirty manors of the Abbey declined from 1895 in 1,346 to 560 in 1350, i.e., by over 70 per cent.[72]

At the end of the 1950s, Postan and Titow published a study of heriots paid on five manors of the bishopric of Winchester, namely Taunton and Wargrave in Somerset and Berkshire, and Meon, Waltham and Farenham in southern Hampshire in the period 1270–1350. Heriots were death duties on customary holdings payable at the death of the tenants and were paid with a good farm animal by those who held significant amounts of land more or less sufficient for subsistence farming, which according to a recent study would require a minimum of 18 acres of land.[73] It was usual that the landless classes did not pay heriots for the obvious reason that they often or normally did not possess any farm animal. However, on the manors mentioned, heriots were paid in the form of small money payments for cottages and for the disposal of tiny plots of land. These heriot registers that appear to be complete after 1270 up to and through the time of the Black Death provide a rare opportunity to approach also the question of the mortality rate of the male rural proletariat and to compare it with the mortality of the customary tenantry. Heriot registers can, of course, only be used to analyse mortality if they relate to a fairly constant and well-known number of tenements and cottages, a requirement that also can be met in this case.

These heriot data indicate a mortality rate in the Black Death among these rural proletarians, mostly adult males, of around 50 per cent.[74] The scholars underline the serious methodological problems associated with this estimate and suggest that it should not be taken as a tenable measure of the mortality. This position reflects that they are taken aback by the sheer size of the mortality they found at a time when there were precious few studies with which they could compare their findings. However, the similarity to other manorial data increases its credibility, and most of those data have been produced after Postan and Titow carried out their pioneering study of heriots at the end of the 1950s. The problem specifically mentioned, that during the epidemic a holding could have changed hand several times owing to the death of subsequent holders is relevant, because it will tend to distort the original cohort of potential heriot payers. As a methodological problem it is related to the problem associated with the institutions of the beneficed parish clergy, which could happen more than once to the same living. However, within the manorial context it does not appear that this phenomenon has been sufficiently frequent during the Black Death to distort the basic data in a serious way.[75] While the need for a parish priest during the Black Death was acute for the whole population, from the landless

[72] Ecclestone 1999: 14.
[73] Kitsikopoulos 2000: 237–61.
[74] Postan and Titow 1958–9: 408; Ohlin 1966: 84–9.
[75] For Winchester manors, see Levett 1916: 77; Ballard 1916: 196. See also, e.g., Hatcher 1970: 102–5.

labourer to the lord of the manor, the need to formalize changes regarding holders of tenements or cottages or tiny plots of land could wait. Thus, in most cases of plural changes of householders, only the surviving holder at the end of the epidemic would eventually pay the heriot. However, there are other problems of source criticism that affect the usefulness of heriot data: what was, for instance, the incidence of heriots paid on retirement rather than death? What about the quality of recording: were heriots really assiduously collected from the landless classes, and what was the incidence of householders who were so dirt-poor and destitute that they had nothing with which they could pay?[76]

English studies on the mortality in the Black Death have used quite varied types of sources, and the great consistency in results is therefore the more remarkable. They are all the more significant because they have a wide distribution around the country, and because they relate overwhelmingly to the countryside where the vast majority of the English population lived.

First, the comprehensive studies of the mortality among the beneficed parish clergy constitute a valuable source material. Thorough discussion of the many source-critical and epidemiological factors bearing upon these studies have clarified that the mortality estimates for this upper-class social category of male adults at the diocesan level must tend to be significant underestimations. The real mortality rate must have been noticeably higher than the estimated 45 per cent, and 50 per cent is a moderate adjustment.

It was predicted on the basis of this comprehensive source-critical and epidemiological discussion that the mortality would be higher among the manorial populations than among the beneficed parish clergy. Mortality data on the ravages of the Black Death come from 51 manors distributed widely within England and 28 townships in County Durham and the county of Northumberland. These studies show an average mortality rate among the customary tenantry of about or at least close to 55 per cent. Use of the standard assumption on the reduction in average household size between the pre-plague and the immediate post-plague populations indicates that the tenant population was reduced by 60 per cent. In addition, it must be assumed that the landless classes suffered significant supermortality, especially from secondary catastrophe effects owing to poor(er) standards of nursing care during illness, breakdown of care for healthy children, and economic hardship in the aftermath of the epidemic. Thus, the general population mortality in England appears to have been of the order of magnitude of 62.5 per cent. This conclusion on the mortality in England caused by the Black Death fits remarkably well into the general European picture. This estimate of the English mortality rate in the Black Death is of special interest and significance, because it is the only available general mortality rate at the national level of analysis and because it is based on rural data.

The reason the English society and manorial economy could cope with such a tremendous loss of population must be the great overpopulation of the English countryside that has been emphasized by so many English agricultural historians. Postan studied the social composition of 104 English manors in the thirteenth century and found that

---

[76] Hatcher 1986: 22.

tenants with ten acres and less formed more than one-half of the population on all estates except those of St Peter's, Gloucester, where manorial sources conceal from our view large numbers of tenants' sub-tenants [. . .] Taken as a whole, the smallholding population of thirteenth-century villages was very numerous, frequently more numerous than the middling group and some- times more numerous than the rest of the village taken together.[77]

In Tim Lomas' more recent words:

the Durham evidence seems to support the view that much of the population was surplus to the economy by the mid-fourteenth century and that the plague of 1348–9 was more purgative than calamitous in its economic effects.[78]

As mentioned above, it has been estimated in a recent study that an average tenant household would need 18 acres to scrape by on subsistence farming, i.e., without supplementing the income in some way. Also this scholar underscores the very high proportion of the rural population that had less land at its disposal.[79] Postan's finding that tenants holding less than 10 acres represented more than half the manorial households puts the social conditions in a dramatic social perspective.

Surviving households among the smallholding and landless classes happily took up vacant tenements and moved into the ranks of the customary tenantry, young men and women married and did the same thing, and surviving tenants added vacant land to their tenements. Thus, little land was left unused, although it could now be used more extensively with a somewhat higher emphasis on animal husbandry and a less extreme emphasis on arable husbandry, also because there was no longer any need to maximize calorific production. It is also clear that not all vacated tenements were taken up by new households. Despite the great pre-plague population surplus in the form of large landless classes, mortality was greater among the tenantry than the survivors among the proletarian classes could replace.

Medieval man had no intellectual basis for understanding the demographic effects of the Black Death's ravages on the structures of the rudimentary English market economy. Their basic reaction was instinctively traditionalistic: the landlords expected, the surviving tenantry expected and the influx of happy new tenants from the landless classes expected that the customs of the tenurial system would remain unchanged. The new tenants had few or no objections to taking on the customary obligations of the tenant class, labour services, rents, fines, and so on. Only gradually did the new economic realities dawn upon the social classes of English society. Some

---

[77] Postan 1966: 622. Postan here defines smallholders as 'men whose holdings were as a rule too small for true subsistence farming. At the bottom of the group were to be found the all-but-landless villagers possessing little more than the cottages in which they lived. Some of the men in the nethermost stratum were servants who may not even have possessed any cottages but resided under their masters' roof. On the other hand, the top of the group comprised men whom the documents might describe as "ferlingers", i.e. holders of quarter virgates of customary land, who need not have fallen much short of the "middling" villagers in output and in standard of life.'

[78] T. Lomas 1984: 260. As this book was nearing completion the same point was strongly emphasized by Kitsikopulos 2000: 237–61.

[79] Kitsikopoulos 2000: 237–61.

of these processes have recently been excellently uncovered by John Hatcher,[80] but this is only an exciting beginning of the in-depth study of this problem. The mechanisms and processes of adjustment and societal change triggered by the Black Death should be put more at the centre of manorial studies in the future.

[80] Hatcher 1994.

33

How Many Died in the Black Death?

Up to now, scholars have generally assumed on quite flimsy grounds, usually a few urban data and the mortality of English parish priests, that one-fourth or one-third of Europe's population perished in the Black Death. The impressive number of new local studies published in the last four decades of the previous century constitutes a completely new opportunity for assessing the demographic effects of the Black Death. This work has produced remarkable and even startling results.

However, these mortality data are also characterized by comprehensive limitations. For most of the vast area ravaged by the Black Death, there are no mortality data. In the case of Spain, Italy and France, comprehensive data are obtainable, but only at regional levels, for the Kingdom of Navarre, Tuscany, Provence and the County of Savoy. Only in the case of England has it been possible to establish an approximate national mortality rate.

The mortality data are based on a great variety of sources that all involve their own source-critical problems, which have to be addressed carefully in order to ascertain their validity or usability and their suitability for fusion with other mortality data into generalized mortality rates. Uncertainty is the steady companion of all attempts to produce demographic estimates on the basis of sources from pre-statistical times, sources that never were intended to be used for this purpose – margins of uncertainty is a key term. In the first half of the fourteenth century, some Italian city states were developing registrations of their populations for various purposes that take on the character of censuses. However, generally the most important type of source used in these mortality studies is tax registers of various types that involve an array of source-critical issues relating to the proportion of untaxed population, tax evasion, and so on. Only in England is the main type of source manorial records, which, however, involve source-critical issues of their own, as do institutions of beneficed parish clergy.

There are also some dissimilarities in the social-class composition of the populations that are registered in the various sources used, but this does not really represent as much a problem as an opportunity to acquire valuable insights into various aspects and nuances in the complexity of social structures. Such insights improve the quality of social analysis and contribute to the upgrading of the validity and tenability of the generalizing conclusions inferred from the data. The one real problem in this context is a clear preponderance of urban studies in Italian and French studies of the Black

Death, which raises problems of representativeness because the great majority of the populations lived in the countryside.

The results obtained in this section on mortality have two conspicuous features, namely the extreme level of mortality caused by the Black Death, and the remarkable similarity of the levels of mortality in such widespread and diverse regions as the Kingdom of Navarre and Catalonia in Spain, Tuscany and the Piedmont in Italy, Provence, the County of Savoy and the Languedoc in France, and England. With the exception of Tuscany and possibly the Piedmont where the general mortality rate may have been around five percentage points lower, the discernible differences are so small that they by and large are safely located within the margins of uncertainty.

Perhaps the precocious modernization of northern Italy and the political structure there gave certain advantages. Modernization entailed greatly improved administrative capabilities, while the political divisions into city states and communes gave practicable and surveyable population size, which stimulated local identification and solidarity, and political responsibility and sensitivity to population needs. The grave population pressures in the first half of the fourteenth century had inspired responsible governments to record the totality of the population, i.e., the taking of censuses, in order to enable them to provide relief and succour, especially to the poor and destitute, in times of dearth and famine. Thus, in northern Italy, political and social structures suitable to handle grave crises had been developed that could also make a significant difference in the case of such a unique catastrophe as the Black Death. Certainly, it has never been my objective to show that the mortality in the Black Death was similar around Europe, for a continent characterized by such great variation should be expected to exhibit comprehensive variation also in relation to the Black Death. However, as it seems, great similarity could be the case.

The great mass of data on mortality caused by the Black Death have been produced on the basis of local studies of various types. In order to obtain a more generalized picture of the total mortality in the Black Death, these studies must be fused into generalized data taking into consideration various problems of source-criticism, the methodology of demography, history and social science, and the epidemiology of plague. The foundation of our knowledge on mortality in the Black Death is the quite numerous data that are based on registers recording taxpaying and rentpaying householders. These householders are not representative of the general population for several demographically and sociologically important reasons. First, they represent overwhelmingly male and adult categories of persons; secondly, they represent the economically better-off taxable and rentpaying social classes in towns and countryside. With few exceptions, the poor, destitute, propertyless and landless classes of labourers, sub-tenants, seasonal workers and suchlike people that constituted the proletariat of medieval society are left out, because they could not bear any tax assessment and, consequently, were not worthwhile to record.

Nonetheless, the estimates of mortality among taxpaying or rentpaying householders provide good data on a substantial proportion of local populations. These data can serve as a base for further studies of the mortality that involve larger parts of the population. This work must be based on some standard assumptions that necessarily will be open to discussion and further development or refinement. First, in the case of an epidemic disease that swept away 45–65 per cent of the population, there can be no doubt that the households of the surviving householders would have tended to have lost members in the plague, often to a degree that would endanger the stability and continuity of the household. In this book, it has been argued in favour of a cautious standard assumption on this point to the effect that average household size was reduced from 4.5 members in the countryside and 4 members in urban centres before the plague to 4 persons and 3.5 persons, respectively, on the morrow of the Black Death. This is probably a marked underestimation, but takes our notions of the level of mortality in the right direction. The significance of this standard assumption can be illustrated by pointing out that in the case of a mortality rate among house-holders of around 50 per cent, use of these household multipliers will indicate that the mortality rate in the corresponding household population would have been about 5 percentage points higher, i.e., around 55 per cent.

In addition, it must be assumed that the proletarian classes suffered at least signifi-cant supermortality as a result of the debilitating effects of malnutrition and undernutrition on the immune system and the higher degree of exposure to rats and rat fleas brought about by lower standards of housing and poorer indoor hygienic standards. A rough and ready consideration of the significance of these factors as applied above indicates that the mortality level among the general population was about 7.5 percentage points higher than estimated for taxpaying or rentpaying house-holders. It could be argued quite well in favour of a somewhat higher addition, prefer-ably around 10 percentage points.

Table 38 shows the generalized mortality rates for the taxpaying and rentpaying householders, for the population segments they constitute together with their house-holds, and for the general population. The quality of the data are uneven, the esti-mates for Catalonia and Languedoc, for instance, being based on only a few data. The best estimates relate to Provence, the County of Savoy (comprising also the eastern districts of the Swiss canton of Valais) and England, while the estimate for the Kingdom of Navarre has quite a good evidential basis as well. Some interesting data fall out of the table, especially the mortality estimates for parish priests in Barcelona and England and the estimates for 'men able to bear arms' in Bologna and Siena. Vari-ation in the comprehensiveness of the basic registration with respect to the recording of poor and destitute households make for some variation in the rightwards progres-sion of figures between the columns.

Table 38 shows that over half of the populations in the regions and countries for which there are data of useful quality and numbers died in the Black Death, probably around 60 per cent. Most of this mortality was due to plague disease, and a significant or substantial amount was due to secondary catastrophe effects. If these data are representative of the Black Death's ravages elsewhere in Europe, and Europe's popu-lation at the time was around 80 million persons, as commonly believed, 50 million of them died in the Black Death. This is a truly mind-boggling, horrifying and even unnerving result to all persons with their elementary sensibilities intact. It even over-shadows the horrors of the Second World War, and it is twice as many persons as were murdered by Stalin's regime in the Soviet Union.

This level of mortality indicates that ensuing plague epidemics did not over time reduce the European populations by much. Their main function appears to have been the cutting down of the population growth achieved since the previous epidemic, and thus to keep down the size of populations in towns and countryside and, by

Table 38. Mortality in the Black Death according to region and country (%)

Region and country	Tax- and rentpaying householders	Tax- and rentpaying population	General population
Kingdom of Navarre	55–60	60–65	60–65
Catalonia	(71)	(74)	(60–70)
'Spain'	55–60	60–65	60–65
Florence			60
Tuscany			50–60
Piedmont	42	50	52.5
'Italy'			50–60
Provence	54.5	60	60
Languedoc and Forais	50–55	55–60	60
County of Savoy	50–55	55–60	60
'France'	50–55	55–60	60
England	55	60	62.5
Synthesis	50–55	55–60	60

consequence, in Europe. Presumably this was also the case where plague appeared elsewhere according to the same pattern, for instance in North Africa, the Middle East and the Near East for which there are no usable mortality data.

The best data on the late-medieval population decline comes from England and Norway. In England mainstream scholarly opinion holds that the population was reduced from a pre-plague population of around six million[1] to a late-medieval population minimum of 2–2.5 million from the mid-fifteenth century to the beginning of the sixteenth century,[2] i.e., is a decline of between 66.67 and 58.33 per cent, around or somewhat above the level of 60 per cent that is indicated by the data on the mortality in the Black Death. This implies a decline in the number of inhabitants of 3.5–4 million persons in the period 1348–1450/1500, and a decline in the Black Death of 3.6 million persons. In the case of England, the order of magnitude of the mortality caused by the Black Death is known, the only country for which such information is available, and in view of this information it appears that the English population had not diminished by much between the onslaught of the Black Death and the ensuing 100–150 years.

Within the present-day Norwegian territory, more than 95 per cent of the population lived on 64,000 tenements or more or less privately owned holdings, which, using a common term, will be designated individual settlements (detached or semi-detached). These settlements contained almost no 'undersettlers' (sub-tenancies) and few living-in servants, labour families or joint families. Around 1500 the number of individual settlements had tumbled to 23,000–24,000, i.e., a decline of 62.5–64 per cent.[3] At both points in time, the population was quite stationary, but, because, at the latter point, there were good vacant holdings to be taken up everywhere, the average number of persons that inhabited these individual settlements

[1]   See p. 124, n. 2.
[2]   Hatcher 1977: 69; Smith 1978: 202. Cf. Cornwall 1970: 39–44.
[3]   Sandnes 1981: 94; Marthinsen 1996: 157.

must be assumed to have sagged slightly, probably from about 4.5 persons to 4.25 persons.[4] Furthermore, the scholar who has performed the estimate of the number of individual settlements in pre-plague society indicates that this estimate is probably on the low side. For both these reasons, a slightly higher late-medieval population decline is indicated, which corresponds to the highest reaches of the range of decline estimated in the case of England. The similarity of these dramatic developments is again striking, and suggests pronounced similarity in causation and pattern of developments.

Interestingly, this could be the case also in Southern Europe. It is possible to make some rough estimates for Catalonia that could suggest a population decline of the order of magnitude of 60–65 per cent in the period 1347–1497.[5] Thus, at the present stage of research, the contours of a cross-European similarity in the size and temporal pattern of the late medieval decline of populations can be discerned.

Hopefully, there is still sufficient unused late-medieval source material in Europe to enlarge upon and deepen our insights into these developments.

---

[4] See above, pp. 269–70, n. 46.

[5] The point of departure is records of households in Catalonia made in 1359–60 and in 1497, respectively, and which are of the same type. Within the Catalan borders of the time there were registered 85,822 and 60,570 households, respectively. Iglésias 1959: 254–5. Without going into source-critical problems, but assuming comparability over time, one could make the following probably reasonable assumptions: half of all households had succumbed to the Black Death, corresponding to a loss of population of 55 per cent when the standard assumption on the decline in average household size is taken into account; in the 11–12 years 1349–1359/60 the number of households had increased by 10 per cent. This means that that the number of households on the morrow of the Black Death was 78,000, on the eve of the Black Death 153,000, corresponding to populations of roughly 300,000 and 665,000 persons, respectively, when we take into account that urban households were smaller than rural households (pre-plague household average of 4.35 and post-plague average of 3.85).

In 1497, the number of recorded households was 60,570, corresponding to a population of 263,500 persons. This implies a decline of 60 per cent. If the population of Catalonia at this point had begun to grow like the populations in Italy and France, the nadir of the late-medieval population decline could have been even somewhat lower. These figures are interestingly similar to those presented above.

Part Five
The Black Death: Its Impact
on History

34

A Turning Point in History?

The Black Death has often been called 'a turning point in history', although usually without persuasive arguments being provided in support of such a sweeping statement.[1] Conspicuously, the historical period that the arrival of the Black Death heralded is still called the Late Middle Ages or the Late Medieval period, which means that it is primarily designated as and, consequently, considered as the societal and cultural continuation of the High Middle Ages and as having the characteristic societal and cultural features of medieval European civilization. On the other hand, the term *late* medieval characterizes it as the final period of the Middle Ages, the period when medieval societal and cultural features petered out and lost their character as the prevailing systemic features. This implies that the Late Medieval period also comprised profound structural changes and transformations that contained the societal requirements for the development of a qualitatively new societal system and, as such, definitionally, of a new historical period, namely the Early Modern period.

Such societal shifts are engendered by the accumulation of slow but profound or basic changes in economic, technological, social, demographic, political, cultural and mental structures and in the way they interact in the production of the social processes of societal transformation. In this case, it is implied that the Late Medieval period was characterized by increasing changes of the main structures of society in the direction of modernization, the accumulation of systemic changes that in the end moulded the framework of a qualitatively different social formation or societal system. In other words, as a historical period the Late Middle Ages is not only medieval, but increasingly modern, and it is this amalgam of the medieval and early modern systemic features that lends the Late Medieval period its distinctive character.

This is the central historical meaning of the concept of the Renaissance, a distinct social system that develops in the course of the Late Middle Ages with continuity into the Early Modern period, when, however, its constituent medieval features are slowly suppressed and supplanted by the further development of the Early Modern structural developments until, some time in the first half of the seventeenth century, Early Modern society takes on a clear-cut form. The famous artistic achievements of the Renaissance are 'only' the elite cultural expressions of a more generally vibrant and innovative historical

---

[1] See *The Black Death. A Turning Point in History*, 1971; and Hatcher 1977: 33.

social formation. All people living in the Renaissance were Renaissance men or women, because their lives and minds were formed by a specific social formation.

Actually, this process started in the High Middle Ages, with the greatest powerhouse of structural change in northern Italy, especially the city state of Florence, and a smaller one in Flanders. At the heart of the matter was the development of a capitalist market economy, first as trade and financial capitalism, then, in the thirteenth century, began the investment of fortunes with this background in the basic development of modern banking and insurance and of large-scale proto-industrial manufacturing.

On the social scene, these epoch-making developments were reflected in the rise of a capitalist class of proto-industrial entrepreneurs, of the proto-industrial proletariat and of salaried classes of clerks and office workers that created a new and Early Modern social fabric, the 'birth' of class society in its Early Modern form. This took place in the northern Italian and partly also in the Flemish proto-industrial centres at the end of the High Middle Ages and the beginning of the Late Middle Ages. These profound economic and social developments triggered an explosive growth in primary and secondary educa-tion,[2] and in the foundation of universities, because the capitalist entrepreneurs needed employees with various educational attainments for their capitalist businesses and ventures. They needed people who could write business letters and set up and under-stand contracts, preferably both in foreign languages and in Latin, and who could keep or audit accounts, relate to prices and costs in often violently gyrating markets, and fill active and constructive roles in the continuous endeavours to develop and rationalize produc-tion and organization. The political leaders and governments needed personnel with much the same qualifications in order to strengthen the capabilities and efficiency of their emerging early modern state administrations, and they needed employees educated in regional and Roman law. There was a strong shift from religious education to secular and humanistic education based on classical ideals, which also opened the doors of the mind to scientific exploration of reality. These developments continued unabated throughout the Late Medieval period. At the end of this short historical period the number of univer-sities had trebled, although the population had been more than halved.

The dramatic population fall caused by the Black Death and maintained by later plague epidemics lent new dynamic powers to some of these trends and stimulated the developments in specific ways, while levels of mortality never previously experi-enced gave the period other important characteristic features. The previous long-run trend of roughly the period 1150–1320 had been characterized by a relatively stronger rise in the prices of basic foodstuffs like grain and beans than in other foods and a concomitant falling trend in real incomes engendered by long-run population growth and consequent increasing population pressures on the agricultural resources. As population growth dwindled or even changed into a slight decline in the early decades of the fourteenth century, the fall in real incomes, the relative increase in the prices of basic foodstuffs, and the increase in rents and fines ended and may also have changed into a slight reversal.[3] The arrival of the Black Death and the ensuing plague epidemics abruptly reversed these long-term trends, and landlords, wealthy peasants and urban employers suddenly had to compete for labourers, workers or tenants. The

2   See, for instance, Herlihy and Klapisch-Zuber 1978: 563–78.
3   Miller and Hatcher 1978: 27–69; Abel 1978: 27–50; Abel 1980a.

all-but-landless classes and the classes of smallholders whose holdings were as a rule too small for true subsistence farming were even depleted twice over, by the Black Death and subsequent epidemics and, next, by the taking up of vacant good tenements and consequent social rise into the ranks of the middling peasantry. Consequently, rents and fines fell strongly in the long term and both agricultural and urban real wages increased correspondingly. This was 'the golden era of the wage worker', as Wilhelm Abel called it. It was the 'golden era' of poor people in the countryside as well. Inevitably, these developments also left losers, all those who possessed or owned more land than they could cultivate themselves with the help of their household, namely the lords of the manors and the 'village rich', the yeomen and franklins and the wealthier peasants who had gained greatly from the inexhaustible pool of very cheap manpower before the plague, saw their incomes diminish, and in the long term fall disastrously.

Thus, the Black Death and ensuing plague epidemics brought about a strong diminution of the proletarian classes and a strong relative growth of the classes of the middling peasantry, while the owners of the means of production lost great parts of their incomes and tended to slide downwards on the social ladder. These two disparate economic and social developments in post-Black Death society implied a profound change towards less glaring social inequalities.

Strongly rising levels of real wages for ordinary people both in town and country and a long-term strong decline in the levels of rents and fines for the customary tenantry, in other words, a sharp reduction in the extraction of surplus production by the upper classes and social elites, meant strongly increased purchasing power for the lower classes, raising correspondingly the level of consumption and changing the pattern of consumption into a much wider range of consumer goods.

This pattern of development and change fits nicely into a Malthusian explanatory model. However, the abrupt reversal of this situation caused by the Black Death and maintained by the ensuing plague epidemics did not affect the economic and social scene in accordance with the Malthusian explanatory model. The Black Death reduced the population far below any Malthusian readjustment between the level of population size and the resources for the feeding of the population within the framework of prevailing technology (a process that can be studied over much of Europe in the High Middle Ages and in the period 1600–1750). The economic dynamics of a dramatic fall in population created correspondingly dramatic changes in the economic and social parameters, from quite stationary, harshly depressed living standards for ordinary people in the decades prior to the Black Death, to dramatic improvements in the following hundred years. As estimated by Phelps Brown and Hopkins, real wages for building workers in England were as high in the mid-fifteenth century as at the end of the nineteenth century, and appreciably higher than during the First World War. It has been shown that this was also the case for agricultural labour.[4] The Black Death cut down the size of the European populations to a much lower level than warranted by the pre-plague population crisis and the need for a readjustment of the numbers of people and the amount of available productive land with the prevailing agricultural technology. The mortality effects of the subsequent plague

---

[4] Phelps Brown and Hopkins 1962: 179–96; Hatcher 1977: 48–52.

epidemics is the reason that the vast numbers of vacant good tenements that came into being did not function as a basis for rapid sustained long-term population growth that over time would reverse the specific late medieval trend and re-establish the pre-plague economic and social scene, much as happened in large regions of Europe around 1600 after about a hundred years of population growth. As a long-term situation, the great imbalance between people and resources created a high and consistent demand for manpower by those having at their disposal unused or underused resources in the form of land or of productive equipment and shops, which translated into a great improvement in the material well-being of ordinary people. The 'golden age of bacteria'[5] and the 'golden age of the wage worker' were in a causal relationship.

It also meant that the pattern of demand and consumption changed. After having satisfied a basic demand for consumption of energy in the form of grain-based or bean-based, cheap, calory-rich foods, people still had an economic surplus that they could use to increase their consumption of other foodstuffs that tasted better, that increased their sense of well-being or their enjoyment of life. In short, people ate more meat and butter, drank more beer and wine, socialized more and spent more time in taverns and inns. When they still had an economic surplus, they could buy more stylish and colourful clothing or cloth, ready-made fashionable shoes, ornaments and finery, household goods, bedding and household utensils, improve their housing, and so on. While the prices of grain or flour fell strongly over time, the real prices of meat, butter, beer and wine, building materials, and suchlike, tended only to sag.

In its turn, this long-term pattern of demand and consumption meant the break-through of mass production of cheap consumer goods at which first the Dutch and, next, the English proved themselves much better than the Italians, for reasons that cannot be commented on here, but which in the course of the fifteenth and sixteenth centuries shifted the economic and financial centre in Europe from Italy to the Low Countries and England.

On the other hand, the greatly increased cost of labour provided an impetus for the development of more efficient production, better equipment and productive machinery, better organization of work, rationalization, and so on, that would not have been there with plentiful cheap labour. While, for instance, the technology of the water-powered saw mill had been developed in the early thirteenth century,[6] it came into widespread use only in the Late Middle Ages.

As mentioned above, neither the upper classes nor the lower classes had any real or rational understanding of the effects on the economic system of a huge diminution of the population; nobody had any inkling that this was going to be a long-term feature and would be one of the main characteristic or constituting features of the Late Middle Ages as an historical period. All sorts of people related to the aftermath of the Black Death in a traditionalistic perspective, everybody expecting that everything would shortly revert to its pre-plague status, and life would soon be what it was assumed always to have been. At first, new tenants and labourers alike accepted

---

5 Thrupp 1965: 118; Smith 1988: 208–9.
6 White 1962: 82, 118.

customary contracts or wages according to pre-plague standards. Only slowly did it dawn upon them that the economic and social scene had changed profoundly. At first, as excellently demonstrated by Hatcher in a recent paper, the economic and social adjustments tended to take on a concealed or veiled character in the face of partly adamant resistance on the part of the magnates and gentry.[7] The decline of the traditional medieval economic and social system was a gradual process shaped by the interaction between the new economic and demographic realities with mental customary structures: serfdom disappeared and the relationships between peasants, labourers, workers, artisans and their landlords or employers took on increasingly the character of a market-oriented system where the levels of rents and wages were formed by demand for and supply of manpower. Thus, the new demographic situation hastened the breakdown of the feudal economic system and the rise of capitalist market economy, especially in Western Europe.

The crucial point in this context is that the sharp decline in the European populations caused by the Black Death and maintained by subsequent plague epidemics triggered economic and social responses of long-term profound significance, at least in the meaning that such processes were speeded up, the pace and dynamics of societal change and transformation increased. It also gave increased impetus to technological innovation and strengthened the emphasis on goods and products for general consumption within a more clearly consumer-oriented market economy: consumer society had its first breakthrough.

For the same basic reasons, the kings, princes, city states and urban governments improved and professionalized their administrations, seeking to cut costs, increase the efficiency of taxation and improve the provision of public services.

As the economic and social realities of great demographic contraction increasingly became transparent, the great ecclesiastical landowners, the religious houses and the magnates and gentry, had to realize that the cost of labour had increased greatly, whereas their ability to pay higher wages had declined as strongly with the fall of rents and fines; in short, that their real incomes had diminished precipitously and even catastrophically. The yeomen and franklins and substantial tenants found that they no longer could afford to hire farmhands or maids or employ resident servants, and faced social degradation into the ranks of the middling tenantry, which survived on the proceeds of their own work. There was really only one positive solution: the Hundred Years War lasted for 113 years because it was in the interest of the kings and the warrior classes (including the yeomen) and of parts of the merchant classes to keep the war going. It justified the levying of war taxes that ended in their purses, and the spoils of war could also contribute to improving their economic situation and making it more easy to maintain their particular lifestyle, social prestige and social status. When the English were forced to return home at the middle of the fifteenth century, they found similar employment in the War of Roses.

In the Nordic countries, the political elites of prelates and noblemen organized a union of Denmark, Sweden and Norway in 1397 (the Kalmar Union) in order to defend their privileges and political power against the expansion of the dukes and

---

[7] Hatcher 1994.

noblemen of the northern German Duchy of Mecklenburg for much the same basic reasons.

In Spain, the 'hidalgos', i.e., the lesser nobility or the gentry, who likewise found themselves in desperate financial straits caused by the effects of the great population decline, could engage with greater enthusiasm in wars against the Muslims in the Kingdom of Granada. When these wars eventually succeeded in the final conquest of the city of Granada in 1492, the king and the queen were so enthusiastic that they granted Columbus the money to discover the western sea route to India, which actually led to the European discovery of America (or rather the definite discovery, as the Vikings had discovered America almost 500 years earlier). The hidalgos could go on with their trade of war and earn the spoils of war there, now acquiring the name of 'conquistadors', conquerers.

The ravages of the Black Death also affected culture and mentality in specific ways. There was a new obsession with death in art and literature, even with the art of dying.[8] The distinguished French historian Emmanuel Le Roy Ladurie focuses on these aspects of the impact of plague in his great work on the peasantry of Languedoc:

> after 1665, for the ordinary people of the Languedoc the plague was no more than a bad memory, soon only a grandfather's story. It is the end of the plague psychology established after the fourteenth century, and in which were blended obsession with mass death, a sense of sinfulness (the plague, punishment for sins) and also, from Boccaccio (Florence, 1348) to Samuel Pepys (London, 1665), a compensating and unbridled desire for sexual pleasures. This mentality retreats after the age of the plagues to make room for the more peaceful emotions – in which security wins over anxiety – which are one of the multiple constituents of the modern mind.[9]

Such an epochal catastrophe as the Black Death and the return of plague epidemics transformed the tendencies of religious fanaticism and intense prejudice that were evident in pre-plague European society into religious panic. Large groups of flagellants wandered from town to town scourging themselves in order to save their souls and alleviate the Lord's wrath, believing in the mortification of the flesh as suitable penance for men's sins. As the Black Death approached new areas or towns, flagellation movements flared up and could take on the character of mass flagellation.[10]

The flagellants played also an active role in another type of panicky and far more malignant reaction to the Black Death, namely the persecution of Jews.[11] Also anti-Jewish sentiments had been strongly on the increase in the century preceding the Black Death, probably stimulated by the increasingly hard times for the great majority of ordinary people, and a consequent increasing susceptibility to notions of scapegoats. The Jews had been forced to leave both England and France in the decades around 1300, many settling in Germany or the Low Countries. The Black Death trig-

---

[8]   See, for instance the papers by Bernardo, Lerner, Polzer, and Wenzel in *The Black Death*, 1982.
[9]   Le Roy Ladurie 1966: 554. My translation from French.
[10] Cohn 1970: 127–47; Ziegler 1970: 89–111.
[11] Cohn 1970: 139; Hoeniger 1881.

gered violent persecutions of Jews over large parts of Europe, especially in Germany and the Low Countries, but also in Spain and other places where they had been permitted to stay. In the intense religious mind of medieval man, it was generally thought that epidemic disease was God's way of punishing people for their moral depravity and grave sins. One such grave sin could be that they allowed people that did not worship Christ or God in the required way to stay among them. Because the Jews in many places also functioned as pawnbrokers and moneylenders, activities that were prohibited for Christians by the Catholic Church, persecution, exiling and murdering of Jews could also serve personal economic motives. Many people found it hard to imagine that the Lord would really punish them so severely for their sins; they were after all only human beings. They developed instead the theory that the great mortality was caused by Jews and other 'enemies of Christendom' that poisoned their wells and other sources of drinking water.[12]

One may wonder how it could be that contemporaries did not observe that the mortality of the Jews in the Black Death was as great as for others. Pope Clement VI, for one, attempted to stop the persecution of the Jews, but without success. He issued two bulls against it, and when these proved ineffectual, he finally condemned the flagellants in 1349.[13]

Surviving Jews fled to Eastern Europe where they were allowed to stay by rulers anxious to include in their populations persons with great skills both in the financial sphere and as artisans and jewellers. Thus, the Black Death had two main functions in this context: tragically it transformed the process of increasing exiling and eviction of Jews from countries in Western Europe into a sort of medieval holocaust with extensive and indiscriminate murder of Jews; and it hastened the movement of Jews into Eastern Europe where their descendants were, to a large extent, annihilated in a new and even far more violent holocaust 600 years later.[14]

Summing up, it should be clear that the Black Death was an event of great historical importance. It put its stamp on the economic and social scene, the living standards of the masses improved greatly, while the upper classes and social elites saw their incomes fall and their charmed way of life being undermined. It also put its stamp on the period's religious mentality and outlook on life.

It hastened the development and transformation of European medieval society and civilization into its (early) modern historical form. By creating a great deficit of labour it speeded up economic, technological, social and administrative modernization, which especially in the capitalist centres in northern Italy and partly in Flanders found expression in a more secular and urban culture associated with the Renaissance. It also hastened the breakdown of feudal economic structures and mentalities and the rise of a prevailing dynamic capitalist market economy and concomitant innovative and dynamic attitudes and mentalities. Thus, the seeming paradox that late-medieval culture and mentality comprised both obsession with death and

---

[12] See also above pp. 178, 281–2
[13] Ziegler 1969: 96–8.
[14] The best presentation and discussion of the Flagellants and the persecution of the Jews is still Hoeniger 1881, and Ziegler 1970: 87–111.

salvation, fascination with economic and social opportunities, and the secularization of economy and art.

This could be taken as the start of the increasing compartmentalization of religion in the European mind as a characteristic feature of the modernization and rationalization of European society and culture, in which religious notions were retreating into a steadily more clear-cut spiritual role aimed at salvation. Religion's role in shaping and defending the social and economic structures of society and explaining worldly events like good or bad harvests, epidemics and disease, good luck or bad health, economic or social misfortune, and personal tragedy, and so on, receded under a slowly increasing pressure from the increasing rationality of the modernizing European mind and the developing alternative scientific approaches and explanations. The improving ability of rational observation permitted a better understanding of how plague was disseminated and the rudimentary development of modern epidemiology.

It was this development that, as shown by Carlo M. Cipolla, from the mid-sixteenth century allowed the Italians to develop efficient anti-epidemic organisations and health boards in order to combat plague. This was no longer considered an attempt to avoid God's will, but an expression of the responsibilities of governments to protect and help their inhabitants. In the seventeenth century the administrative means developed by the Italians spread over Europe, and plague disappeared gradually over the century. The Europeans had succeeded in combating an awesome, gruesome and invisible enemy of uncomprehended nature. The greatly increased administrative capabilities of the Early Modern political structures made it possible to set up efficient anti-epidemic organizations, plague hospitals and health boards. Thus, the combating of plague gave a strong impetus to the notion that governments had responsibilities for the welfare of their peoples. What over time would become national health systems was born as organizations primarily aimed at protecting populations from invasion of plague epidemics, at combating the spread of plague if the first line of defence, namely the quarantine organisations, failed, and at providing assistance and succour to the diseased and their families.

Bibliography

German and Nordic personal names and place names may include letters not used in English that are entered alphabetically according to the following phonetic rules: Å/å = AA/aa; Ä/ä, Æ/æ = AE/ae; ü = y; Ø/ø, Ö/ö = Oe/oe; ð = d.

Abel, W. 1955. *Die Wüstungen des ausgehenden Mittelalters*. Stuttgart: Gustav Fischer Verlag
———— 1978. *Agrarkrisen und Agrarkonjunktur im Mitteleuropa vom 13. bis zum 19. Jahrhundert*. Berlin: Verlag von Paul Parey. 3rd edn [first pub. 1935]
———— 1980a. *Agricultural Fluctuations in Europe from the Thirteenth to the Twentieth Centuries*. London: Methuen & Co.
———— 1980b. *Strukturen und Krisen der spätmittelalterlichen Wirtschaft*. Stuttgart: Gustav Fischer Verlag.
Aberth, J. 1995. 'The Black Death in the diocese of Ely: The evidence of the bishop's register', *Journal of Medieval History*, 21: 275–287
The Agrarian History of England and Wales. 1988. Vol. 2. H.E. Hallam (ed.). Cambridge: Cambridge University Press
Ahnlund, N. 1953. *Stockholms Historia före Gustav Vasa*. Stockholm: P.A. Nordstedt & Söners Förlag
Akiander, M. 1849. *Utdrag ur ryska annaler*. Helsinki: Simelii arfvingar
Alberch i Fugueras, R. and Castells i Calzada, N. 1985. *La població de Girona (segles XIV–XX)*. Girona: Institut d'estudis Gironins
Alexander, J.T. 1980. *Bubonic Plague in Early Modern Russia*. Baltimore: The Johns Hopkins University Press
Andenmatten, B. et Morerod, J.-D. 1987. 'La Peste à Lausanne au XIVᵉ siècle (1348/49, 1360): étude de Chapitre cathédral et des testaments vaudois', *Etudes de lettres. Revue de la Faculté des lettres de l'Université de Lausanne*, 2/3: 19–49
Annales Danici medii ævi. 1920. E. Jørgensen (ed.). Copenhagen: Selskabet for Udgivelse af Kilder til dansk Historie
Armitage, P., West, B. and Steedman, K. 1984. 'New Evidence of Black Rat in Roman London', *London Archaeologist*, 4: 375–383
Astill, G. and Grant, A. 1991. 'The Medieval Countryside: Efficiency, progress and change', in: *The Countryside of Medieval England*: 213–261
Aubry, M. 1983. 'Les mortalités lilloises (1328–1369)', *Revue du Nord*, 65: 327–432
Audisio, G. 1968. 'La peste en Auvergne au XIVᵉ siècle', *Revue d'Auvergne*, 82: 257–265
Ballard, A. 1916. 'The Manors of Witney, Brightwell, and Downton', in: *Oxford Studies in Social and Legal History*, Vol. 5. *The Black Death on the Estates of the See of Winchester*: 181–220
Ballesteros Rodriguez, J. 1982. *La peste en Cordoba*. Cordoba: Estudios Cordobeses. Publicaciones de la Excma. Diputatión Provincial de Córdoba
Baltazard, M, Bahmanyar, P., Mostachfi P et al. 1960. 'Recherches sur la peste en Iran', *Bulletin of WHO*, 23: 141–154
Baratier, E. 1961. *La démographie provençale du XIIIᵉ au XVIᵉ siècle*. Paris: SEVPEN

Barbadoro, B. 1931. 'Finanza e demografia nei ruoli fiorentini d'imposta del 1352', *Atti del congresso internazionale per gli studi sulla poplazione*. Roma: 615–619

Barnes, A.M., Quan, T.J. and Poland, J.D. 1985. 'Plague in the United States, 1984', *Morbidity and Mortality Weekly Report*, 34: 9SS–14SS

Bartsocas, C.S. 1966. 'Two Fourteenth-century Descriptions of the "Black Death" ', *Journal of the History of Medicine and Allied Sciences*, 21: 394–400

Battara, P. 1935. 'La popolazione di Firenze dal XIV al XVI secolo', *Economia. Rivista di economia corporativa e di scienze sociali*, 14: 345–354

Before the Black Death. Studies in the 'Crisis' of the Early Fourteenth Century. 1991. Manchester: Manchester University Press

Belletini, A. 1973. 'La popolazione italiana dall'inizio dell'era volgare ai giorni nostri. Valutazioni e tendenze', in: *Storia d'Italia*, Vol. 5: 489–532

Benedictow, O.J. 1985a. 'The Milky Way in History: Breast feeding, antagonism between the sexes and infant mortality in Medieval Norway', *Scandinavian Journal of History*: 19–53

—— 1985b. 'Some Social and Medical Factors which affect the Reliability of Statistical Data on Plague Epidemics. The Italian scene', *Middelalderforum. Forum mediaevale*, 11: 182–193

—— 1987. 'Morbidity in Historical Plague Epidemics', *Population Studies*, 41: 401–431

—— 1988. 'Breast Feeding and Sexual Abstinence in Early Medieval Europe and the Importance of Protein-calorie Malnutrition (Kwashiorkor and Marasmus)', *Scandinavian Journal of History*, 13: 167–206

—— 1992. 'Pestepidemiers spredningskraft i tynt befolkete landistrikt. Kan pest forklare befolkningsnedgangen i Norge i seinmiddelalderen?', in: *Liv og helse i middelalderen*. (Onsdagskvelder i Bryggens Museum, no. 6.) Bergen: Bryggens Museum: 80–101

—— 1996a. *Plague in the Late Medieval Nordic Countries. Epidemiological Studies*. Oslo: Middelalderforlaget. 2nd rev. edn [reprint of 2nd edn, 1993]

—— 1996b. *The Medieval Demographic System of the Nordic Countries*. Oslo: Middelalderforlaget [first pub. 1993; a significantly expanded 2nd edn. appeared in 1996, referred to here as 1996b]

—— 1996c. 'The Demography of the Viking Age and the High Middle Ages in the Nordic Countries', *Scandinavian Journal of History*, 21: 151–182

—— 2002. *Svartedauen og senere pestepidemier i Norge. Pestepidemienes historie 1348–1654*. Oslo: Unipub

Benjamin, B. 1955. 'Quality of Response in Census Taking', *Population Studies*, 8: 288–293

Bennassar, B. 1969. *Recherches sur les grandes épidémies dans le Nord de l'Espagne à la fin du XVIe siècle*. Paris: SEVPEN

Bennett, J.M. 1987. *Women in the Medieval English Countryside: Gender and Household in Brigstock Before the Plague*. Oxford: Oxford University Press

Bergquist, H. 1957. 'Skeletal Finds of Black Rat from the Early Middle Ages', *Archaeology of Lund*, Lund, 1: 98–103

Bernardo, A.S. 1982. 'The Plague as Key to Meaning in Boccaccio's *Decameron*', in: *The Black Death*: 23–38

Bernström, J. 1969. 'Råttor och möss', *Kulturhistorisk leksikon for nordisk middelalde*, Vol. 14. Oslo: Gyldendal Norsk Forlag: 577–583

Berthe, M. 1976. *Le comté de Bigorre. Un milieu rural au bas Moyen Age*. Paris: SEVPEN

—— 1983. 'Famines et épidémies dans le monde paysan au Navarre aux XIVe et XVe siècles', *L'Académie des inscriptions et belles lettres. Compte rendus de seances*: 299–314

—— 1984. *Famines et épidémies dans les campagne navarraises à la fin du moyen âge*. Paris: SFIED. Vols 1–2

Bibikova, V.A. 1977. 'Contemporary Views on the Interrelationships Between Fleas and the Pathogens of Human and Animal Diseases', *Annual Review of Entomology*, 22: 23–32

Bibikova, V.A. i Alekseyev, A.N. 1969. 'Zarazhennost' i blokoobrazovanie v zavisimosti ot kolichestva popavshikh v blokh mikrobov chumy' [= Contagiousness and formation of blockage as variables of the number of plague microbes ingested by fleas], *Parazitologiya*, 8: 196–202

Bibikova, V.A. i Klassovskiy, L.N. 1974. *Peredacha chumy blokhami* [= Transmission of plague by fleas]. Moscow: Meditsina

Biraben, J.-N. 1974. 'Les pauvres et la peste', in: *Études sur l'historie de la pauvreté*. Vol. 2: 505–518

———— 1975. *Les hommes et la peste en France et dans les pays européens et méditerranéens*. Paris: Mouton. Vols 1–2

———— 1979. 'La Peste Noire en terre d'Islam', *L'histoire*, 11, April: 30–40

———— 1988. 'L'hygiène, la maladie, la mort', in: *Histoire de la population française*: 421–462

Biraben, J.-N. et Le Goff, J. 1969. 'La Peste dans le Haut Moyen Age', *Annales Économies Sociétés Civilisations*, 24: 1484–1510

The Black Death. 1982. D. Williman (ed). New York: State University of New York at Binghamton (Center for Medieval & Early Renaissance Studies)

The Black Death. A Turning Point in History? 1971. W.M. Bowsky (ed). New York: Holt, Rinehart & Winston, Inc.

Blanc, G. et Baltazard, M. 1945. 'Recherches sur le mode de transmission naturelle de la peste bubonique et septicémique', *Archives de l'Institut Pasteur du Maroc*, 3, Cahier 5: 173–354 [14 plates]

Block, M.G. 1711. *Atskillige Anmærkningar Œfwer nærwarande Pestilentias Beskaffenhet, Motande, Botande Och Utrotande Uti Östergœtland*. Linköping: published by the author

Blockmans, W.P. 1980. 'The Social and Economic Effects of Plague in the Low Countries 1349–1500', *Revue Belge de Philologie et d'Histoire (Belgisch Tijdschift voor Philologie en Geschiedenis)*, 58: 833–863

Blondheim, S.H. 1955. 'The First Recorded Epidemic of Pneumonic Plague: the Bible, *I Samuel VI*', *Bulletin of the History of Medicine*, 29: 337–345

Bocquet, A. 1969. *Recherches sur la population rurale de l'Artois et du Boulonnais pendant la période bourguignonne (1384–1477)*. Arras: Mémoires de la Commission Départementale des Monuments Historiques de Pas-de-Calais, No. 13

Bodenheimer, F.S.1935. *Animal Life in Palestine*. Jerusalem: L. Mayer

———— 1960. *Animal and Man in Bible Lands* (Collection de travaux de l'Académie internationale d'histoire des sciences, No. 10.). Leiden: E.J. Brill

Bøhm, T. 1999. *En demografisk analyse av bondehushold og gårdsbefolkningens størrelse og sammensetning på Østlandet 1520–1660*, Cand. Phil. Diss., Department of History, University of Oslo

Boessneck, J. and Von den Driesch, A. 1979. 'Die Tierknochenfunde mit Ausnahme der Fischknochen', in: *Eketorp. Befestigung auf Öland/Schweden. Die Fauna*. Vol. 3: 24–421

Bois, G. 1976. *Crise du féodalisme. Economie rurale et démographie en Normandie orientale du début du XIVe au milieu du XVIe siècles*. Paris: Presses de la fondation nationale des sciences politiques/Editions de l'École des hautes études en sciences sociales

Boucher, C.E. 1938. 'The Black Death in Bristol', *Transactions of the Bristol and Gloucestershire Archaeological Society*, 60: 31–46

Boudet, M. and Grand, R. 1902. 'Étude historique sur les épidémies de peste en Haute-Auvergne (XIVe –XVIIIe siècles)', *Revue de la Haute-Auvergne*, 4: 44–299

Bowsky, W.M. 1964. 'The Impact of the Black Death upon Sienese Government and Society', *Speculum*, 39: 1–34

Bradley, L. 1977. 'The Most Famous of All English Plagues: A detailed analysis of the Plague at Eyam 1665–6', in: *The Plague Reconsidered*: 63–94

The British Encyclopedia of Medical Practice. 1938. London: Buttersworth & Co. Vol. 9

Brondy, R. 1988. *Chambéry. Histoire d'une capital, vers 1350–1560*. Lyon: Presses Universitaires de Lyon

Brondy, R., Demotz, B. and Leguay, J.-P. 1984. *La Savoie de l'an mil à la Réforme (XIᵉ–début XVIᵉ siècle)*. Ouest-France

Bruns, F. 1900. *Die Lübecker Bergenfahrer und ihre Chronistik*. (Hansische Geschichtsquellen, New Series, Vol. 2.) Berlin: Pass & Garleb

Brygoo, E.-R. 1966. 'Épidémiologie de la peste à Madagascar', *Archives de l'Institut Pasteur Madagascar*, 35: 9–147

Bucher, S. 1979. 'Die Pest in der Ostschweiz', *Neujahrsblatt Herausgegeben vom Historischen Verein des Kantons St Gallen*. St Gallen, Vol. 119

Bulst, R. 1977. 'Der Schwarze Tod. Demographische, wirtschafts- und kulturgeschichtliche Aspekte der Pestkatastrophe von 1347–1352. Bilanz der neueren Forschung', *Saeculum*, 30: 45–67

Burkle, F.M. 1973. 'Plague as seen in South Vietnamese Children. A chronicle of observation and treatment under adverse conditions', *Clinical Pediatrics*, 12: 291–298

Burnet, F.M. and White, D.O. 1972. *Natural History of Infectious Disease*. Cambridge: Cambridge University Press. 4th edn

Burroughs, A.L. 1947. 'Sylvatic Plague Studies. The vector efficiency of nine species of fleas compared with *Xenopsylla cheopis*', *The Journal of Hygiene*, 45: 371–396

Butler, T. 1972. 'A Clinical Study of Bubonic Plague', *The American Journal of Medicine*, 53: 268–276

——— 1983. *Plague and Other Yersinia Infections*. New York: Plenum Medical Book Co.

Cabrillana, N. 1968. 'La crisis del siglo XIV en Castilla: La Peste Negra en el obispado de Palencia', *Hispania*, 109: 245–258

The Cambridge Economic History of Europe. 1966. Vol. 1. *The Agrarian Life of the Middle Ages*. Cambridge: Cambridge University Press. 2nd edn

Campbell, B.M.S. 1984. 'Population Pressure, Inheritance and the Land Market in a Fourteenth-century Peasant Community', in: *Land, Kinship and Life-Cycle*: 87–134

Capmany y de Montpalau, A. 1962. *Memorias históricas sobre la marina, comercio y artes de la antiqua ciudad de Barcelona*. Barcelona. Vol. 2

Carpentier, É. 1962. *Une ville devant la peste: Orvieto et la Peste Noire de 1348*. Paris: Université de Paris, Imprimerie Nationale

Carrasco Perez, J. 1973. *La población de Navarra en el siglo XIV*. Pamplona: Universidad de Navarra

Carreras Panchon, A., Mitre Fernandez, E. and Valdeón, J. 1980. 'La peste negra', *Historia*, 4: 47–71

Cazelles, R. 1962. 'La peste de 1348–1349 en langue d'oil. Épidémie prolétarienne et enfantine', *Bulletin philologique et historique du Comité des travaux historiques et scientifiques (jusqu'en 1610)*: 293–305

Centenaire du Séminaire d'histoire Médiévale l'Université Libre de Bruxelles 1876–1976. 1977. Bruxelles: La Renaissance du Livre

Chiapelli, A. 1887. 'Gli ordinamenti sanitari del comune di Pistoia contro la pestilenza del 1348', *Archivio Storico Italiano*, 20, Dispensa 4ª: 3–21

Christie, A.B., Chen, T.H. and Elberg, S.S. 1980. 'Plague in Camels and Goats: Their role in human epidemics', *Journal of Infectious Diseases*, 141: 724–726

The Chronicle of Pskov: see Pskovskaya Letopis'

Chun, J.W.H. 1936. 'Clinical Features', in: Wu, Chun, Pollitzer et al., *A Manual for Medical and Publich Health Workers*: 309–333

Cipolla, C.M. 1973. *Cristofano and the Plague. A Study in the History of Public Health in the Age of Galileo*. Berkeley: University of California Press

———— 1974. 'The Plague and the Pre-Malthus Malthusians', *The Journal of European Economic History*, 3: 277–284

———— 1976. 'The Origin and Development of the Health Boards', in: *Public Health and the Medical Profession in the Renaissance*: London: Cambridge University Press: 11–66

———— 1979. *Faith, Reason, and the Plague in Seventeenth-century Tuscany*. Ithaca, New York: Cornell University Press

———— 1981. *Fighting the Plague in Seventeenth-Century Italy*. Madison: The University of Wisconsin Press

Cipolla, C.M. et Zanetti, D.E. 1972. 'Peste et mortalité différentielle', *Annales de démographie historique*: 197–202

Civiltá ed economia agricola in Toscana nei secc. XIII–XV: Problemi della vita delle campagne nel tardo medioevo. 1981. Pistoia: Centro Italiano di Studia Storia e d'Arte Pistoia. Ottavo Convegno Internazionale

Coale, A.J. and Demeny, P, with Vaughan, B. 1983. *Regional Model Life Tables and Stable Populations*. New York: Academic Press. 2nd edn

Cohn, N. 1970. *The Pursuit of the Millennium. Revolutionary Millenarians and Mystical Anarchists of the Middle Ages*. Oxford: M.T. Smith. 2nd edn

Comba, R. 1977. 'Vicende demografiche in Piemonte nell'ultimo medioevo', *Bollettino storico–bibliografico subalpino*, 75: 39–125

Commanay, C. 1963. *Recherches démographiques dans la châtellenie d'Aiguebelle (d'après les comptes de subside de 1333 à 1451)*. Unpublished thesis, École des Chartes (Microfilm at the Archives Départementales de Savoie, 1 Mi 84 R 1.)

Contamine, P. 1976. *La vie quotidienne pendant la guerre de cent ans. France et Angleterre (XIVe siécle)*. Paris: Hachette

Conti, E. 1966. *I catasti agrari della repubblica fiorentina*. Roma: Istituto storico italiano per il medio evo

Cornwall, J. 1970. 'English Population in the Early Sixteenth Century', *Economic History Review*, 2nd Series, 23: 32–44

Coulanges, P.1989. 'La peste à Tananarive (de son apparition en 1921 à sa resurgence en 1979', *Archives de l'Institut Pasteur du Madagascar*, 56: 9–35

Coulton, G.G. 1947. *Medieval Panorama. The English Scene from Conquest to Reformation*. Cambridge: Cambridge University Press

The Countryside of Medieval England. 1988. A. Grenville and A. Grant (eds.). Oxford: Basil Blackwell

Creighton, C. 1891. *A History of Epidemics in Britain*. Cambridge: The University Press. Vol. 1

'Cronaca senese attribuita ad Agnolo di Tura del Grassso'. 1934. In: *Cronache senesi*

Cronache senesi. 1934. A. Lisini and F. Iacometti (eds.), *Rerum Italicarum Scriptores*, New Series, 15, Part 6

Da Costa Roque, M. 1979. *As pestes medievais europeias e o 'Regimento proueytoso contra ha pestelença'. Lisboa, Valentim Fernandes [1495–1496]. Tentativa de interpretação à luz dos conhecimentos pestologicos actuais*. Paris: Fundação Calouste Gulbenkian Centro Cultural Português

Dahlbäck. G. 1988. *I medeltidens Stockholm* (Stockholmsmonografiker utgivna av Stockholms stad). Stockholm

Danmark i Senmiddelalderen. 1994. P. Ingesman and J.V. Jensen (eds.). Århus: Aarhus Universitetsforlag

Danmarks Riges Breve. 1958–63. 3rd Series, Vols 1–3. Copenhagen: E. Munksgaards Forlag AS

Davis, D.E. 1986. 'The Scarcity of Rats and the Black Death: An ecological history', *Journal of Interdisciplinary History*, 16: 455–470

Davis, R.A. 1989. 'The Effect of the Black Death on the Parish Priests of the Medieval Diocese of Coventry and Lichfield', *Historical Research*, 62: 85–90

Davis, V. 1998. 'Medieval Longevity: The experience of members of religious orders in Late Medieval England', *Medieval Prosopography*, 19: 111–124

Death in Towns. Urban Responses to the Dying and the Dead, 1000–1600. 1992. Leicester: Leicester University Press

De Boer, D.E.H. 1978. *Graaf en grafiek. Sociale en economische ontwikkelingen in the middeleeuwse 'Noordholland' tussen ±1345 en ±1415*. Leyden

De Lavigne, R.L. 1971. 'La peste noir et la commune de Toulouse: Le témoignage du livre des matricules des notaires', *Annales de Midi*: 413–429

Delille, G. 1974. 'Un problème de démographie historique: Hommes et femmes face à la mort', *Melanges de l'École française de Rome*, 86: 419–443

Del Panta, L. 1980. *Le epidemie nella storia demografica italiana (secoli XIV–XIX)*. Torino: Lescher editore

Demotz, B. 1975. 'Ugine au moyen âge', in: *Histoire d'Ugine*: 25–118

Denecke, D. 1986. 'Straße und Weg im Mittelalter als Lebensraum und Vermittler zwischen entfernten Orten', in: *Mensch und Umwelt im Mittelalter*: 207–223

Desertion and Land Colonization in the Nordic Countries c. 1300–1540. 1981. Stockholm: Almqvist & Wiksell International

Despy, G. 1977. 'La "Grande Peste Noire de 1348": a-t-elle touché le roman pays de Brabant?', in: *Centenaire du Séminaire d'histoire Médiévale l'Université Libre de Bruxelles 1876–1976*: 195–217

Dewindt, E.W. 1972. *Land and People in Holywell-cum-Needingworth. Structures of Tenure and Patterns of Social Organization in an East Midlands Village*. Toronto: Pontifical Institute of Mediaeval Studies

Diplomatarium Danicum. 1958–63. 3rd Series, Vols 1–3. Copenhagen: E. Munksgaards Forlag AS

Diplomatarium Norvegicum. 1849–1976. Christiania-Oslo. I–XXII

Diplomatarium Suecanum. 1853–65. Stockholm: Nordstedt & Söner. Vols 4–5

D'Irsay, S. 1926. 'Notes to the Origin of the Expression: Atra Mors', *Isis*, 8: 328–332

——— 1927. 'Defense Reactions during the Black Death 1348–1349', *Annals of Medical History*, 9: 169–179

Dodgshon, R.A. 1981. *Land and Society in Early Scotland*. Oxford: Oxford University Press

Dörbeck, F. 1906. *Geschichte der Pestepidemien in Russland*. Breslau: J.U. Kern's Verlag

Dols, M.W. 1977. *The Black Death in the Middle East*. Princeton: Princeton University Press

——— 1978. 'Geographical Origin of the Black Death', *Bulletin of the History of Medicine*, 52: 112–113

——— 1982. 'Al-Manbiji's "Report of the Plague": A treatise on the Plague of 764–65/1362–64 in the Middle East', in: *The Black Death*: 65–75

Doñate Sebastia, J.M. 1969. 'Datos negativos, referidos a la Plana de Castellón, en relacion con la peste negra de 1348', *VIII Congreso de historia de la Corona de Aragón, Valencia 1967*, II. 1 (*La Corona de Aragón en el siglo XIV*). Valencia: 27–43

Drivon, J. 1912. 'La peste noire à Lyon', *Lyon Médical*, 118: 859–869

Dubled, H. 1969. 'Le épidémies de peste à Carpentras et dans le Comtat Venaissin', *Provence historique*, 75

Dubois, H. 1988a. 'L'essor médiéval', in: *Histoire de la population Française*: 207–266

——— 1988b. 'La dépression (XIVᵉ et XVᵉ siècles)', in: *Histoire de la population Française*. 313–366

Dubuis, P. 1979, 'Démographie et peuplement dans le diocèse de Sion au moyen âge', *Revue suisse d'histoire*, 29: 144–158

——— 1980a. 'Le rôle du facteur démographique dans les crises du bas moyen âge: la vision des victimes', *Revue suisse d'histoire*, 30: 390–401

——— 1980b. 'L'épidémie de peste de 1349 à Saint-Maurice d'Agaune', *Études de Lettres. Bulletin de la Faculté des lettres de l'Université de Lausanne* , 1: 3–20

——— 1990. *Une économie alpine à la fin du Moyen Age. Orsières, l'Entremont et les régions voisines, 1250–1500.* Saint-Maurice: Université de Lausanne, Faculté des lettres. Vols 1–2

Dufourcq, C.-E. 1970–1. 'Les relations de la péninsule ibérique et de l'Afrique du nord au XIVᵉ siècle', *Anuario de estudios medievales*, 7: 39–65

Duparc, P. 1962. 'Évolution démographique de quelques paroisses de Savoie depuis la fin du XIIIᵉ siécle', *Bulletin philologique et historique (jusqu'à 1610) du comité des travaux historiques et scientifiques.* [Année 1962, pub. 1965.]: 247–277

Durliat, P.M. and Pons i Marqués J. 1959. 'Recerques sobre el moviment del port de Mallorca en la primera meitat del segle XIV', *Congreso de Historia de la Corona de Aragón, en Cerdeña 1957.* Madrid: 345–363

Dyer, C. 1980. *Lords and Peasants in a Changing Society. The Estates of the Bishopric of Worcester, 680–1540.* Cambridge: Cambridge University Press

——— 1986. 'English Peasant Buildings in the Later Middle Ages (1200–1500)', *Medieval Archaeology*, 30: 19–45

Ecclestone, M. 1999. 'Mortality of Rural Landless Men before the Black Death: the Glastonbury head-tax lists', *Local Population Studies*, 63: 6–29

Eketorp. Befestigung auf Öland/Schweden. Die Fauna. 1970. J. Boessneck et al. (eds.). Stockholm: Royal Academy of Letters, History and Antiquities. Vol. 3

Emery, R.W. 1967. 'The Black Death of 1348 in Perpignan', *Speculum* , 42: 611–623

Eskey, C.R. and Haas, V.H. 1940. 'Plague in the Western Part of the United States', *Public Health Bulletin*, No. 254: 29–82

Essays in Economic History. 1962. E.M. Carus-Wilson (ed.) London: Edward Arnold. Vol. 2

Estrade, F. 1935. 'Observations relatives à la biologie de Xenopsylla cheopis en Emyrne', *Bulletin de la Société de pathologie exotique*, 28: 293–298

Études sur l'historie de la pauvreté. 1974. E. Mollat (ed.). Paris: Publications de la Sorbonne. Vol. 2

Falsini, A.B. 1971. 'Firenze dopo il 1348. Le conseguenze della peste nera', *Archivio Storico Italiano*, 129: 425–496

Fedorov, V.N. 1960a: *see* Fyodorov

Fenyuk, B.K. 1960. 'Experience in the Eradication of Enzootic Plague in the North–West Part of the Caspian Region of the USSR', *Bulletin of the WHO* , 23: 263–273

Feroci, A. 1892. *La peste bubonica in Pisa nel medio evo ed il 1630. Notizie tolte da documenti inediti.* Pisa: Pubblicate da Antonio Feroci

Finlands historia. 1993. Esbo: Schildts Förlag. Vol. 1

Fisher, J.L. 1943. 'The Black Death in Essex', *Essex Review*, 52: 13–20

Fiumi, E. 1950. 'La demografia fiorentina nelle pagine di Giovanni Villani', *Archivio Storico Italiano*, 108: 78–158

——— 1961. *Storia economica e sociale di San Gimignano.* Florence

——— 1962. 'La popolazione del territorio volterrano-sangimignanese ed il problema demografico dell'età comunale', in: *Studi in onore di Amintore Fanfani*: 249–290

——— 1968. *Demografia, Movimento urbanistico e classi sociali in Prato dall'età comunale ai tempi moderni.* Florence: Leo S. Olschki, Editore

Fletcher, J.M.J. 1922. 'The Black Death in Dorset, 1348–1349', *Proceedings of the Dorset Natural History and Antiquarian Field Club*, 43: 1–14

Flinn, M.W. 1981. *The European Demographic System*. Brighton: The Harvester Press

Fößel, A. 1987. 'Der "Schwarze Tod" in Franken 1348–1350', *Mitteilungen des Vereins für Geschichte der Stadt Nürnberg*, 74: 1–76

Fourastié, J. 1972. 'From the Traditional to the "Tertiary" Life Cycle', in: *Readings in Population*: 29–38

Fournée, J. 1978. 'Les normands face à la peste', *Le pays Bas-Normand. Société, d'art et d'histoire*, 71, No. 1: 3–145

Fourquin, G. 1964. *Les campagnes de la région parisienne à la fin du moyen âge, du milieu du XIIIe siècle au début du XVIe siècle*. Paris: Presses Universitaires de France

Frank, R. 1973. 'Marriage in Twelfth- and Thirteenth-century Iceland', *Viator* 4: 473–484

Fritzner, J. 1954. *Ordbog over Det gamle norske Sprog*. Oslo: Trygve Juul Møllers Forlag. Vol.2, 2nd edn

Fyodorov, V.N. 1960a. 'Plague in Camels and its Prevention in the USSR', *Bulletin of the WHO*, 23: 275–281

——— 1960b. 'The Question of the Existence of Natual Foci of Plague in Europe in the Past', *Journal of Hygiene, Epidemiology, Microbiology and Immunology*, 4: 135–141

Gad, T., Berulfsen, B. and Kilström, B.I. 1963. 'Jøder', *Kulturhistorisk leksikon for nordisk middelalder*. Oslo: Gyldendal Norsk Forlag. Vol. 8: 73–78

Gaspari, F. 1970. 'La population d'Orange au XIVe siècle', *Provence Historique*, No. 120, 20: 215–218

Gasquet, F.A. 1908. *The Black Death of 1348 and 1349*. London: George Bell and Sons. 2nd edn

Gautier-Dalché, J. 1962. 'La peste noire dans les états de la Couronne d'Aragon', *Bulletin hispanique*, 64: 65–80

Gelting, M. 1991. 'The Mountains and the Plague: Maurienne, 1348', *Collegium Medievale*, 4: 7–45

Girard, G. 1943. 'Les ectoparasites de l'homme dans l'épidémiologie de la peste', *Bulletin de la Société de pathologie exotique et de ses filiales*, 36: 4–43

——— 1959. 'Considerations sur l'épidémiologie de la peste', *Revue de médécine et d'hygiène d'outre-mer*, No. 281, Oct.: 114–120

Gottskálks Annáll. 1888. In: *Islandske Annaler indtil 1578*: 297–378

Grandison, K.G. 1885. 'Bilaga: Magnus Erikssons itinerar', in: *Studier i hanseatisk–svensk historia*

Grandson, A. 1957. 'A Fourteenth Century Chronicle from the Grey Friars at Lynn', *The English Historical Review*, 72: 270–278

Gras, P. 1939. 'Le registre paroissial de Givry (1334–1357) et la peste noire en Bourgogne', *Bibliotheque de l'École des chartes*, 100: 295–308

Greenwood, M. 1911. 'On Some of the Factors which Influence the Prevalence of Plague', *The Journal of Hygiene*. Plague Supplement I, 12: 62–151

Greslou, N. 1973, *La Peste en Savoie*. Chambéry

Guilleré, C. 1984. 'La peste noire à Gérone (1348)', *Annals Institut d'Estudis Gironins*, 27: 87–140

Gwynn, A. 1935. 'The Black Death in Ireland. Studies', *An Irish Quarterly Review*, 24: 25–42

Gyug, R. 1983. 'The Effects and Extent of the Black Death of 1348: New evidence for clerical mortality in Barcelona', *Medieval Studies*, 45: 385–398

Haeser, H. 1882, *Lehrbuch der Geschichte der Medicin und der Epidemischen Krankheiten*. Jena. Vol. 3

Hajnal, J. 1965. 'European Marriage Patterns in Perspective', in: *Population in History*. 101–143

Hallam, E.H. 1957–8. 'Some Thirteenth-century Censuses', *The Economic History Review*, 2nd Series, 10: 340–361

———— 1988. 'Population Movements in England, 1086–1350', in: *The Agrarian History of England and Wales*. Vol. 2: 508–593

Halsberghe, R. 1983. 'Étude historiographique des "Récits d'un Bourgeois de Valencienne" (1253–1366)', *Revue du Nord*, 65: 471–479

Hamarkrøniken (Om Hammer). 1895. In: *Historisk-topografiske Skrifter om Norge og norske Landsdele, forfattede i Norge det 16de Aarhundrede* G. Storm (ed.). Christiana: Det norske historiske Kildeskriftfond: 117–146

Hanawalt, B. 1977. 'Childrearing among the Lower Classes of Late Medieval England', *Journal of Interdisciplinary History*, 8: 1–22

———— 1986. *The Ties that Bound: Peasant Families in Medieval England*. New York: Oxford University Press

Hankin, E.H. 1905. 'On the Epidemiology of Plague', *Journal of Hygiene*, 5: 48–83

Hansen, J. 1912. *Beiträge zur Geschichte des Getreidehandels und der Getreidepolitik Lübecks* (Veröffentlichungen zur Geschichte der Freien und Hansestadt Lübeck, Vol. 1). Lübeck: Verlag Max Schmidt.

Harvey, B. 1993. *Living and Dying in England, 1100–1540*. Oxford: Clarendon Press

Harvey, P.D.A. 1965. *A Medieval Oxfordshire Village: Cuxham, 1200–1400*. Oxford: Oxford University Press

Hasund, S. 1920. *Ikring Mannedauden. Ei liti sogestudie*. Kristiania: Grøndahl & søn

Hatcher, J. 1970. *Rural Economy and Society in the Duchy of Cornwall, 1300–1500*. Cambridge: Cambridge University Press

———— 1977. *Plague, Population and the English Economy 1348–1530*. London: Macmillan Education [four reprints 1982–7]

———— 1986. 'Mortality in the Fifteenth Century: Some New Evidence', *The Economic History Review*, 2nd Series, 39: 19–38

———— 1994. 'England in the Aftermath of the Black Death', *Past & Present*, No. 144: 3–35

Havstad, L.A. 1975. *Mandtallet i Norge 1664–1666 benyttet til Fremstilling af Aldersforholdene*. Tillægshefte til Videnskabs-Selskabets Forhandlingerfor 1874. Christiania

Hawkins, D. 1990. 'The Black Death and the New London Cemeteries of 1348', *Antiquity*, 64: 637–642

Helgeandsholmen. 1000 år i Stockholms ström. 1983. G. Dahlbeck (ed.). Stockholm: Liber Förlag

Henderson, J. 1992. 'The Black Death in Florence: Medical and communal responses', in: *Death in Towns*: 136–150

Herlihy, D. 1970. 'The Tuscan Town in the Quattrocento: A demographic profile', *Medevalia et Humanistica*, 1: 81–109

———— 1981. 'The Problem of the "Return to the Land" in Tuscan Economic History of the Fourteenth and Fifteenth Centuries', in: *Civiltá ed economia agricola in Toscana*: 401–416

Herlihy, D. and Klapisch-Zuber, C. 1978. *Les toscans et leurs familles. Une étude du catasto florentin de 1427*. Paris: Editions de l'École des hautes études en sciences sociales

Herrlinger, R. 1955. 'Die geschichtliche Entwicklung des Begriffes "Pest" ', *Deutsches medizinisches Journal*, 6: 696–699

Higden, R. 1865. *Polychronicon Ranulphi Higden Monachi Cestrensis*. C.A. Babington (ed.). London

Higounet-Nadal A. 1988. 'La croissance urbaine', in: *Histoire de la population française*: 267–311

Hirst, L.F. 1938. 'Plague', in: *The British Encyclopedia of Medical Practice*. Vol. 9: 675–698

———— 1953. *The Conquest of Plague*. Oxford: Clarendon Press

Histoire de la Catalogne. 1983. J. Nadal Farreras et P.H. Wolff (eds.). Barcelona: Privat

Histoire de la France rurale. 1975. Vol. 2. G. Duby et A. Wallon (eds.). Paris: Seuil

Historie de la France urbaine. 1980. Vol. 2. G. Duby (ed.). Paris: Seuil

Histoire de la population française. 1988. Vol. 1. Paris: Presses Universitaires de France

Histoire d'Ugine. 1975. R. Devos (ed.). Annecy: Mémoires et documents publiés par l'Académie Salésienne 48 bis

An Historical Geography of England and Wales. 1978. R.A. Dodgshon and R.A. Butlin (eds.). London: Academic Press

Hoeniger, R. 1881. *Gang und Verbreitung des schwarzen Todes in Deutschland von 1348–1351 und sein Zusammenhang mit den Judenverfolgungen und Geisselfahrten dieser Jahre.* Berlin: Buchdruckerei von Eugen Grosser

Hoensch, J.K. 1987. *Geschichte Böhmens von der slavischen Landnahme bis ins 20. Jahrhundert.* Munich: Verlag C.H. Beck

Hollingsworth, T.H. 1969. *Historical Demography.* London: The Sources of History Limited

Homenaje a Jaime Vicens Vives. 1965. Barcelona: Universidad de Barcelona, Facultad de filosofía y letras

Howell, C. 1983. *Land, Family and Inheritance in Transition. Kibworth Harcourt, 1280–1700.* Cambridge: Cambridge University Press

Howell, M. and Ford, P. 1986. *The Ghost Disease and Twelve other Stories of Detective Work in the Medical Field.* Harmondsworth: Penguin Books

Hurst, J.G. 1988. 'Rural Building in England and Wales: England', in: *The Agrarian History of England and Wales.* Vol. 2: 854–930

Ibs, J.H. 1994. *Die Pest in Schleswig-Holstein von 1350 bis 1547–48.* (Kiler Werkstücke, Reihe A: Beiträge zur schleswig-holsteinischen und skandinavischen Geschichte, 12.) Frankfurt-am-Main: Peter Lang

An Icelandic–English Dictionary. 1975. Oxford: Clarendon Press. 2nd edn

Iglésies, P.J. 1959. 'El poblament de Catalunya durant els segles XIV i XV', in: *VI Congreso de Historia de la Corona de Aragón en Cerdeña 8 a 14 Diciembre 1957.* Madrid: 247–270

Ilmoni, I. 1846. *Bidrag till Nordens Sjukdomshistoria.* Helsinki: J. Simelii arfvingar. Vol. 1

Indian Plague Research Commission. 1907. Reports on Plague Investigations in India. XXV. 'Observations in the Punjab Villages of Dhand and Kasel', *The Journal of Hygiene,* 7: 895–985

Industrialization in Two Systems: Essays in Honor of Alexander Gerschenkron. 1966. H. Rosovsky (ed.). New York: John Wiley & Sons, Inc.

Infections in Children. 1982. R.J. Wedgwood, S.D. Davis, C.G. Ray et al. (eds.). Philadelphia: Harper & Row

Infectious Diseases. 1983. P.D. Hoeprich (ed.). Philadelphia: Harper & Row

Innsikt og Utsyn. Festskrift til Jørn Sandnes. 1996. Trondheim: Historisk institutt, Norges teknisk-naturvitenskapelige universitet

Inventaire du Trésor de St-Nizier de Lyon 1365–1373. Listes des sépultures de la paroisse Saint-Nizier de Lyon. 1346–1348. 1899. G. Guigue (ed.). Lyons: Société des bibliophiles Lyonnois

Islandske Annaler indtil 1578. 1888. G. Storm (ed.). Christiana: Det Norske Historiske Kildeskriftfond [reprint: Oslo, 1977]

James, B.T. 1998. 'The Black Death in Berkshire and Wiltshire', *The Hatcher Review,* 5: 11–20

——— 1999. 'The Black Death in Hampshire', *Hampshire Papers,* 18, Dec.: 1–28

——— 2001. 'Years of Pestilence', *British Archaeology,* 61, Oct.: 8–13

Jessopp, A. 1922. 'The Black Death in East Anglia', in: *The Coming of the Friars and other Historic Essays.* London: T. Fisher Unwin. 19th imp. 166–261 [first pub. 1888]

Jochens, J.M. 1985. 'En Islande médiévale: A la recherche de la famille nucléaire', *Annales ESC*: 95–112

——— 1995. *Women in Old Norse Society.* Ithaca, New York: Cornell University Press

Jouet, R. 1972. 'Autour de la Peste Noire en Basse-Normandie au XIVe siècle', *Annales de Normandie*, 22: 265–276

Kern, H.P. 1969. 'La Peste Negra y su influjo en la provisión de los beneficios ecclesiásticos', in: *VIII Congreso de historia de la Corona de Aragón, Valencia 1967*, II. 1 (*La Corona de Aragón en el siglo XIV*). Valencia: 71–83

Khoroshkevich, A.L. 1963. *Torgovlya Velikogo Novgoroda s pribaltikoy i zapadnoi Evropoy v XIV–XV vekakh* [Great Novgorod's Trade with the Countries around the Baltic Sea and Western Europe in the Fourteenth and Fifteenth Centuries]. Moscow: Izdatel'stvo Akademii Nauk SSSR

Kinch, J. 1869. *Ribe Bys Historie og Beskrivelse*. Copenhagen: G.E.C. Gad

Kitsikopoulos, H. 2000. 'Standards of Living and Capital Formation in Pre-plague England: A Peasant Budget Model', *The Economic History Review*, 53: 237–261

Klein, H. 1960. 'Das Große Sterben von 1348–49 und seine Auswirkung auf die Besiedlung der Ostalpenländer', *Mitteilungen der Gesellschaft für Salzburger Landesgeschichte*, 100: 91–170

Klimenko, V.S. 1910. 'O chumnykh epidemiyakh v Rossii' [On plague epidemics in Russia], *Voienno-medisinskiy Zhurnal*, 229: 659–663

Kolsrud, O. 1907–13. 'Den norske Kirkes Erkebiskoper og Biskoper indtil Reformationen', in: *Diplomatarium Norvegicum*. Kristiania [= Oslo]. Vol. 17, Pt II: 177–360

Lalla, R. 1999. *Hanseatene og Svartedauden*. Norges Landbrukshøgskole: graduate thesis presented at the Institute for Economy and Social Sciences

Land, Kinship and Life-Cycle. 1984. R.M. Smith (ed.). Cambridge: Cambridge University Press

Lange, C. 1862. 'Den sorte død', *Dansk maanedsskrift*, 2: 81–129

Langer, L.N. 1976. 'Plague and the Russian Countryside: Monastic Estates in the Late Fourteenth and Fifteenth Centuries', *Canadian–American Slavic Studies*, 10: 351–368

Leads from the MMWR. 1984. 'Plague Pneumonia – California', *Journal of American Medical Association*, 252: 1399–1400

Lechner, K. 1884. *Das Große Sterben in Deutschland in den Jahren 1348 bis 1351 und die folgenden Pestepidemien bis zum Schluss des 14. Jahrhunderts*. Innsbruck: Verlag der Wagner'schen Universitätsbuchhandlung

Lepiksaar, J. 1965. 'Djurrester från det medeltida Ny Varberg', *Varbergs Museum*, Årsbok. 16: 73–102

—— 1969. 'Nytt om djur från det medeltida Ny Varberg', *Varbergs Museum*, Årsbok. 20: 37–68

—— 1975. 'Über die Tierknochenfunde aus den mittelalterlichen Siedlungen Südschwedens', in: *Archaeozoological Studies*: 230–239

Lerner, R.E. 1982. 'The Black Death and Western European Eschatological Mentalities', in: *The Black Death*: 77–106

Le Roy Ladurie, E. 1966. *Les paysans de Languedoc*. Paris: SEVPEN

—— 1981a. 'A Concept: The unification of the globe by disease (fourteenth to seventeenth centuries', in: *The Mind and Method of the Historian*: 28–83, 292–297 [originally published in French in 1973: *Revue suisse d'histoire*, 23: 627–696]

—— 1981b. *The Mind and Method of the Historian*, tr. Sian and Ben Reynolds. Brighton: The Harvester Press

—— 1988. 'Postface: Démographie et histoire rurale en perspective', in: *Histoire de la population Française*: 513–524

Levett, E.A. 1916. 'The Black Death on the Estates of the See of Winchester', in: *Oxford Studies in Social and Legal History*. Vol. 5. *The Black Death on the Estates of the See of Winchester*. Oxford: 1–220

Levron, J. 1959. 'Les registres paroissiaux et d'état civil en France', *Archivum*, 9: 55–100

Lindal, S. 1976. 'Ægteskab', in: *Kulturhistorisk leksikon for nordisk middelalder*. Vol. 20. Oslo: Gyldendal Norsk Forlag: 495

Livi Bacchi, M. 1978. *La société italienne devant les crises de mortalité*. Florence: Universitá di Firenze, Dipartimento Statistico

Lock, R. 1992. 'The Black Death in Walsham-le-Willows', *Proceedings of the Suffolk Institute of Archaeology and History*, 37: 316–337

Lögmanns–annáll. 1888. *Islandske Annaler indtil 1578*: 231–296

Lomas, R. 1989. 'The Black Death in County Durham', *Journal of Medieval History*, 15: 127–140

Lomas, T. 1984. 'South-East Durham: Late fourteenth and fifteenth centuries', in: *The Peasant Land Market*: 253–327

López de Meneses, A. 1956. 'Documentos acerca de la peste negra en los dominios de la Corona de Aragón', in: *Estudios de Edad Media de la Corona de Aragón*, 6: 291–447

———— 1959. 'La peste negra en las Islas Baleares', in: *VI Congreso de Historia de la Corona de Aragón, en Cerdeña 8 a 14 dicembre 1957*. Madrid: 331–344

———— 1965. 'La peste negra en Cerdeña', in: *Homenaje a Jaime Vicens Vives*: 533–541

———— 1968–71. 'Datos acerca de la peste negra en Vic.', *AUSA*, 6: 280–285

Loschky, D. and Childers, B.D. 1993. 'Early English Mortality', *The Journal of Interdisciplinary History*, 24: 85–97

MacArthur, W.P. 1925–6. 'Old-Time Plague in Britain', *Transactions of the Royal Society of Tropical Medicine and Hygiene*, 19: 355–372

———— 1949. 'The Identification of some Pestilences recorded in the Irish Annals', *Irish Historical Studies*, 6: 169–188

———— 1952. 'The Occurrence of the Rat in Early Europe. The Plague of the Philistines', *Transactions of the Royal Society of Tropical Medicine and Hygiene*, 46: 209–212, 464

———— 1959. 'The Medical Identification of some Pestilences of the Past', *Transactions of the Royal Society of Tropical Medicine and Hygiene*, 53: 423–439

Mansa, F.V. 1840. 'Pesten i Helsingør og København i 1710 og 1711', *Historisk Tidsskrift* [Denmark], 1: 477–574

Maréchal, G. 1980. 'De Zwarte Dood the Brugge (1349–1351)', *Biekorf: Westvlaams Archief voor Geschiedenis, Oudheidkunde en Folklore*, 80: 377–392

Marshall, J.D, Jr, Joy, R.J.T., Ai, N.V. et al. 1967. 'Plague in Vietnam 1965–1966', *American Journal of Epidemiology*, 86: 603–616

Martens, I. 1989. 'Middaldergårder i Fyresdal – arkeologiske registreringer og historiske kilder', *Collegium Medievale*, 2: 73–90

———— 1990. 'Å bu oppunder fjell. Fjellbygder i Telemark før Svartedauen', *Telemark Historie*, 11: 70–81

Marthinsen, L. 1996. 'Maksimum og minimum. Norsk busetnadshistorie etter DNØ', in: *Innsikt og Utsyn. Festskrift til Jørn Sandnes*: 144–182

Mattmüller, M. 1987. *Bevölkerungsgeschichte der Schweiz*. Vol. 1. Basle and Frankfurt: Verlag Helbing & Lichtenhahn

Maur, E. 1987. 'Sterblichkeit in den böhmischen Ländern im 14. Jahrhundert.', in: *Symposium Bevölkerungsbiologie der Europäischen Völker im Mittelalter. Sborník Národního Muzea v Praze. Acta Musei Nationalis Pragae*. 43 B: 160–165

McIntosh, M.K. 1986. *Autonomy and Community: The Royal Manor of Havering, 1200–1500*. Cambridge: Cambridge University Press

McNeill, W.H. 1979. *Plagues and Peoples*. Harmondsworth: Penguin Books

Med kjønnsperspektiv på norsk historie. Fra vikingtid til 2000–årsskiftet. 1999. I. Blom and S. Sogner (eds.). Oslo: Cappelen Akademisk Forlag

Megson, B.E. 1998. 'Mortality among London Citizens in the Black Death', *Medieval Prosopography*, 19: 125–133

Meinsma, K.O. 1924. *De Zwarte Dood 1347–1352*. Zutphen

Mensch und Umwelt im Mittelalter. 1986. B. Herrmann (ed.). Stuttgart: Deutsche Verlags-Anstalt

Meyer, K.F. 1957. 'The Natural History of Plague and Psitticosis', *Public Health Reports*, 72: 705–719

———— 1961. 'Pneumonic Plague', *Microbiological Reviews* [= *Bacteriological Reviews*], 25: 249–261

Miller, E. and Hatcher, J. 1978. *Medieval England. Rural Society and Economic Change 1086–1348*. London and New York: Longman

Miscelanea Jose M.ª Lacarra. Estudios de historia medieval. 1968. Zaragoza: Universidad de Zaragoza

Mollat, H. 1963. 'Notes sur la mortalité à Paris au temps de la Peste Noire d'après les comptes de l'œuvre de Saint-Germain-L'Auxerrois', *Le Moyen Age*, 18: 505–527

Monumenta historica Norvegiæ. Latinske Kildeskrifter til Norges Historie i Middelalderen. 1880. G. Storm (ed.). Kristiania

Mueller, R.C. 1979a. 'Aspetti sociali ed economici della peste a Venezia nel Medioevo', in: *Venezia e la peste 1348–1797*: 71–76

———— 1979b. 'Peste e demografia. Medioevo e Rinascimento', in: *Venezia e la peste 1348–1797*: 93–96

Myrdal, J. 1994. *Kvinnor, barn och fester i medeltida mirakelberättelser*. Skara: Skaraborgs länsmuseum

Nada Patrone, A.M. and Naso, I. 1981. *Le epdiemie del tardo medioevo nell'area pedemontana*. Turin: Centro Studi Piemontese

Nadal Farreras, J. 1983. 'La vraie richesse: les hommes', in: *Histoire de la Catalogne*: 61–74

Naturens liv i ord och bild. 1928. L.A. Jägerskiöld och T. Pehrson (eds.). Stockholm: Bokförlaget Natur och Kultur. Vol. 2

Neumayr, A., Makazarini, L. und Potuzhek, O. 1964. 'Zur Geschichte der Pestepidemien in Wien', *Wiener Zeitschrift für innere Medizin und ihre Grenzgebiete*: 259–281

Neveux, H. 1975. 'Déclin et reprise: la fluctuation biséculaire 1330–1560', in: *Histoire de la France rurale*. Vol. 2: 19–183

Nielsen, H. 1970. 'Sjællandske krønike', in: *Kulturhistorisk leksikon for nordisk middelalder*. Oslo: Gyldendal Norsk Forlag. Vol. 15: 325–326

Nohl, J. 1961. *The Black Death. A Chronicle of the Plague. Compiled from Contemporary Sources*. London: Unwin Books [2nd repr. 1971]

Nordisk Kultur. 1934. Vol. 16B. Oslo: Aschehoug & Co.

Norris, J. 1977. 'East or West? The Geographic Origin of the Black Death', *Bulletin of the History of Medicine*, 51: 1–24

———— 1978. 'Response', *Bulletin of the History of Medicine*, 52: 114–120

Norske Regnskaber og Jordebøger fra det 16de Aarhundrede. 1887–1983. H.J. Huitfeldt-Kaas (utg.). Christiania. Vols 1–5

Nybelin, O. 1928. 'Den svarta råttan och den bruna', in: *Naturens liv i ord och bild*. Vol. 2: 850–857

Øye. I. 1999. 'Kvinner, kjønn og samfunn. Fra vikingtid til reformasjon', in: *Med kjønnsperspektiv på norsk historie*: 17–82

Ohlin, G. 1966. 'No Safety in Numbers: Some pitfalls of historical statistics', in: *Industrialization in Two Systems*. 68–90. [This pioneering paper is so important that it has been reprinted in another work, *Essays in Quantitative Economic History*, 1974]

Orrman, E. 1981. 'The Progress of Settlement in Finland during the Late Middle Ages', *The Scandinavian Economic History Review*, 29: 129–142

———— 1996. 'Ett försök att beräkna bebyggelsens omfattning i Finland vid utgången av högmedeltiden', in: *Innsikt og Utsyn. Festskrift til Jørn Sandnes*: 125–143

Otway-Ruthven, A.J. 1968. *A History of Medieval Ireland*. London and New York: Routledge

Oxford Studies in Social and Legal History. 1916. Vol. 5. *The Black Death on the Estates of the See of Winchester*. P. Vinogradoff (ed.). Oxford: Clarendon Press

Page, F.M. 1934. *The Estates of Crowland Abbey. A Study in Manorial Organization*. Cambridge: Cambridge University Press

Palm, L.A. 1999a. 'Stormaktstidens dolda systemskifte – från tonårsäktenskap til sena giften', *Historisk tidskrift*, 119: 55–90

———— 1999b. 'Household Size in Pre-industrial Sweden', *Scandinavian Economic History Review*, 47: 78–90

———— 2000. *Folkmängden i Sveriges socknar och kommuner 1571–1997. Med särskild hänsyn till perioden 1571–1751*. Stockholm [English summary, pp. 129–131]

The Peasant Land Market in Medieval England. 1984. P.D.A. Harvey (ed.). Oxford: Clarendon Press

Pelc, A. 1938. *Ceny v Krakowie* [The Prices in Krakow]. Krakow

Peters, E. 1940. 'Das große Sterben des Jahres 1350 in Lübeck und seine Auswirkungen auf die wirtschaftliche und soziale Struktur der Stadt', *Zeitschrift des Vereins für Lübeckische Geschichte und Altertumskunde*, 30: 15–148

Petrie, G.F., Todd, R.E., Skander, R. et al. 1924. 'A Report on Plague Investigations in Egypt', *The Journal of Hygiene*, 23: 117–150

Phelps Brown, E.H. and Hopkins, S.V. 1962. 'Seven Centuries of the Prices of Consumables, compared with Builders' Wage-Rates', in: *Essays in Economic History*: 179–196

Philip, W.M. and Hirst, L.F. 1917. 'A Report on the Outbreak of the Plague in Colombo, 1914–1916', *The Journal of Hygiene*, 15: 527–564

Pickard, R. 1947. *The Population and Epidemics of Exeter in Pre-Census Times*. Exeter: published by the author

Pini, A.I. and Greci, R. 1976. 'Una fonte per la demografia storica medievale: "Le venticinquine" bolognesi (1247–1404)', *Rassegna degli Archivi di Stato*, 36: 337–417

Pladevall, A. 1961–3. 'La disminucio de poblament a la Plana de Vich a mijans del segle XIV', *AUSA*, 4: 361–373

The Plague Reconsidered. A New Look at its Origins and Effects in 16th and 17th Century England. 1977. Matlock: Local Population Studies

Poland, J.D. 1983. 'Plague', in: *Infectious Diseases*: 1227–1237

Pollitzer, R. 1954. *Plague*. Geneva: WHO

———— 1960. 'A Review of Recent Literature on Plague', *Bulletin of the WHO*, 23: 313–400

Pollitzer, R. and Li, C.C. 1943. 'Some Observations on the Decline of Pneumonic Plague Epidemics', *Chinese Medical Journal*, 61: 212–216

Pollitzer, R. and Meyer, K.F. 1961. 'The Ecology of Plague', in: *Studies in Disease Ecology*: 433–590

Polzer, J. 1982. 'Aspects of the Fourteenth–Century Iconography of Death and the Plague', in: *The Black Death* : 107–130

Poos, L.R. 1985. 'The Rural Population of Essex in the Later Middle Ages', *The Economic History Review*, 2nd Series, 38: 515–530

———— 1986. 'Population Turnover in Medieval Essex: The evidence of some early-fourteenth-century tithing lists', in: *The World We Have Gained* : 1–22

———— 1991. *A Rural Society after the Black Death: Essex 1350–1525*. Cambridge: Cambridge University Press

Poos, L.R. and Smith, R.M. 1984. ' "Legal Windows Onto Historical Populations?" Recent research on demography and the manor court in Medieval England', *Law and History Review*, 2: 128–152

———— 1985. ' "Shades Still on the Window". A Reply to Zvi Razi', *Law and History Review*, 3: 409–429

Population in History. 1965. D.V. Glass and D.E.C. Eversley (eds.). London: Edward Arnold

Porquet, L. 1898. *La peste en Normandie*. Vire: Imprimerie René Eng

Portela Silva, E. 1976. *La región del obispado de Tuy en los siglos XII a XV. Una sociedad en la expansión y en la crisis*. Santiago de Compostela

Postan, M.M. 1950. 'Some Economic Evidence of Declining Population in the Later Middle Ages', *The Economic History Review*, 2nd Series, 2: 328–344

—— 1966. 'Medieval Agrarian History in its Prime: England', in: *Cambridge Economic History of Europe*. Vol. 1: 549–632

—— 1972. *The Medieval Economy and Society. An Economic History of Britain, 1100–1500*. Berkeley and Los Angeles: University of California Press

Postan, M.M. and Titow, J. 1958–9. 'Heriots and Prices on Winchester Manors', *The Economic History Review*, 2nd Series, 11: 392–415

Postles, D. 1992. 'Demographic Change in Kibworth Harcourt, Leicestershire in the Later Middle Ages', *Local Population Studies*, 48: 41–48

Pounds, N.J.G. 1974. *An Economic History of Medieval Europe*. London and New York: Longman

Prat, G. 1952. 'Albi et la Peste Noire', *Annales du Midi*, 64: 15–25

Prevenier, W. 1983. 'La démographie des villes du comté de Flandre aux XIIIe et XIVe siècles', *Revue du Nord*, 65: 255–275

Pskovskaya Letopis'. [The Chronicle of Pskov.] 1837. Moscow

Quadeer, I., Nayar, K.R. and Baru, R.V. 1994. 'Contextualizing Plague. A Reconstruction and an Analysis', *Economic and Political Weekly*, 29, No. 47, 19 Nov.: 2981–2989

Rafto, T. 1958. 'Englandshandel', in: *Kulturhistorisk leksikon for nordisk middelalder*. Oslo: Gyldendal Norsk Forlag. Vol. 3: 658–665

Rasmussen, C.P. 1994. 'Kronens gods', in: *Danmark i Senmiddelalderen*: 69–87

Ravensdale, J. 1984. 'Population Changes and the Transfer of Customary Land on a Cambridgeshire Manor in the Fourteenth century', in: *Land, Kinship and Life-Cycle*: 197–225

Razi, Z. 1980. *Life, Marriage and Death in a Medieval Parish. Economy, Society and Demography in Halesowen 1270–1400*. Cambridge: Cambridge University Press

—— 1985. 'The Use of Manorial Court Rolls in Demographic Analysis. A Reconsideration', *Law and History Review*, 3: 191–200 [cf. Poos and Smith, 1984, 1985]

—— 1987. 'The Demographic Transparency of Manorial Court Rolls', *Law and History Review*, 5: 523–535 [cf. Poos and Smith, 1984, 1985]

Readings in Population. 1972. W. Petersen (ed.). New York: Macmillan

Recommendations of the Advisory Committee on Immunization Practices. 1966. 'Prevention of Plague', *Morbidity and Mortality Weekly Report*. Vol. 45, 13 Dec.: 1–4

Reed, W.P., Palmer, D.L., Williams, R.C. et al. 1970. 'Bubonic Plague in the Southwestern United States', *Medicine*, 49: 465–486

Rees, W. 1923. 'The Black Death in England and Wales, as exhibited in Manorial Documents', *Proceedings of the Royal Society of Medicine* (Section of the History of Medicine), 16: 27–45

Regesta Norvegica. 1979. Vol. 5: 1337–1350. Oslo: Norsk Historik Kjeldeskrift-Institut

Regesta Norvegica. 1993. Vol. 6. H. Kjellberg (ed.). Oslo: Riksarkivet

Reichstein, H. 1974. 'Bemerkungen zur Verbreitungsgeschichte der Hausratte (Rattus rattus Linné, 1758) an Hand jüngeren Knochenfunde aus Haithabu', *Die Heimat*, 81: 113–114

—— 1987. 'Archözoologie und die prähistorische Verbreitung von Kleinsäugern', *Sitzungsberichte der Gesellschaft Naturforschender Freunde zu Berlin*, 27: 9–21

Riley, H.D. 1982. 'Plague and Other Yersinsia Infections', in: *Infections in Children*: 746–768

Rogghe, P. 1952. 'De Zwarte Dood in de Zuidelijke Nederlanden', *Belgisch Tijdschift voor Philologie en Geschiedenis (Revue Belge de Philologie et d'Histoire)*, 30: 834–837

Rosén, J. 1962. 'Jordejendom', in: *Kulturhistorisk leksikon for Nordisk Middelalder*. Oslo: Gyldendal, Norsk Forlag. Vol. 7: 658–661

Rossiaud, J. 1980. 'Crises et consolidations', in: *Histoire de la France urbaine*: 413–614

Rotelli, C. 1973. *Una campagna medievale. Storia agraria del Piemonte fra il 1250 e il 1450*. Turin: Giulio Einaudi editore

Rubio Vela, A. 1979. *Peste negra, crisis y comportamientos sociales en la España del siglo XIV. La ciudad Valencia (1348–1401)*. Granada: Universidad de Granada

Russell, J.C. 1948. *British Medieval Population*. Albuquerque: The University of New Mexico Press

———— 1962. 'The Medieval Monedatge of Aragon and Valencia', *Proceedings of the American Philosophical Society*, 106: 483–504

Sandnes, J. 1971. *Ødetid og Gjenreisning*. Oslo: Universitetsforlaget

———— 1981. 'Settlement Developments in the Late Middle Ages (approx. 1300–1540)', in: *Desertion and Land Colonization*: 78–114

Santamaría Arández, A. 1969. 'La peste negra en Mallorca', in: *VIII Congreso de historia de la Corona de Aragón, Valencia 1967, II. 1 (La Corona de Aragón en el siglo XIV)*. Valencia: 103–125

———— 1970–1. 'Mallorca en el siglo XIV', *Anuario de estudios medievales*, 7: 165–236

Schevill, F. 1961. *History of Florence*. New York: Ungar

Schofield, R. 1977. 'An Anatomy of an Epidemic: Colyton, November 1645 to November 1646', in: *The Plague Reconsidered*: 95–132

Sellers, M. 1913. 'Social and Economic History', in: *The Victoria History of the County of York*.

Sevillano Colom, F. 1974. 'La demografia de Mallorca a traves del impuesto del morabati: siglos XIV, XV y XVI', *Boletín de la Sociedad Arqueologica Luliana*, 34: 233–273

Shirk, M.V. 1981. 'The Black Death in Aragon, 1348–1351', *Journal of Medieval History*, 7: 357–368

Shrewsbury, J.F.D. 1971. *A History of Bubonic Plague in the British Isles*. Cambridge: The University Press

Sigurðsson, J.V. 1995. 'Forholdet mellom frender, hushold og venner på Island i fristatstiden', *Historisk tidsskrift* (Norway): 311–330

Simpson, W.J. 1905. *A Treatise on Plague*. Cambridge: Cambridge University Press

Sivéry, G. 1965. 'Le Hainaut et la Peste Noire', *Mémoires et publications de la Société des sciences, des arts et des lettres du Hainaut*, 79: 431–447

———— 1966. 'La Peste Noire et l'épidémie de 1400–1401 dans le Hainaut. Questions de methodologie', *Annales de la Société Belge d'histoire des hôpitaux*, 4: 51–65

Slack, P. 1977. 'The Local Incidence of Epidemic Disease. The case of Bristol 1540–1650', in: *The Plague Reconsidered*: 49–62

Smith, R.M. 1978. 'Population and its Geography in England 1500–1730', in: *An Historical Geography of England and Wales*: 199–237

———— 1988. 'Human Resources', in: *The Countryside of Medieval England*: 189–212

———— 1991. 'Demographic Developments in Rural England, 1300–48: A survey', in: *Before the Black Death*: 25–77

Sobrequés Callicó, J. 1966. 'La peste negra en la Península Ibérica', *Anuario de estudios medievales*: 67–102

Stampfli, H.R. 1965–6. 'Die Tierreste aus der römischen Villa "Ersigen–Murain" in Gegenüberstellung zu anderen Zeitgleichen Funden aus der Schweiz und dem Ausland', *Jahrbuch des Bernischen Historischen Museums in Bern*, 45–46: 449–469

Steen, S. 1934. 'Veiene og leden i Norge', in: *Nordisk Kultur*. Vol. 16B: 217–228

Sticker, G. 1908. *Abhandlungen aus der Seuchengeschichte und Seuchenlehre. Die Pest.* Giessen: Alfred Töpelmann. Vol. 1, Pt 1

Storia d'Italia. 1973. Turin: Einaudi. Vol. 5

Stouff, L. 1962. 'Trois dénombrements de la population arlésienne aux XIIIe, XIVe et XVe siècles', *Bulletin philologique et historique du Comité des travaux historiques et scientifiques (jusqu'en 1610)*: 275–292

Studi in onore di Amintore Fanfani. 1962. Milan: Dott. A. Guiffrè editore. Vol. 1

Studi in onore di Armando Sapori. 1957. Milan: Istituto Editoriale Cisalpino

Studier i hanseatisk–svensk historia. 1885. Stockholm: Kungl. Boktryckeriet. Vol. 2

Studies in Disease Ecology. 1961. J.M. May (ed.). New York: Hafner Publishing Co.

Svenskt Diplomatarium. 1878–1959. Stockholm: Riksarkivet. Vol. 6

Techen, F. 1926. *Die Bürgersprachen der Stadt Wismar.* Leipzig

Teichert, M. 1985. 'Beitrag zur Faunengeschichte der Hausratte. *Rattus rattus* L.', *Zeitschrift für Archäologie*, 19: 263–269

Thompson, A.H. 1911. 'Registers of John Gynewell, Bishop of Lincoln, for the Years 1347–1350', *The Archaeological Journal*, 68: 301–360

———— 1914. 'The Pestilences of the Fourteenth Century in the Diocese of York', *The Archaeological Journal*, 71: 97–154

Thrupp, S. 1962. *The Merchant Class of Medieval London.* Ann Arbor: The University of Michigan Press. 2nd edn

———— 1965. 'The Problem of Replacement Rates in Late Medieval England', *The Economic History Review*, 2nd Series, 14: 101–119

Titow, J.Z. 1969, *English Rural Society, 1200–1350.* London: George Allen & Unwin

Törnblom, L. 1993. 'Medeltiden', in: *Finlands historia*: 271–426

Trenchs Odena, J. 1969. 'La diocesis de Tarragona y la peste negra: los cargos de la catedral', in: *VIII Congreso de historia de la Corona de Aragón, Valencia 1967*, II. 1 (*La Corona de Aragón en el siglo XIV*). Valencia: 45–64

———— 1972–3. 'El Monasterio de Ripoll y la Peste Negra de 1348', *Anales del Instituto de Estudios Gerundenses*, 21: 103–115

———— 1974. 'Documentos vaticanos de los años de la peste negra referentes a la diócesis de Lérida', *ILERDA*, No. 35: 203–10

———— 1978. 'El Reino de Valencia y la peste de 1348. Datos para su estudio', *Estudios de Historia de Valencia*: 23–71

———— 1980. 'Documentos pontificios sobre la peste negra en la diócesis de Gerona', *La diócesis de Gerona y la peste de 1348*. Escuela Española de Historia y Arqueología en Roma (Cuadernos de Trabajos). Rome: 183–204

———— 1981. 'La epidemia de peste de 1348 y las diócesis de Huesca y Tarazona', *Zurita.Cuadernos de historia*, 39–40: 197–204

Tucco Chala, P. 1951. 'Notes sur la peste noire de 1348 en Béarn', *Revue régionaliste des Pyrénées*, 111–112: 80–85

Ubieto Arteta, A. 1975. 'Cronología del desarrollo del la peste negra en la Península Ibérica', *Cuadernos de historia. Anexos de la revista Hispaña*, 5: 47–66

Udovitch, A.L. 1971. 'Egypt: Crisis in a Muslim Land', in: *The Black Death. A Turning Point in History?*: 122–125

Ulsig, E. 1991. 'Pest og befolkningsnedgang i Danmark i det 14. århundrede', *Historisk tidsskrift* (Denmark), 91: 21–43

———— 1994. 'Review paper of O.J. Benedictow, *Plague in the Late Medieval Nordic Countries*', *Historisk tidsskrift* (Norway), 73: 94–104

Urkundenbuch der Stadt Lübeck (Codex diplomaticus Lubeccensis). 1870. Lübeck: Aschenfeldt. 1st Series, Vol. 3

Van Loghem, J.J. und Swellengrebel, N.H. 1914. 'Kontinuierliche und metastatische Pestverbreitung', *Medical Microbiology and Immunobiology*, 77: 460–481

Van Werveke, H. 1950. 'De Zwarte Dood in de Zuidelijke Nederlanden (1349–1351)', *Medelingen van de Koninklijke Vlaamse Acadademie voor Wetenschappen, Letteren en Schone Kunsten van België*, Klasse der Letteren, No. 3, 12

―――― 1953–4. 'Noogmaals De Zwarte Dood in de Nederlanden', *Bijdragen voor de Geschiedenes der Nederlanden*, 8: 251–258

Vasil'yev, K.G. i Segal, A.E. 1960. *Istoriya epidemiy v Rossii* [History of epidemics in Russia]. Moscow: Gosudarstvennoye izdatel'stvo meditsinskoy literatury

Velimirovich, B. and Velimirovich, H. 1989. 'Plague in Vienna', *Review of Infectious Diseases*, 11: 808–825

Venezia e la peste 1348–1797. 1979. Venice: Commune di Venezia, Marsilio Editori

The Victoria History of the County of Cambridge and the Isle of Ely. 1948. L.F. Salzman (ed.). London: Oxford University Press

The Victoria History of the County of York. 1913. W. Page (ed.). London. Vol. 3

Vilar, P. 1962. *La Catalogne dans l'Espagne moderne.* Paris: SEVPEN. Vol. 1

Vilkuna, K. 1969. 'Råttor och möss', in: *Kulturhistorisk leksikon for nordisk middelalder.* Oslo: Gyldendal Norsk Forlag. Vol. 14: 583–584

Von Brandt, A. 1964. *Regesten der Lübecker Bürgertestamente des Mittelalters.* Vol. 1, 1278–1350. Veröffentlichungen zur Geschichte der Freien und Hansestadt Lübeck, No. 18. Lübeck

―――― 1973. 'Mitteralterliche Bürgertestamente', Neuerschlossene Quellen zur Geschichte der materiellen und geistigen Kultur. *Sitzungsberichte der Heidelberger Akademie der Wissenschaften, phil.-hist. Klasse*, Jahrgang 73, Abteilung 3. Heidelberg

Vretemark, M. 1983. 'Svartråttan – snyltgäst och pestspridare', in: *Helgeandsholmen.1000 år i Stockholms ström*: 294, 467

Wakil, A.W. 1932. *The Third Pandemic of Plague in Egypt.* (The Faculty of Medicine, Publication No. 3). Cairo: The Egyptian University

Watts, D.G. 1998. 'The Black Death in Dorset and Hampshire', *The Hatcher Review*, 5: 21–31

Welty, T.K., Grabman, J., Kompare, E. et al. 1985. 'Nineteen Cases of Plague in Arizona', *Clinical Medicine*, 142: 641–646

Wenzel, S. 1982. 'Pestilence and Middle English Literature: Friar John Grimestone's poems on death', in: *The Black Death*: 131–159

White, Lynn, Jr. 1970. *Medieval Technology and Social Change.* Oxford: Oxford University Press

WHO Expert Committee on Plague. 1970

Wilson, F.P. 1963. *The Plague in Shakespeare's London.* Oxford: Oxford University Press.

Wolff, P. 1957. 'Trois études de démographie médiévale en France méridionale', in: *Studi in onore di Armando Sapori*: 493–503

―――― 1959. 'Un grand commerce mediéval: Les céréales dans le bassin de la Mediterranée occidentale. Remarques et suggestions', in: *VI Congreso de historia de la Corona de Aragón, en Cerdeña 8 a 14 dicembre 1957.* Madrid: 147–164

Wood-Legh, K.L. 1948. 'Ecclesiastical History', in: *The Victoria History of the County of Cambridge and the Isle of Ely*: 141–196

The World We Have Gained. Essays presented to Peter Laslett on his Seventieth Birthday. 1986. L. Bonfield, R.M. Smith and K. Wrightson (eds.). Oxford: Basil Blackwell

Wrigley, E.A. and Schofield, R.S. 1981. *The Population History of England, 1541–1871. A Reconstruction.* Cambridge: Cambridge University Press [2nd edn 1989]

Wu, C.Y. 1936. 'Insect Vectors', in: Wu, Chun, Pollitzer et al. *Plague. A Manual for Medical and Public Health Workers*: 249–308

Wu, L.-T. 1913–14. 'First Report of the North Manchurian Plague Prevention Service', *The Journal of Hygiene*, 13: 237–290, plus 10 pp. with plates

——— 1922–3. 'The Second Pneumonic Plague Epidemic in Manchuria, 1920–21', *The Journal of Hygiene*, 21: 262–288

——— 1926. *A Treatise on Pneumonic Plague*. Geneva: League of Nations, Health Organization

——— 1927–8. 'Recent Knowledge on Pneumonic Plague', *North Manchurian Plague Prevention Service, Reports*, 6: 55–92

——— 1936a. 'Historical Aspects', in: Wu, Chun, Pollitzer et al. *Plague. A Manual for Medical and Public Health Workers*: 1–55

——— 1936b. 'Epidemiological Factors', in: Wu, Chun, Pollitzer et al. *Plague. A Manual for Medical and Public Health Workers*: 383–423

Wu, L.-T., Chun, J.W.H., Pollitzer, R. and Wu, C.Y. 1936. *Plague. A Manual for Medical and Public Health Workers*. Shanghai Station: National Quarantine Service

Zabalo Zabalegui, F.J. 1968. 'Algunos datos sobre la regresión demográfica causada por la peste en la Navarra del siglo XIV', in: *Miscelanea Jose M.ª Lacarra*: 81–87

Zaddach, B.I. 1971. *Die Folgen des Schwarzen Todes (1347–1351) für den Klerus Mitteleuropas*. Stuttgart: Gustav Fischer Verlag

Ziegler, P. 1970. *The Black Death*. Harmondsworth: Pelican Books [first pub. 1969]

Zwanenberg, D.V. 1970. 'The Last Epidemic of Plague in England? Suffolk 1906–1918', *Medical History*, 14: 62–74

Index

(1) The *Index* has the following sections: *Subject Index, Geographical names and peoples, Name Index.*

(2) Medieval and classical persons are registered according to Christian names, modern persons according to surnames.

(3) For medical and epidemiological terms see also *Glossary* xiv–xvi.

(4) German and Nordic personal names and place names may include letters not used in English that are entered alphabetically in the *Index* according to the following phonetic rules: Å/å = AA/aa; Ä/ä, Æ/æ = AE/ae; ü = y; Ø/ø, Ö/ö = Oe/oe; ð = d.

(5) In order to make titles of annals and chronicles and similar types of sources more immediately and generally comprehensible, they have been translated into English in the text and are entered according to the English translation in the *Index.*

(6) Page references to specific mortality rates in countries, regions, local societies in the section of the *Index* called *Geographical names and peoples* are marked with the letter M, as are entries on mortality rates among special social categories of persons.

Subject Index

Geographical names and peoples

Name index

(1) Persons in the running text (not authors of fn.s)
(2) Medieval and classical persons are entered according to Christian name, except in a few cases of persons who are systematically known by their surnames; modern persons are entered according to surname.
(3) Regarding special letters, see introduction to Index, no. 4.